Nationalizing the Body

Nationalizing the Body

The Medical Market, Print and Daktari Medicine

Projit Bihari Mukharji

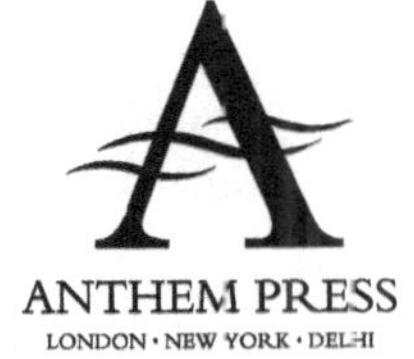

ANTHEM PRESS
LONDON · NEW YORK · DELHI

Anthem Press
An imprint of Wimbledon Publishing Company
www.anthempress.com

This edition first published in UK and USA 2011
by ANTHEM PRESS
75-76 Blackfriars Road, London SE1 8HA, UK
or PO Box 9779, London SW19 7ZG, UK
and
244 Madison Ave. #116, New York, NY 10016, USA

British Library Cataloguing in Publication Data
A catalogue record for this book is available from the British Library.

Library of Congress Cataloging in Publication Data
A catalog record for this book has been requested.

ISBN-13: 978 0 85728 995 7 (Pbk)
ISBN-10: 0 85728 995 0 (Pbk)

This title is also available as an eBook.

For

Ma, Dadabhai and Dima

—in gratitude for blessings past,
in anticipation of joys to come.

CONTENTS

List of Illustrations		ix
Acknowledgements		xi
Introduction		1
Chapter I.	Healers in Context: Forgotten Pioneers	35
Chapter II.	Daktari Prints: The World of Bengali Printing and the Multiple Inscriptions of *Daktari* Medicine	75
Chapter III.	Contagious Nationalism: Contagion and the Actualization of the Nation	111
Chapter IV.	Political Plague: Diagnosing a Neo-Hindu Modernity	147
Chapter V.	Endemic Commerce: Cholera and the Medical Market	179
Chapter VI.	*Dhatu Dourbalya*: Diagnosing the Rhizoid Pathologies of Weakness	213
Conclusion		249
Notes		261
Bibliography		311
Index		337

LIST OF ILLUSTRATIONS

I. Caricature of exploitation of patients by reputed *daktars* by H. Guha in Sri Nripendrakumar Basu, "*Parasparik Haran*" (The Mutual Robbery), *Swasthya Samachar* 16, no. 1 (1927): 30. 71

II. Advertisement for *Sahaj Daktari Shikhya*, *Gupta Press Dairektari Panjika for 1322 BS.* 103

III. Plate 6, *Harbola Bhnar* (The Ventriloquizing Jester: Journal of Cartoons and Caricatures) 1, no.1 (1874). 107

IV. "Paripak Jantrabali" (The Instruments of Digestion) in Dr Rameshchandra Roy, "Koshtoshuddhi" (Cleaning the Bowels), *Swasthya Samachar* 17, no. 4 (1928): 98. 127

V. "Katipay Khadya-sthita Upakaraner Satakara Pariman" (The ingredients of a few foodstuff expressed in percentages) in Chunilal Basu, Village Sanitation and a Manual of Hygiene (Calcutta: np, 1931): 186. 128

VI. "*Swasthyadharma Sangha Bidyapithe goto Kartiker Goshthashthami dibasey Go-Pujar par Sampadak nija hastae gabhi-paricharja karitechhen*" (The Editor personally bathing cows at the recent cow-worship festival organized by the *Swasthyadharma Sangha* school on the occasion of Goshthashthami) *Swasthya Samachar* 16, no. 1 (1927): 18–19. 131

VII. A contemporary popular representation of the work of Sister Nivedita and the Neo-Hindu monks during the Calcutta Plague, available at www.uttishthata.org, accessed on 24th October 2008. 163

VIII. "Jaipur Hat (Jessore) Station-e Kolerar Tika Laibar Janya Janasamagamer Chitra" (A Picture of the crowd gathered to receive vaccination against Cholera at the Jaipur Hat Station in Jessore), *Swasthya Samachar* 17, no. 2 (1928): Unnumbered page. 187

IX. Advertisement for Nerve Pills, Gupta Press Dairektari Panjika for 1322 BS. 219

X. Advertisement for Prameha Chintamani, Nutan Panjika (1896). 229

XI. Advertisement for Amritasagar Salsa, Gupta Press Dairektari Panjika for 1322 BS. 244

XII. Advertisement for HD Manna Co-operative Salsa, Nutan Panjika (1901). 245

XIII. Advertisement for Mahashakti Salsa, Gupta Press Dairektari Panjika for 1322 BS. 246

ACKNOWLEDGEMENTS

Like most creatures of the mind, the precise date of the birth of the idea of this book is today difficult to identify. As Ideas have developed into Positions and Positions been honed to Arguments, numerous suggestions, corrections, digressions and directions have egged it on. Not all of those incitements can be acknowledged and it must suffice to acknowledge only the handful of people whose imprint on this book has been indelible.

Foremost among these is Prof. David Arnold. His work had been the beacon which first attracted me to the history of medicine in colonial India and—as any reading of this book will show—his remains the master narrative along which I have plotted all other work, including my own present effort. During the three years of my doctoral work at The School of Oriental and African Studies SOAS—and since—I have found in him one of the most patient and perceptive readers of my work. His numerous suggestions and many more criticisms, have, I believe, inestimably enhanced my work.

My debt to Prof. Majid Hayat Siddiqi is as profound as it is to Prof. Arnold. It was under Prof. Siddiqi at JNU that I made my first hesitant forays into historical research. His personal charisma and trenchant refusal to fit into fashionable academic boxes have educated me no less than his insistence on the rigour of research without lapsing into the lap of naïve empiricism.

Though I have never had the honour of being a student of Prof. Gautam Bhadra, I have learnt as much from him as I have from anybody else. Not only has his infectious enthusiasm for the marginalized archives of Bengali history proved to be one contagion too strong for me to resist, but I have found in his stubborn opposition to the imposition of alien analytical categories upon historical documents and his consequent insistence on the use of immanent categories of analysis, one of the most scrupulously democratic ethics of academic praxis.

During my undergraduate years at Presidency College, Calcutta, the erudition and charisma of Prof. Rajat Kanta Ray and Prof. Subhas Ranjan Chakrabarty were a source of immense inspiration and excitement. Their brilliant examples were crucial in awakening my interest in History.

The friendship, suggestions and encouragement of Prof. David Hardiman has been a source of great joy and inspiration.

Prof. Sabyasachi Bhattacharya at Jawaharlal Nehru University (JNU) and Dr Daud Ali at SOAS have also taught me much. At various junctures, their support and encouragement have proved crucial to the sustenance and completion of my research. Their capacity to express the most complex of arguments in the most accessible of idioms is something I have greatly admired and tried to mimic—I know not with what degree of success.

Prof. Francis Robinson and Dr Crispin Bates have been unrestrained in their support and generous with their time whenever I have turned to them for support or advice.

Dr Biswamoy Pati, whom I first met under the seemingly 'hostile' environment of an MPhil viva voce, has proved to be a pillar of friendship, trust and support ever since. Prof. Mark Harrison's searching review of my doctoral work has allowed me to express my arguments with greater clarity. Dr Pratik Chakrabarti's comments on some earlier draft chapters have also been most helpful.

I must also acknowledge my debts to Prof. KN Panikkar, Prof. Neeladri Bhattarcharya, Prof. Heeraman Tiwari and Prof. Tanika Sarkar at JNU and Prof. Peter Robb and Dr Shabnum Tejani at SOAS. From all of them I have learnt much which I have used here.

A brief stint as a Research Fellow under Prof. Ashis Nandy forced me to seriously rethink the protocols of historical truth I had adhered to, and this rethinking has immeasurably deepened my understanding of the past in all its varied forms.

During my fieldwork in Dhaka I learnt much from Prof. Sirajul Islam and Prof. Sonia Nishat Amin. Prof. Islam's erudition and readiness to help and Prof. Amin's infectious enthusiasm and liberality made my research in Dhaka both rewarding and enjoyable.

My colleagues and students at Southampton and Newcastle have influenced this work in myriad ways. Their conversations, queries and comments have at various times suggested and instigated my research in new directions.

My particularly long *addas* with Guy Attewell and Matti Pohjonen have immensely enriched me and my work. Guy's nuanced vision and Matti's ceaseless theorization has infiltrated more corners of my mind and work than I can ever hope to acknowledge. I have also found much crisp wit and a host of new ideas from Markus Daeschel, Bodhisattva Kar and Prabhat Kumar.

I have benefited immensely from the interest, suggestions and guidance of Kaushik Roy.

My research has also greatly benefited from the archival knowledge of Abhijit Majumdar of the Centre for Studies in Social Sciences Calcutta (CSSSC) and Asim Mukhopadhyay of the National Library. Their devotion to their craft as well as the sheer depth of their interest is a source of inspiration. To Abhijit Majumdar in particular I owe much. I also remain in the debt of the members of staff at the British Library, SOAS Library, Wellcome Library and the Newcastle Library. Binaybhushan Ray's and Kalyan Basak's generosity in sharing their personal collections with me has humbled and helped me immensely.

The material for this book was collected over the course of several years, in which time I have had the honour of holding different fellowships. These fellowships have made this book possible through their munificence. I gratefully acknowledge my debts to the Indian Council of Historical Research, to the trustees of the Felix Fellowship Trust, the Central Research Fund of the University of London and the trustees of the Wellcome Trust.

I must also express my deepest gratitude to Alexander Beecroft and Tej PS Sood of Anthem Press for their interest, patience and care in the materialization of this book.

Beyond the call of History, I have found much delight in the company of Vivek Boray, Andrew Nelson, Anshuman Rane, Christoph Sprung, Christian Oesterheld, Nitin Sinha, Santanu Banerjee, Tanmoy Das, Ishan Dutt, Supaul Chandra, Sunanda 'Bobby' Sarkar and Saurabh 'Fonke' Dutta. My debt to Arka Paul deserves a special mention here. His encyclopaedic knowledge of cinema and his helpfulness in all maters have together been a source of much pleasure. I must also thank Monami Mukherjee for her hospitality and friendship during my stay in Southampton.

During the course of numerous rushed research trips to London, Anshuman and Amanda and Arka and Debopriya and Sudip Mazumder have sustained me with bed, board and wine. Without their generosity much of this research would never have happened.

Parama Sarkar's friendship and companionship sustained me through some of the toughest times in my life. My debt to her is immense.

In Boria Majumdar I have found the firmest and the most dependable friend. At various moments of crisis and despondency, he has stood like a bulwark of reliability and steadfastness.

Amit Maity has been more than a brother, and his presence through thick and thin has made the *thin* less depressing and the *thick* more enjoyable.

Samar Nag's timely help and subsequent friendship has proved to be a source of great pleasure. The breadth of his liberality has been matched only by the stimulating width of his intellectual interests.

Uncle Haider and Aunt Anna lovingly welcomed me into their home upon my first arrival in the UK. Their hospitality and love made settling in to life as a research-student in England much less traumatic than it might otherwise have been.

One of my most significant debts of gratitude is to Prof. Waltraud Ernst. I have resisted the temptation to acknowledge my debt to her alongside my other professional debts, simply because she has been much more than a professional colleague. As the exigencies of post-colonial labour flows have turned the colonial metropole into the destination rather than source of exile, it is Waltraud who has made the exile look less alien. She has truly been a friend, philosopher and guide.

Amongst my immediate family, my greatest debt is to Dadabhai whose tales of far-away lands were the source of my earliest dreams. It is his memory and that of those early dreams which first stoked my curiosity and draws me still to the long-lost lands of the past.

As we travelled along the meandering rivulets of the past in Dadabhai's boat of stories, it was Dima who kept our strengths up for the daily adventures through her timely ministrations. My debt to her, too is profound.

It will be a source of lasting regret that neither Thampadada nor Thampa nor Baba could see my work. Their influence, I am sure, permeates this work in more ways than I am conscious off.

To Ma: I owe everything that I am. It would be pointless to acknowledge her debt separately for the writing of this book. Suffice it to say that her love and affection have been what has made my life possible.

As Ma's love made life possible, Monjita's love has made it enjoyable. Her collaboration has been immense all through the journey of this book, from an amorphous set of ideas to a tangible reality. She has intellectually and materially sustained me and my work through much, and I hope she finds something worth her efforts in this book.

Needless to say, I remain solely to blame for all faults that remain.

Nationalizing the Body

INTRODUCTION

Meeting the *Daktars*

This book is about *daktari* medicine. Simply put, *daktari* medicine was the name given to the medicine practised by *daktars*. But who exactly were the *daktars*?

The term itself, as we shall see in Chapter I, did not emerge until the second half of the nineteenth century. Even then they did not constitute a single homogenous group but were rather a composite group made up of many heterogeneous elements whose social status and pedagogical background both differed widely. Yet, after the 1860s the word *daktar* clearly referred to people who were thought to practise 'western' medicine. John Iliffe's comprehensive study *East African Doctors: A History of the Modern Profession* mentions the development of similar vernacular designations for some early African practitioners of 'western' medicine. In some cases the terms used to refer to them drew upon older 'indigenous' vocabularies, such as *mganga* or *omusawo* or, as in the Kenyan *dakitari*, the term was, like in Bengal, a vernacularization of the English 'doctor'.[1]

To what extent these *daktars* drew upon earlier traditions of South Asians practising 'western' medicine cannot now be ascertained with any degree of certainty. This much, however, is certain: South Asia had been exposed to 'western' medicine for at least two centuries before the term *daktar* emerged as a socially significant identity. Numerous European medical travellers such as Francois Bernier, Niocolao Manucci, Garcia d'Orta and John Ovington, visited Mughal South Asia.[2] There is also evidence to suggest that contemporary South Asian physicians were engaged in a dialogue with some of these early European doctors. Through this dialogue, South Asian physicians adopted some European drugs and practices. Some of the early European doctors like Manucci even set themselves up for a while in independent medical practice.

As Deepak Kumar points out, this climate of exchange and dialogue began to change with the 'colonial watershed'.[3] Yet, in another way, the transformation of Europeans from itinerant adventurers first to temporarily settled traders (in factories at Surat, Hughli, etc.) and later into a political power also spurred another level of medical exchange. As a group of settled people in South Asia, they were in need of regular medical help. Even when they had a few European doctors in their employ, these doctors needed helpers, assistants, Dressers, etc. With the emergence of the Europeans as a political power, they also developed an ever-growing retinue of South Asian employees—particularly soldiers—the health of which also needed attention. From the seventeenth century onwards, therefore, we come to hear of South Asians being employed at various English trading posts. In the late 1630s and early 1640s, for instance, one Adhar Bhatt is mentioned as "our *banyan* doctor" in records pertaining to the Surat Factory. In Bengal, the earliest references to a South Asian physician employed by the English comes from Strenshyam Master's diaries, which mention one Nilkanth or Nilchand practising at the Hughli Factory around 1676. Similarly, in 1740 one Numshivia, in a petition to the company, mentions that he and his father, Shevandavadum, had been employed for over 50 years as physicians at Fort St David near Cuddalore on the east coast of India.[4] There is, however, no way of ascertaining what kind of medicine these early Indian practitioners practised on their European patients. Though there is every reason to believe that they would have picked up some 'western' medical practices and ideas in the course of their employment, it remains possible that they practised according to purely 'indigenous' traditions.

A more clear evidence of South Asian practice of 'western' medicine is available in 1701 in Bombay, where reference is made to a 'black hospital assistant.' Later, the names of Balloo and Morar Purvoe are found in relation to the European medical establishment in Bombay. Purvoe is also referred to as a 'Hospital Mate'—a designation till then reserved for Europeans. From the middle of the eighteenth century there also began the practice of employing South Asian physicians for 'native' regiments of the English army.[5] That at least some of these early 'native' doctors in the army enjoyed a degree of proximity to European army doctors of the time can be seen from a letter of recommendation written in 1797. One Dr Fraser had, in the letter, appraised the Calcutta Medical Board of the services of a 'Native Doctor' named Ramnath—a Brahmin—who had served with credit with the Second Native Infantry at Kishanganj for over twenty-six years. Fraser heartily recommended Ramnath to the board for the grant of a pension.[6] By the end of the century, a right to such pensions for South Asian medical subordinates had become fairly institutionalized. The proximity to European physicians undoubtedly resulted in some degree of medical exchange as well. Writing in the 1760s, John Peter Wade's detailed case histories frequently mentions him leaving the patient in the hands of a 'Compounder' with instructions for treatment.[7]

By 1792 a 'native hospital' had been established in Calcutta and several South Asians were employed in it to practise 'western medicine'.[8] These practitioners were usually referred to as 'Native Dressers' or 'Black Doctors'. Apart from these there were numerous others who worked as Dressers, Compounders, Hospital Mates, etc., in both military and civil capacities. In time, in Madras, these South Asian medical subordinates came to be referred to more or less uniformly as 'Native Dressers', while in Bengal they were generally referred to as 'Black Doctors'.

Socially, unlike in the case of East Africa—where the earliest practitioners of 'western' medicine tended to be social outcasts—in South Asia the early practitioners came from two relatively prominent groups. Either they were Eurasians like Domingo Vancloster de Roza at Madras or Nicola, the 'Native Dresser' at Patna, or they were Brahmins like Adhar Bhatt and Ramnath. These latter possibly had some hereditary connection with medicine. Numshivia's petition in 1740 ,for example, mentioned not only him having followed his father in medical practice, but, indeed, the immediate object of the petition was to obtain a subordinate medical position for his son. By 1812, the Governor General approved of a plan to recruit boys from the Upper and Lower Orphan and Free schools to become 'Compounders' and 'Dressers'.[9] Eventually these recruits were expected to rise to the position of 'Apothecary' and 'Sub-Assistant Surgeon'. Ten years later, in 1822, the Government established the Native Medical Institution.[10] The classes for the NMI were to be held at both the Sanskrit College and the Calcutta Madrasa. The syllabi were to be a mixture of some 'western' medical ideas and some classical 'indigenous' medical traditions.[11] Clearly, both the location of the classes and the syllabi were intended to draw recruits from the upper echelons of South Asian society. By 1833 a proposal was made to produce doctors of a higher grade of training who would be given the titles of Sub-Assistant Surgeon and comprise the 'Civil Sub-Medical Department'.[12] They were also to be paid at a higher scale. These Sub-Assistant Surgeons were to be posted at the ever-increasing public dispensaries that were being opened throughout the land.

By 1835 this scheme was superseded by the establishment of the Calcutta Medical College (CMC). There is no evidence to bear out the assertion by some scholars that, 'initially, only lower castes and classes came to study in the College for the job of Compounder in the district dispensaries'.[13] In fact, the Government Order No. 28 of 28 January 1835 that finally approved the foundation of the Medical College, explicitly mentioned that, 'the benefits of the college shall be open to all classes of native youths between the age of fourteen and twenty…*provided they possess respectable connections* [emphasis added] and conduct…'.[14] The first batch of CMC graduates, in 1838—Umacharan Seth,

Dwarkanath Gupta, Rajkrista Dey and Nabinchandra Mitra—all came from the upper castes. Gupta was of the *Vaidya* caste and Dey and Mitra were from the *Kayastha* caste. These two castes, together with the Brahmins, made up the topmost echelon of the Bengali caste hierarchy. None of them become Compounders; instead, they were all posted as Sub-Assistant Surgeons at a monthly pay of Rs 100.[15] These Sub-Assistant Surgeons became both the most commonly seen Indian faces of 'western' medicine as well as the sources of further dissemination of 'western' medicine through their training of numerous apprentices, Compounders, Dressers, etc. Most of these early Sub-Assistant Surgeons working in North and East India were ethnically Bengalis. Of the first available list of Civil Sub-Assistant Surgeons in 1840, out of a total of eleven, eight were ethnic Bengalis, of whom at least two were Brahmins. By 1845, as the total number of Sub-Assistant Surgeons employed at various dispensaries across northern and eastern India increased to twenty, the total number of Bengalis went up to fifteen, of whom at least one was a Brahmin and another a Bengali Muslim. Of the remaining five, one was Indo-Portuguese, one Indo-Jewish who later converted to Christianity, two upper Indian Hindus (including one Brahmin) and another, a Muslim who was in all probability from upper India.[16] Not all of these were graduates of the CMC. Some old graduates of the NMI were also recruited, such as Syed Enayat Hossein of Lucknow. However as Seema Alavi points out, 'respectability', 'family background' and elite social status were crucial in the choice of candidates. The company was also willing to pay higher salaries for such candidates.[17]

Sub-Assistant Surgeons at the Beginning of 1840

Dispensary	Sub-Assistant Surgeon
Dhaka	Nabinchandra Pal
Chittagong	Rajkrista Chatterjee
Puri	Neelmani Datta
Murshidabad	Panchanan Sreemani
Patna	Rameshwar Awasthi
Benares City Hospital and Secrole	Iswarchandra Ganguly
Allahabad	Shyamacharan Datta
Kanpur	Ramnarayan Das
Bareilly	Jadabchandra Seth
Delhi	R Hemming
Moradabad	Vacant
Agra	Umacharan Seth

Source: V/26/732.

Sub-Assistant Surgeons at the Beginning of 1845

Dispensary	Sub-Assistant Surgeon
Bhabanipur	Kalachand Dey
Murshidabad	Panchanan Sreemani
Puri	Neelmani Datta
Chittagong	Gohur Khan
Dhaka	EJ Lazarus
Patna	Rameshwar Awasthi
Benares	Iswarchandra Ganguly
Farrukhabad	Sadhucharan Mullick
Kanpur	Ramnarayan Das
Allahabad	Jadabchandra Dhara
Agra	Dharmadas Bhose
Mathura	Maheshchandra Naun
Bareilly	Jadabchandra Seth
Jabbalpur	Shyamacharan Datta
Moradabad	Tarachand Pyne
Shahjahanpur	L De Souza
Delhi	Chiman Lal
Lucknow	Syed Enayat Hussain
Hughli	Badanchandra Choudhury
Gaya	Shyamacharan Sircar

Source: V/26/735.

Having started in 1835 with a batch of 50 students, by 1873 the CMC had 1,226 students. The courses had also been greatly diversified by the 1870s. Initially, graduates of the college were awarded a diploma. After the founding of the Calcutta University in 1857, however, it started awarding a degree of Doctor of Medicine (MD) and a licence for medicine and surgery (LMS). By 1860 a baccalaureate degree in medicine (MB) was added. The duration of study had also been extended from the initial three years to four years in 1840 and five years in 1845. Apart from a military class where instruction was imparted in Hindustani, by 1852 a Bengali Class was also added to the college. Of the 1,226 students in 1873, 635 students were studying in the Bengali class, out of which 421 were paying students.[18]

By 1849 the employment of these Sub-Assistant Surgeons came to be regulated by new, detailed service rules. According to these rules, Sub-Assistant Surgeons with less than seven years in service earned Rs 100 per month, those between seven and fourteen years earned Rs 150 and those above fourteen years earned Rs 200.[19] By 1863, they became eligible for pension. From March 1874 the title of Sub-Assistant Surgeon was replaced by Assistant Surgeon.

In 1898 another higher rank of Senior Assistant Surgeon at a pay of Rs 300 was created and some Civil Surgeoncies were reserved for them.[20] After 1912, they also became eligible for annual increments of Rs 10 until their pays reached Rs 300.[21]

After 1860, however, the ever-growing numbers of Bengali class medical graduates and the low salaries offered to them in the government service, as well as the limited opportunities for career advancements, seemed to have driven an increasing number of qualified men away from government service and into private medical practice. This in turn had led to a crisis of qualified manpower at the lower end of state's medical establishment, which led to the increasing employment of 'locally trained native doctors'. These were usually men without a college education who had learnt medicine through a period of apprenticeship, self-study or, in a few cases, had qualified for a lesser position as a Hospital Assistant or Compounder.[22] The designation of Hospital Assistant, which had with numerous changes been in vogue since the 1820s and described a lesser position than the Assistant Surgeon, was replaced in 1910 by Sub-Assistant Surgeon—the title which had fallen into disuse since 1874. Thus both Civil and Military Hospital Assistants after 1910 were described as Sub-Assistant Surgeons.[23]

The change in designation reflected the intellectual attainments of the class. The insinuation of the earlier designation was that these men were mere practical helps. In practice they had long been skilled medical personnel in their own right, often being given independent charge of important medical missions—especially at times of epidemics—and themselves giving ample proof of a vibrant intellectual culture. In 1907 for instance, when the *Indian Medical Gazette* announced a special cash prize for the best essay on plague prophylaxis, P. S. Ramachandrier of Mysore—a Hospital Assistant and the energetic editor of the *All-India Hospital Assistant's Journal* won the prize beating a host of Assistant Surgeons who had also entered the fray. Even the second prize was claimed by First Grade Civil Hospital Assistant Annadacharan Sircar.[24]

Of the three medical services—the covenanted, the Uncovenanted and the Subordinate—South Asians were present in all three branches since the 1850s. The number of South Asians in the covenanted service remained low throughout the nineteenth century since Soorjo Coomar Goodeve Chuckerbutty entered it, despite European opposition, at the first open entrance examinations. By 1905 only 5 percent of the covenanted service was occupied by Indians.[25] The Uncovenanted and the Subordinate services however, increasingly came to be dominated by South Asians in the nineteenth century. The 1891 Census of India described 3,078 people in Bengal as belonging to the Subordinate Medical Service alone.[26] In 1901, 2914 people in the province were working as matrons, Compounders, nurses, etc. in the hospital, asylum and dispensary services.[27] The vast majority of these lower services comprised South Asians. Both Anil Kumar and Sandeep Sinha argue that racial prejudice was rife within these services and an 'indecent disparity existed between the European medical professionals and their Indian counterparts'.[28] Such racial prejudice undoubtedly did much to prevent the emergence of a homogenized State Medicine.

While some idea of the numbers, nature of practice and social backgrounds of those in various levels of government service can be had, it is well-nigh impossible to find corresponding data for those who practised privately and claimed to use some version of 'western' medicine or other. In 1901, 4,266 people were said to be practising medicine in Bengal 'with diploma, licence or certificate', many of these would have been South Asian graduates of the various medical colleges and classes.[29] Of the nearly 35,000 people practising 'without a diploma', though most claimed to practice indigenous medicines, there were many who, according to H. H. Risley, were in reality 'plucked students of a Calcutta college' and hence practising possibly a bowdlerized form of 'western' medicine.[30]

An objection may here be raised against considering this last category as practising 'western' medicine. Anil Kumar, for instance, refuses to accept the majority of those in private practice dismissing them as 'hybrid quacks of both indigenous as well as alien medical systems'.[31] To delve into this question of which was *really* 'western' medicine and which was not, however, would implicate us in the historically contingent discourse on 'quackery' which had developed in South Asia since the 1880s and eventually produced the Medical Registration Acts around 1913. Issues of professional interest and medical commerce remain entangled with this contentious judgement and it would not be justifiable to unquestioningly draw upon this debate. Indeed, part of the reason why this larger, more popular domain of practice of 'western' medicine has remained hidden from historical analysis is precisely because they have not been considered *proper* 'western' medicine. This judgement, apart from accepting the politically loaded categories of contemporary elite doctors, also essentializes the very identity of 'western' medicine. We will therefore avoid sitting in judgement on this question and include amongst our *daktars* anyone who would have been accepted by his contemporaries as having been a *daktar.*

It must be remembered that this social recognition itself did not homogenize everybody included within it. Even while recognizing many varied people as being *daktars,* contemporaries still distinguished between different levels of *daktars.* Reputations, educational backgrounds, the sort of treatment pursued, social status, fees—everything varied widely. Unlike Iliffe's study, therefore, the present book is not about the development of a profession. It is instead about the development of a socially significant identity. Hospital assistants, MDs from the Calcutta Medical College and the 'plucked students' practising without a licence could not exactly be described as a common professional group. Yet they were all described as *daktar,s* and therefore did share a common social identity. This social identity cannot be solely accessed by reference to professional rules, employment contracts, educational backgrounds, etc.—for these varied widely—instead, the shared social identity can be unpacked in the discursive and practical space in between the self-presentation of these practitioners and the anonymous social images of them. *Daktars* and those close to them presented their identities through introductory, congratulatory and hagiographic texts. Society at large, on the other hand, saw them in terms of popular images found scattered in popular literary presentations of the day. The social identity of the *daktars* emerged in the space between these practices of self-presentation and literary representation.

History of 'Western' Medicine in a Colonial Context

The one question that has dominated conferences, articles and discussions on the history of medicine in a colonial context since the early 1980s has been, 'What is "colonial" about "colonial medicine"?' Though originally asked by Roy Porter, this agenda-defining question is today mostly attributed to Shula Marks restatement of it some ten years after Porter.[32] The singular importance that this one question has come to acquire through repeated restatements has done much to outline the specificities and violence of the colonial context. The extraordinary privileging of this one question in academic agendas, however, has often led to the formulation of colonial medical history in terms of 'an encounter'.

The word 'encounter' continues to be one of the most widely used term in histories of colonial medicine.[33] At the risk of slight oversimplification, this 'encounter-frame' might be said to organize colonial medical history in terms of a narrative of confrontation—a confrontation where two relatively discrete entities meet each other in a zero-sum game for domination.[34] Thus a well-bounded, discrete 'western' medicine meets an equally homogenized and bounded 'indigenous' society. In South Asia, however, the word 'encounter' has a specifically ominous ring to it. It has been regularly used by the media to designate 'false' or 'staged' confrontations wherein state militias (the army and the police) have gunned down 'secessionists', 'communists' and other radicals while in state custody. This widespread popular usage of the term 'encounter' has two axes to it.[35] First, it draws attention to the 'staged' nature of the confrontation and second, it highlights the role of the word ('encounter') in hiding from view an act of one-sided violence. Both these axes will help us unpack the term's usage in the historiography of colonial medicine as well. The conflict between the parties itself is not unreal in this sense of the word 'encounter', but the acting out of that conflict as a single episode of open confrontation is staged to hide from view a unilateral act of (immediately) unprovoked violence. It stages a complex conflict as a single episode of violent confrontation. The 'encounter frame' similarly helps to *stage* medical history as an episodic confrontation of two relatively well-bounded, internally coherent entities (these entities might be either rival 'medical systems', or 'state' and 'society' or categories of belonging such as 'foreign' and 'indigenous') in a violent open clash. Its 'epistemic violence' lies in erasing the numerous levels of long-term mimesis, hybridization, negotiation, etc. between the multiple internal strands that constitute each entity. Such a framework, particularly in South Asian history, is surprising, since in many other areas of historical investigation such reductions of colonial conflict to a single dimension have been discredited since the 1970s.

One of the consequences of this 'encounter frame' has been an internal bifurcation of the field of colonial medicine itself. On the one hand there has emerged a wealth of studies on public health in colonial societies, where the emphasis has been on understanding the relationship between medicine and colonial domination. In South Asia, David Arnold's and Mark Harrison's works have provided some of the best analyses of these connections.[36] On the other hand another rich corpus of studies has emerged on the histories of the 'indigenous medical systems' of India. The works of Brahmanand Gupta and Poonam Bala have played a pioneering role in this area.[37]

These two branches of South Asian medical historiography have also developed their own preferred analytic frames. The more recent studies on 'public health' have developed a Foucaultian analytic framework which accents 'governmentality' and 'bio-power'.[38] The recent histories of 'indigenous medicine', on the other hand, usually adopt a social–historical approach.[39] The most engaging of these, such as Guy Attewell's brilliant work on unani medicine, engages in a robust dialogue with medical anthropology and incorporates within its analytical toolbox, tools developed in a range of disciplinary fields ranging from cultural studies, science studies and postcolonial theory.[40]

This divergence in the analytic framework of the two most important branches of South Asian medical historiography has led to a curious result, especially in the study of 'western' medicine in South Asia. 'Western' medicine's links with *repressive* dimensions of (colonial and more recently postcolonial) power have been explored in depth, while its *productive* role in constituting new subjects and subject-positions have been relatively unexplored. This has also led to disengagement with the intellectual world of early South Asian doctors. Whereas historians of 'indigenous' medicine have engaged intimately with the intellectual milieu of ayurveda, siddha, unani, etc., there has been no comparable exploration of the intellectual milieu of South Asian practitioners of 'western' medicine. This disengagement, in turn, has implicitly reaffirmed the view of 'western' medicine as 'foreign' and having only an external, repressive role in South Asian lives until well into the twentieth century. 'Western' medicine as a metonym for colonial modernity has therefore remained largely a bad word, a factor mediating the capacity of the colonial power to 'control' its subjects.

Scholars working on other colonial and postcolonial locations, such as Megan Vaughan and Warwick Anderson, have noticed a more complex history of 'western' medicine's role in a colonial situation. They have noted that both repressive 'control' and productive 'self-formation' have often been the consequences of colonial medical power.[41] Both Vaughan and Anderson dub their analytical frameworks 'postcolonial'. Anderson has outlined that 'postcolonial' analysis of medical history, need be neither the celebration of the end of colonialism nor remain attached to 'unitary totalities' of 'colonialism', 'colonial discourse', 'the Other', 'orientalism' and 'imperialism'.[42] The 'global' and the 'local' or the 'foreign' and the 'indigenous' are not, within this framework, descriptive commonplaces, but rather historically contingent categories which emerge within particular historical and political contexts and are continually being mutually reorganized. Anderson's postcolonial framework works to 'destabilize or at least challenge the assumption that Western knowledge is objective, authoritative and universally applicable'.[43] It seeks to 'understand the ways in which technoscience is implicated in postcolonial provincializing of "universal" reason, the description of "alternative modernities", and the recognition of hybridities, borderlines and in-between conditions'.[44] Anderson therefore affirms Stacy Leigh Pigg's contention that, 'we now need to find out more about how science and technology travel, not whether they belong to one culture or another'.[45] It is here that Vaughan's pithy statement made in the context of colonial Africa, but equally applicable to colonial South Asia, becomes relevant. 'It should be remembered', wrote Vaughan, 'that biomedicine is practised and interpreted by African doctors, nurses and medical assistants and as a practice is therefore as "African" as any other healing system'.[46] There is, therefore, in Vaughan's analytical scheme, no reason why those kinds of analytical frameworks hitherto reserved for 'indigenous' or 'traditional medical systems' should not be applied to 'western' medicine.[47]

It would be incorrect to conclude that there have been absolutely no attempts to study the provincialization of 'western' medicine and science in colonial South Asia.[48] As Anderson himself has pointed out, the works of scholars like Deepak Kumar have done much to construct a 'usable history of third-world science and technology' and thereby expand the categories of 'science' and 'technology' beyond their Eurocentric registers.[49] In the related field of science studies, the works of Kapil Raj, S. Irfan Habib and Dhruv Raina have similarly highlighted the 'domestication' of 'western science' in South Asia.[50] In medicine particularly, the works of Mridula Ramanna, Kabita Ray, Achintya Kumar Dutta and others have similarly focussed on South Asian practitioners of 'western' medicine.[51]

These studies in the provincialization of 'western' science in general and medicine in particular remain however focussed almost exclusively on individual personalities and particular institutions.[52] There is, unfortunately, in South Asia no work till date comparable to John Illife's comprehensive study of early African practitioners of 'western' medicine.[53] The works of Iliffe, Adell Paton and, most recently, Walter Bruchhausen have done much to bring to light the distinct roles played by Africans in the colonial medical apparatus.[54] They have accented the unique intellectual traditions, political roles and distinct modernities developed by these early African practitioners of 'western' medicine.

These works have provided a set of illustrative ethnographies of African medical modernities. They have provided both the evidence as well as the instantiations of the theses about constant diversification of modernity through the production of multiple distinctive modernities. Vaughan's comment about deploying analytical frames reserved for 'indigenous medicines' in the analysis of 'western medicine' assumes greater importance when set beside these descriptions of multiple modernities. Vaughan clarifies that the Foucaultian impulse, which informed the earlier generation of studies linking 'western' medicine to the 'repressive power' of the colonial state, while being highly enlightening, was not exhaustive. Vaughan rightly contends that Foucault's oeuvre does not constitute a monolithic system and there are different elements within his corpus that are not always exhaustively accessed through a focus upon the repressive capacities of power actualized through a nexus between Power/Knowledge. Instead, suggests Vaughan, that Foucault's propositions about the 'productive' capacities of Power have remained underutilized by historians of medicine. This productive capacity of 'power' had allowed the objectification entailed in the repressive mechanisms of Power since the eighteenth century to double up as a process of subjectification as well. The objectifying tendencies therefore also results in the creation of individuated subjects capable of self-making and control. Instead of a clear-cut and deliberate imposition by one social group upon another, therefore, Power became something constitutive of 'every speech act and movement and practice of day-to-day life'. Power and Resistance are therefore not two distinct and discrete oppositional categories which 'encounter' each other. They are in a certain sense both articulations of Power.

Yet, Vaughan hastens to add, that under colonialism, power's 'productive' capacity for subjectification often remained marginalized by comparison to its more pronounced 'repressive' features.[55] Colonial power often managed to dominate *without* hegemony and therefore differed at times markedly from the European contexts that Foucault's work referred to. Foucault's ideas about power thus—while being capable of illuminating much—do not provide a pre-given blue-print by reference to which we can fully understand the history of colonial medicine. The southern African historian Fredrick Cooper, who is influenced by the work of the Subaltern Studies in South Asia, is hence approvingly quoted by Anderson, when the former urges scholars to, 'analyse in specific situations how power is constituted, aggregated, contested and limited, going beyond the post-structuralist tendency to find power diffused in 'modernity', 'the post-Enlightenment era' or 'western discourse'.[56]

Anderson suggests that a postcolonial framework of analysis in the history of medicine will, therefore—through its insistence on materiality and specificity, act as a counterweight to the propensity of postcolonial theory to lapse into solipsistic textualism and arcane hermeneutics.[57] Read, together with Vaughan's reading of Foucault's 'productive power' and the fascinating recent ethnographies of 'modern medicine' by scholars like Nancy Scheper-Hughes and Lawrence Cohen, who have reoriented critical medical anthropology towards a more rigorous materiality, and we can develop a radical and powerful new research agenda for the history of 'western medicine' in a colonial context.[58] Disengaging from older questions of clear-cut domination and subordination, we might ask new questions about precisely how in specific situations did 'western' medicine 'produce' new kinds of subjects, identities, spaces, objects, etc., and how these came to be organized within a complex and shifting matrix of Power and Resistance.[59]

Within such a framework the 'foreignness' of 'western' medicine is not a pre-given fact but rather a historically contingent narrative-frame. 'Western' medicine hence is not always already an imposition. Instead, it might in itself function as a site of 'resistance'. It might also 'produce' new subjectivities, spaces and objects which can be marshalled for the cause of such 'resistance'. Crucially, however, 'resistance' in this framework always appears within quotes. It is not an 'authentic' project of amelioration, of subordination or liberation.

'Resistance' to colonial domination might, at the same time, itself be a project for the domination of other marginal groups.

Going Beyond State Medicine

In the historiography on South Asian medicine what reinforced the 'encounter-frame' was the belief that despite the precolonial presence of 'western' medicine in South Asia, with the coming of colonialism, 'western' medicine became wholly subsumed within the politics of the colonial state. Pioneering works on the history of medicine in colonial South Asia have asserted its close links with the colonial state—both as an enabling as well as a disabling factor. An exchange between two of the leading historians of colonial South Asian medicine, amply brings out this consensus over the affinity of 'western' medicine and the colonial state. While accepting the fundamental validity of Mark Harrison's contention that the role of 'western' medicine in stabilizing colonial domination was significantly limited by the values, opinions and opposition of the 'indigenous' society as well as by the ground realities of colonial South Asia, Deepak Kumar contends that Harrison's argument is itself 'limited'. Instead, Kumar argues that 'in the given scenario of complete hegemonization, the possibilities of inter-cultural interactions were rather limited. The indigenous systems felt so marginalized that they sought survival more in resistance than in collaboration'.[60] There are two points in Kumar's comments that are worth further investigation. First, did 'western' medicine or, indeed, the colonial state, achieve 'complete hegemonization' over South Asian society? Second, does 'cultural interactions' have to be limited to transactions between rival 'medical systems'?

In politics, as Ranajit Guha has famously pointed out, colonial rule was often sustained by brute force rather than by hegemony.[61] How far is it likely that where hegemony remained incomplete and limited in the realm of politics, it would be complete in the realm of medicine? Partly the perception of complete hegemonization comes from a historiographic focus that continues to privilege state medicine. The complete appropriation of the state's medical apparatus and discourse by 'western' medicine and its consequent deployment in the course of public health measures is therefore seen to constitute a 'complete hegemony'. There are, however, two serious objections to this privileging. First, surely given the limited interest, reach and resources that the colonial state devoted to public health, state medicine could not have exhaustively attended to all the medical needs of the South Asian subjects.[62] Indeed some scholars have gone so far as to suggest that until the end of the First World War, 'western' medicine's impact was limited social–historical to small enclaves.[63] Though this 'enclavist' argument has now been convincingly qualified by authors like Arnold, it would be wrong to gravitate to the other extreme and contend that 'western' medicine had—in the colonial period—achieved a 'complete hegemony'.[64] The focus on state medicine needs to be supplemented by accounts of the thriving medical market.

The medical market as a concept evolved in the 1980s owing to scholars like Roy Porter and Harold Cook.[65] Ever since, the concept has undergone several elaborations. It has hitherto served as an useful organizational *topos* to understand and describe preprofessional medicine. Amongst the reorientations it has allowed in its wake, several have been significant, including the recovery of the patient and the role of commerce in the histories of medicine. Recent scholars, however, have argued that it has now become a descriptive commonplace and is in need of reinsertion into specific historical contexts to retain its utility.[66] The most prominent use of the notion of a medical market has been to study the impact of the market in shaping the identity and content of 'indigenous' medicines.[67] Besides this recent use of the concept to study the marketing of 'indigenous' medicines in an increasingly globalized, its only significant deployment in colonial South Asian medical historiography has been by Pratik Chakrabarti in his recent exploration of eighteenth century 'bazaar medicine'.[68] Sarah Hodges has also recently used it to study the postcolonial context. Hodges points out that the market and the state, within her context, while being separate domains, are not mutually exclusive or oppositional and often operate to shape, influence and supplement each other.[69] Our use follows these leads in contextualizing the medical market within specific historical contexts, rather than treating it as an already defined analytical category and seeks to see the market and the state as mutually reinforcing and supplementary domains rather than as oppositional entities.

Traditionally, the medical market has tended to be seen as an antithesis to the idea of a medical profession. These two concepts and their understandings within medical history are best discussed together. The idea of the *profession* has been in vogue since the 1690s in some form or other amongst historians of medicine. From the mid-twentieth century it came to be heavily influenced by sociologists and sociological theories. Under this influence it was essentialized and seen as having certain fixed criteria. Though opinion varied on what this crucial essence of a profession was—with some proposing 'knowledge' and others suggesting 'power'—consensus, until the 1990s, remained that it had a definite essence.[70] A colonial dimension to this debate arose through the argument that colonial medical professions, since they did not organize themselves from bottom up as was the case in the 'west', but were organized by the state from the top down, were not 'proper' professions.[71] It was within this context that Cook and Porter produced their influential work on medical markets, which sought to capture a more 'fluid', less 'regulated' world of medicine, before the onset of professional regulations. Since the 1990s, however, historians—increasingly aware of cross-cultural data and under the influence of historicist ideas—have moved away from this essentialized view of a medical profession and asserted simultaneously the power of the notion of a 'profession' for practitioners in many varied contexts as well as the need to rigorously contextualize what *profession* signified in a specific historical context. This new empirical grounding has implicitly enabled the revisiting of the relationship between medical professions and the medical markets. The question is of importance to us, since, though we do not limit ourselves to a professional group, many of the *daktars* whose works, ideas and practices we will be looking at did think of themselves as a professional group. Journals such as the *Bhisak Darpan*—of which we shall hear often in this book—regularly published model question papers for medical examinations, detailed lists of interhospital transfers and even articles avowedly written to clarify important medical issues for *daktars* 'without degrees' to thereby align their practice with 'qualified' practitioners. The *daktars* clearly used some loose notion of constituting a profession, though the identity often lacked precision and leaned heavily upon the broader social identity. This, however, did not position them outside the medical market. On the contrary, the market was often where the *professional* identity of the *daktar* was most conspicuously performed in the course of debates with non-*daktars*.[72] The market and the medical profession—comprising both *daktars* and their European colleagues—often overlapped and intersected with each other in myriad ways. Recently, Seema Alavi in a richly detailed account of Mughal medicine has proposed the notion of a 'medical labour market'. The concept, in Alavi's usage does not derive from the discussions of the market by medical historians, but is amply suited to describe a part of the medical market which comprises skilled manpower and therefore overlaps with the notions of 'profession'.[73] The colonial government admitted as late as 1913 that the limited efforts it made to control the participation of its medical officers in the market were extremely 'limited and unsatisfactory'. These efforts were, moreover, usually limited to the handful of senior medical officers and teaching staff. At the level at which the majority of *daktars* operated (and here we speak of those in government service), controls were minimal and they could easily combine their usually meagre government salaries with earnings from writing books, publishing journals, selling specifics and, of course, by private practice. In fact, the government itself was aware of many *daktars* having fixed and lucrative annual contracts to act as family physicians to numerous wealthy families.[74] There are also, of course, many examples of *daktars* in government service selling their own specifics or even helping others sell their drugs.[75] A good example of how the medical bureaucracy and the market could be supplemented by each other at various levels can be seen in the case of the drug *Izal*. Ms Newton, Chambers & Co. wrote to the government in January 1905 drawing their attention to an article written by Major J. C. S. Vaughan, a member of the Indian Medical Service (IMS), on the usefulness of the drug in treating tropical dysentery. The government replied that IMS members in Bengal had already noticed the article.[76] In the same month the Inspector General of Civil Hospitals recommended the purchase of 100 lbs of *Izal* for use at the CMC.[77] Such examples clarify that the state and the market existed as domains of autonomous, but often supplementary, action without necessarily opposing or precluding each other.

The concept of medical pluralism is often used as a synonym for the medical market. They are however independent concepts. Medical pluralism repositions the patient—rather than the state—at the centre of medical history. Scholars using the concept have usually highlighted what has come to be known as 'healer hopping', whereby patients, by consulting a wide variety of healers, exercise power even in contexts where biomedical doctors have largely objectified and disempowered the patient.[78] Though medical anthropologists such as Mark Nichter have used notions of 'healer hopping' with great effect to study South Asian health-seeking behaviour, its use in medical historiography remains limited.[79]

The second issue that challenges the thesis about 'complete hegemonization', as well as forcing us to rethink the prevalent conceptualization of 'cultural interactions', pertains to the assumed stability and essentialization of the identity 'western' medicine. In order for one form of medicine to 'completely hegemonize' others, we must assume that these medicines constitute relatively stable, discrete entities.[80] As a wealth of recent studies of the histories of South Asia's classical medical traditions have shown, the identities of these 'systems' were not in themselves stable or discrete. They were being constantly redefined in response to a variety of social, political and cultural developments. At the same time, they were internally highly diverse and differentiated. The same, however, can also be said of 'western' medicine. Partly, the reason for the invisibility of the diversity of 'western' medicine has been the result of a persistent emphasis on reading its history through a small set of governmental files and a handful of English texts written by European or high-ranking South Asian physicians. The close identification of 'western' medicine with the colonial state has therefore been overdetermined by its framing as a 'system' accessible only through erudite writings, policies and governmental deployments/ understandings.

It would, however, be inappropriate to dismiss out of hand this state-centric view of 'western' medicine, without reference to the context in which it was developed. It had arisen largely in response to a previous generation of scholarship that had seen the dissemination of 'western' medicine across the globe as a benign diffusion of a fully constituted medical tradition emanating from the colonial metropoles. Steven Shapin has described this paradigm as one organized around the view of an 'osmotic transfer of ideas from regions of high truth concentration to areas of low truth concentration'.[81] Not only were preexisting conditions—both intellectual and material—ignored in this framework, but, more crucially, it was presented as a benign project of modernity. The politics of colonial science was wholly absent within this framework. Colonisers deploying science appeared here as heroic, benevolent despots rather than as 'macro-parasites'.[82] Moreover, the specificity and the agency of the numerous science workers in the colonies were also zeroed out in these accounts. George Basalla's essay in 1967 attempted to qualify this framework by proposing a three-stage model whereby 'western science' eventually managed to establish independent scientific traditions in the colonies. Yet, both the politics of 'western science' in the colonies as well as the particularities of each distinct colonial situation remained absent from Basalla's model.[83]

It was these broadly diffusionist models from which the historiography began to break away at the beginning of the 1990s. Waltraud Ernst's *Mad Tales from the Raj* in 1991 spoke of the 'politics of control'.[84] Two years later, in 1993, appeared David Arnold's hugely influential book *Colonizing the Body*. Arnold, using a broadly Foucaultian paradigm, argued that the 'the history of western medicine in nineteenth-century India demonstrate[d] the limitations (though certainly not the irrelevance) of a Eurocentric diffusionist model and illustrate[d] the need to relate the history of scientific ideas not only to forces emanating from the metropolis, but also to local constraints and imperatives, political and professional influences, as much as to the evolution of scientific theory and technique'.[85] Where Ernst and Arnold had both repositioned the history of medicine with a view to highlighting the politics of (colonial) medicine, Mark Harrison's *Public Health in British India,* which appeared the following year (1994), faulted the diffusionist model for not being attentive to the specific historical exigencies of colonial South Asia and for ignoring the agency and identity of Anglo–Indian medicine.[86] Despite adopting a variety of theoretical approaches, it was the combined impact of this triple intervention that repositioned the history of 'western' medicine in India from being a mere footnote in the global expansion of 'western' medicine to a subject worthy of independent study.

Where the interventions of Ernst, Arnold and Harrison sought to establish a new importance for the local studies of 'western' medicine, two other books appearing from India in 1991 sought to argue for the importance of global networks and exchanges in the development of these local cultures of science and medicine in colonial India. Deepak Kumar's edited volume entitled *Science and Empire* and Satpal Sangwan's *Science, Technology and Colonization* both brought together scholars who looked at a wide range of scientific theories and practices in terms of their implication in local cultural contexts as well as through their networks of exchange and influence with the extra-local sources.[87] Kumar's later work, *Science and the Raj*, published in 1997, distinguished between 'colonial' and 'metropolitan' science, arguing more explicitly for the autonomy of colonial science.[88] The following year Anil Kumar's *Medicine and the Raj* restated what Harrison, in an impassioned review, identified as a 'Whiggish…commitment to the idea of progress' seeking to demonstrate how the ameliorative potential of 'western' medicine was stunted by colonialism and how Indians progressively appropriated 'western' medicine from the hands of colonialists.[89] In some broad contours, then, it resonated with Deepak Kumar's identification of a certain 'bureaucratic momentum' that kept colonial medicine hitched to the colonial state.

Though these two strands of writing—one located in British academia and the other (mostly) in Indian academia—started from different ends of the global/local axis, both converged on the state as the preferred site of such negotiations. 'Western' medicine, despite all qualifications and localizations, remained, in the end, 'state medicine'. The importance given to the issue of loss of state patronage in the early histories of 'indigenous' medicines under colonialism also helped, by implication, to cement the historiographic link between 'western' medicine and state medicine.[90]

Towards the end of the 1990s there began to emerge other trends, which, in various ways, sought to supplement the state-centric approaches to medical history. These emergent histories might be grouped into three corpuses for heuristic purposes. First, there were histories of ideas and categories, which accented textual genealogies and intellectual networks. The works of Michael Worboys, Arnold and Harrison were important interventions in this regard.[91] Second, there emerged histories that looked at transnational networks that were not directly tied to the state. Histories of medical missions and those of global voluntarist organizations were important components of this trend. The interventions of David Hardiman and Sarah Hodges are worthy of mention in this respect.[92] Finally, a third trend, which at first sight often appears very close to the state-centric approach, but in effect subtly reoriented it, was visible in the many fine-toothed histories of specific institutions and medical projects.

This trend, represented by scholars like Sanjoy Bhattacharya, Mridula Ramanna, Jane Buckingham and others, of bringing out the dissonances between the various layers of the state, served to fracture the monolithic image of the state that had been deployed in earlier works. [93] In 2001 a volume co-edited by Harrison and Biswamoy Pati brought these diverse strands together. The much-cited and immensely influential volume established the new broader scope of history of medicine by reaffirming a commitment to detailed empirical case studies.[94]

Science and the Nation

Arnold's locus classicus, *Colonizing the Body,* had ended with brief comments about how the Indian middle classes had appropriated 'modern science' and medicine and integrated these into the latter's rhetoric of legitimation. This Indian middle class appropriation led—historiographically—to a long tradition of hagiographic and celebratory histories. These histories remained mostly couched within a diffusionist framework and concentrated primarily upon eminent personalities and a few elite institutions. Eminent Indian scientists were cast in this framework as promethean men who brought the fire of scientific modernity to the Indian masses. The hoariest of these studies do not fail to point out that India had in fact had a culture and a tradition of advanced 'science' that predated colonialism by hundreds if not thousands of years. One such recent nationalist history, for example, mentioned 4,000-year-old 'operating theatres' in India that anticipated contemporary knowledge of infection.[95] 'Colonial science' in this narrative framework is the antonym of 'national science', and the identity of both derived, in essence, from the racial identities of their practitioners. One of the most prominent exponents of such historiography, Chittabrata Palit, thus writes that the Indian Medical Service was 'primarily of the white people, by the white people and for the white people'.[96] 'national science', according to Palit, was simply the 'reply' to this 'colonial science'.[97] Even in those accounts of 'national science' where 'nationalism' transcends the reductive chromatic binarism of the 'evil white people' and their 'heroic Others', it often fails to historicize the character and politics of 'national science'. J Lourdusamy's *Science and National Consciousness in Bengal,* for instance, while doing much to accent the importance of the colonial/national 'dialectics' in the lives of some of the most eminent Bengali men of science, remains a largely descriptive study, failing to explore distinctive politics of 'national science'. His conclusion that in the 'given context and period, there was a fluidity and flexibility in the conception of modern science which allowed for the rich and creative expressions in indigenous cultural idioms' remains based primarily upon the assertions of his protagonists ('interlocutors') rather than on a critique of their statements.[98]

From the 1990s, however, a small group of scholars began approaching the nexus between science and nationalism more critically. Part of this critical energy derived from the recognition that the pursuit of technoscientific modernity by the postcolonial nation states in South Asia was often inflicting unprecedented violence upon sections of its own populations. In India, the forced sterilization drives of the late 1970s, the enforced evictions of peasants from the Narmada Valley to make way for hydroelectric projects, the developing market for human organs from the poor and, finally, the nuclear race between India and Pakistan—all brought home the malevolent capacities of the compact between science and nation state.[99] Moreover, as the nation state enjoyed a far stronger hegemony than its colonial predecessor, the sites and positions of resistance to its violence had also been limited.

From these scholars who sought to critically disengage the nation, state power and 'modern science', three significant trends can be observed. The first developed a critique of modern science itself by drawing attention to its structural capacity for alienation and violence. Ashis Nandy's influential edited volume *Science, Hegemony and Violence* stated this position with the greatest aplomb.[100] Of the essays in the volume, Manu Kothari and Lopa Mehta's essay specifically critiqued 'modern medicine' for its capacity for violence.[101] Nandy's book perceptively outlined how 'science' had come to assume an unprecedented charisma in contemporary life and how, if relied on, it could demand and—willy-nilly—obtain immense sacrifices.[102] Nandy's critique, though powerful, engaged the nexus between science and state power, not the nation as such. While exposing some of science's claims to disinterestedness and objectivity, it did not actually explore the politics of 'national science'. Elsewhere, however, Nandy developed a reading of 'national science' that did challenge the essentialist descriptions. In *Alternative Sciences*, Nandy provided a wonderful psycho-biographical reading of two eminent South Asian scientists and their quest for an 'alternative' to 'modern' science.[103] This approach also finds resonance in the writings of Dipesh Chakrabarty, who draws attention to a nexus between the 'scientific' re imagination of the body, modern state power and capitalist systems of exploitation.[104]

Gyan Prakash's *Another Reason* brought together some of these emerging ideas about 'alternate', 'national science' and its relationship to state power. Prakash reintroduced 'imagination' into the history of colonial and national science. Prakash did not agree with those who held that while the Indians had creatively reimagined the 'nation', they had eventually surrendered that nation to a derivative and oppressive state-form. Instead, Prakash held that Indian imaginations of the nation had always been premised upon the eventual nationalization of the state, but that nation state itself was imagined differently.[105] Thus, whereas Partha Chatterjee, for instance, had found a disjuncture between earlier communitarian 'national science' (of men like Rajnarayan Basu) and later state-centred 'national science', Prakash found them to be mutually unopposed.[106] Part of the reason for this disagreement lies, no doubt, in the very different types of authors upon whose writings Chatterjee and Prakash builds their respective arguments. Chatterjee uses the works of men like Rajnarayan Basu and Bankimchandra Chattopadhyay—both of whom were in colonial employment and were not overt political nationalists. Moreover, though both were polyglots, the vast majority of their writings are in Bengali. On the other hand, Prakash's arguments (on this particular issue) are based upon the English writings of two overtly political nationalists—Nehru and Gandhi.

A third approach to exploring the nexus between science and nationalism can be glimpsed in the work of Pratik Chakrabarti. Chakrabarti, following Quentin Skinner, seeks to write a de-centred history of ideas.[107] In his histories, neither nationalism nor science have fixed values; instead they come to assume their values within their specific usages in specific and thoroughly historicized texts. Though Chakrabarti's work, too, concentrates on eminent figures and institutions, by rigorously decentring these figures and institutions, he serves to effectively challenge the heroic essentialist accounts of 'national science' developed by scholars like Palit.

Recent historians of nationalism, however, have taken this trend towards decentring even further. A new generation of scholars such as Benjamin Zachariah, Manu Goswami, Srirupa Roy and others have not only de-centred nationalism, they have also challenged its conception as an 'idea'.[108] Their works have reintroduced a new materiality into the history of nationalism in South Asia. They have drawn attention to the material and practical processes, actions and manoeuvres through which the (postcolonial) nation has been actualized as a set of concrete realities. Such a materialist framework also resonates with the neo-materialism emerging within both the related disciplines of science studies and medical anthropology which remain in dialogue with Medical History.

In Science Studies, the invaluable work of Bruno Latour and more recently Manual DeLanda has done much to neutralize the influence of textually oriented approaches to matters of scientific enquiry.[109] Neomaterialists have restored agency to material objects and tried to see scientific inquiry as a dynamic interplay between material and human capacities. In related moves, medical anthropologists have increasingly turned to the materiality of the transactions they study.[110] Transactions of human body parts, biotrash, etc., have therefore become new areas of interest for them.[111] These developments are in constant dialogue with medical history.[112] There is consequently a new interest in the histories of substances, material objects, etc. [113]

This materialist thrust in both studies on nationalism and on science have thus created a context for renegotiating the transactions between science and the nation, while persisting in the efforts to de-centre nation, science and their mutual relationship.

Nation, Subjectivity and the Community of Affect

Vaughan's emphasis on the 'productive' potential of power had highlighted the ways in which colonial objectification can in turn produce subjectification. Those who are reduced to the level of 'objects' by a dehumanizing imperial gaze, might in turn internalize those very capillaries of power to articulate new subjectivities, in time to be pressed into struggles of empowerment. Yet these new empowering subjectivities are not there to begin with. They are only realized in the course of a certain historical process of internalization, appropriation and actualization. What is it, then, that unites the various agents *at the beginning* of the process?

This question is crucial to us, because part of our story lies well before the emergence of an articulated sense of nationalism. Why do the *daktars* show clear evidence of sympathy for their fellow countrymen, even before a clearly articulated sense of nationalism has emerged? Even later—once overt nationalism has emerged—unlike many of the stalwarts of science, whom historians have hitherto studied, the low-level medical functionaries we study were not always keenly politicized nationalists. While it is highly likely that some of them would have had nationalist sentiments, there is no way of knowing with certainty whether all of them would have had such sentiments. Yet during divisive episodes such as the Calcutta plague, the *daktars* remained staunchly sympathetic to countrymen and their intellectual and practical response to the events around them amply reflected this sympathy. How then are we to explain their participation in a project which eventually realized the nation as a set of real bodies, spaces, sentiments, etc.?

There was, we will argue, a sense of community even before the nation emerged as a well-articulated identity. Rajat Kanta Ray has called this the 'felt community'. Ray argues that this 'felt community' predated the nation and continued to exist alongside it.[114] Such a contention is borne out by at least one contemporary witness. Rabindranath Tagore, in his reflective essay entitled 'What is a Nation?' ('Nation Ki?'), mentioned that, ultimately, the nation is an 'animate identity' (*sajeeb satta*). It had, according to him, two axes—memories of what was believed to be a shared past and common will to stay together. It was these two axes that together eventually actualized a nation.

This 'felt' affinity to the larger community, on the part of the *daktars*, would no doubt have been strengthened by the racial prejudice they were subjected to even when working within the government medical services. This prejudice had material consequences for the subordinate South Asian medical staff in the form of lower salaries, lack of opportunities for promotion, etc. Despite repeated petitions their pleas for better service conditions were not fulfilled until the end of the first decade of the twentieth century.[115] All this would undoubtedly have reinforced their identifications with their countrymen over and above any espirit de corps they shared with their European colleagues. Yet the identification of *daktars* with fellow Bengalis or Indians cannot be wholly reduced to the consequence of lower salaries and lack of promotion. Even the best respected and most prosperous of *daktars* expressed their sympathies for their countrymen in their actions and their writings, during the plague upheaval. The affective community would have been constituted through the participation of the *daktars* in spheres of shared 'beliefs, [and] of marriage and a sense of inhabiting the same moral realm'.[116] It is at the level of this emotional identification that we must turn to locate the difference between *daktari* medicine and that practiced by their European colleagues. In fact, Ashis Nandy, highlighting the social nature of emotions and their centrality to scientific work has pointed out that in societies which draw upon 'their versions of the eternal verities, the blueprints of newer national identities…science becomes the battleground where the community's ambitions confronts its backlogs, and the scientist becomes a microcosm where the community's adaptive capabilities challenge the creative power of the individual'.[117] The emotional matrix which informs scientific work is therefore not a 'personal' or 'individual' matter in the scientist/doctor's mind. Its roots lie in the socio-cultural resources through which subjectivities are formed and taught to cope with adaptive challenges. More acutely, in societies caught in the throes of nationalist reinvention, these adaptive challenges are necessarily politicized ('battlegrounds').

Significantly, however, this 'felt community' does not have clearly defined boundaries. While it is usually implicitly operationalized at the level of everyday activities, it does not exist at the level of a well-defined reality capable of clear articulation. Moreover it is capable of changing its shape and size in response to other historically contingent developments. The process whereby this diffuse sense of commonness comes to be clearly defined and articulated is the process of actualizing the nation. The active verb 'nationalizing' in the title of this book designates precisely this process of actualization of the nation.[118]

The existence of such a 'felt community' also raises another important issue. Vaughan's study while accenting the 'productive' capacities of power, had also indicated the limits of traditional Foucaultian categories in a colonial situation. She had pointed out that the governmental practices of the colonial state were distinct from those of European states and they had not encouraged the emergence of fully individuated subjects. The onus had rather been on the control of groups and hence the new subjectivities that developed often reinforced and reformatted new group identities rather than promoted individuation.

Arguing along a wholly different intellectual route, scholars such as Sunil Khilnani, Sudipta Kaviraj, Partha Chatterjee and others have also arrived at a comparable conclusion.[119] These scholars have questioned the clear-cut and exhaustive dichotomy of state and Civil Society that is often thought to define the political lives of 'modern' subjects. The associational forms and calculative rationality premised on individual self-interest, which are seen to be the cornerstones of these two domains, do not—in South Asia—exhaust the political lives of the subjects. The rigorously individuated subjects are often said to be absent. Conventional readings of Foucaultian notions of biopower are premised upon the power to control and discipline individual bodies. Individuals comply with the directives of power, not because they are threatened by death (as Foucault says was previously the case), but because they want to live. Life itself is controlled through the 'anatomopolitics of the human body' and the 'biopolitics of population'. If the Foucaultian model and its categories are adhered to, how then are we to understand the decisions of a man who accepts the likelihood of death from plague, yet refuses to hospitalize his plague-ridden wife because it will violate *purdah*? Where Foucault speaks of the 'investment of the body, its valorization and the distributive management of its forces', our *daktars* throughout subjugated the body to the operation of the will.[120] This will was not akin to the animator of the 'ascetic morality' (sometimes called the 'protestant ethic') which Foucault found. The will that the *daktars* spoke of could intervene to cure by subverting the usual mechanisms of the body. It was a force that could bring about the extraordinary in the context of bodily health and thereby render any anatomopolitics of body redundant. The will bore the signature of Being and thereby dominated the body.

It is undoubtedly partly in response to this awareness of the limitations of some conventional readings of Foucaultian categories—owing to the differential subjectivity observed in South Asia—that some contemporary medical anthropologists such as Lawrence Cohen and Joseph Alter have sought to develop the concept of 'biomorality' rather than 'biopolitics'.[121]

The term was first deployed by McKim Marriott and had then been attached to Marriott's notions of a 'dividual' (as opposed to 'individual') subject.[122] Though the concept has since been developed along many fruitful new directions, its fundamental difference from 'biopower' (as we understand it), is that it eschews the calculative rationality of self-interest premised upon individuated subjects devoted to the preservation of *biological* life. Thus while biopower functions because an 'individual' internalizes a certain logic of calculating self-interest aimed at furthering *biological* life, biomorality is premised upon a logic that calculates self-interest quite differently.[123] To elucidate with an example, while one subject might calculate self-interest by considering the best means of avoiding the infection of plague, for another, the necessary actions involved in avoiding such infection (violation of *purdah,* caste rules, etc.) might, in effect, mean jeopardising another kind of (after) life and the interests tied to such (after) life. The latter's logic of calculation might therefore lead her to believe that infection and even consequent death are actually preferable.

As we shall repeatedly see in this book, the *daktari* discourse promoted a 'technology of selfhood'. This *daktari* 'technology of selfhood', however, ran contrary to those 'technologies of selfhood' described by Nicholas Rose that produce more docile and manageable subjects. The *daktars,* by cultivating an almost narcissistic onus on the 'sovereign will' of the subject, produced, instead, subjects who were, if anything, *less* manageable.[124] In certain instances, the difference becomes obvious. The *daktari* support for the carnivalesque festivities of *Chodok* including the life-threatening "hook-swinging"—which had long been a law-and-order problem, not to mention one endangering individual life—is one conspicuous case in point.[125] The large-scale communal gatherings for the singing of hymns—which the *daktars* also supported—was another example of effectively fashioning subjects *less* rather than more manageable.

'System', Archives and the Vernacularization of Modernity

The reason these differences between *daktari* medicine and state medicine do not usually get noticed by historians is the lasting belief that 'western' medicine constitutes a 'system'. Kumar, for instance, in the introduction to his influential book *Disease and Medicine,* wrote that, 'There were several areas in which western and indigenous systems could have collaborated but did not. The former put emphasis on the cause of the disease, the latter on *nidana* (treatment)'.[126] Similarly, Palit mentions that the 'relationship between western and Indian systems of medicine has been an important issue in medical history'.[127]

Arnold first drew attention to the history of this popular image of the medical traditions as 'systems' by historicizing the image in the context of the revival of 'indigenous' medicines.[128] From its very outset, therefore, the historicization of the concept of 'medical *systems*' has pertained to the history of 'indigenous' rather than 'western' medicine. Yet this literature on 'indigenous' medicines has developed some very astute insights into the concept that might, with profit, be applied to the history of 'western' medicine. The concept of 'medical *systems*' has been historicized along two slightly different routes. First, scholars have understood it as a long-term process whereby disparate medical practices and ideas are reformatted into a coherent *system*. In this rendition, the 'system' as such is real and has some fixed characteristics, and the acquisition of this status is a historically contingent process. Rachel Berger's recent doctoral work on ayurveda in north India takes such an approach.[129] This approach is close—though not identical—to the way nineteenth-century authors understood the 'medical systems'.[130] An alternative route has been taken by Guy Attewell in his history of unani tibb. Attewell's brilliant critique, which follows up Arnold's earlier comments, instead of accepting fixed criteria for 'systems', questions what a 'system' might come to mean in a given context. He goes further and explores the politics of such a systemic frame. What Attewell thus seeks to question is not just when and how unani became 'systematized', but also why was it *presented* as a 'system' and what exactly did it mean to say that unani was a 'system'. In seeking to answer this question, he argues that, 'the use of the word "system"...consolidates the impression of continuity, connoting internal coherence, discreteness, completeness and homogeneity'.[131] Arnold makes two further points in this respect. First, he contends that what makes these 'systems' appear as 'systems might not be internal to them. They may in effect be 'part-systems' immersed within 'a much wider set of norms, beliefs and expressions'. Second, he suggests that the 'system' might be seen differently from different angles. A practitioner might emphatically see himself as belonging to a 'system' and yet, without qualms, mix an eclectic range of medical ideas and practices in everyday treatment, while the patient might not even 'see' a 'system', seeing instead only a practitioner skilled in curing particular types of afflictions.[132] While Attewell highlights the epistemic politics built in to the image of the 'system' and its deployment in the nineteenth century, Arnold exteriorizes the identity of the system.

Once we accept these analytical manoeuvres as valid, there is no reason to not apply the same criteria to judge 'western' medicine in colonial South Asia. Once again, what forestalls such a reappraisal is the close identification of 'western' medicine with the state and the implicit acceptance of the politically loaded discourse on quackery into the analytical framework. A curious analytical double vision therefore persists in the study of 'western' and 'indigenous' medicines. Though some erudite and scholarly traditions of ayurveda or unani often displayed a high degree of internal coherence and opposed 'quackery' (usually anything that deviated from the normative coherence) with vigour, these are usually seen as only one strand within a complex milieu of 'indigenous' healing. Yet, in the case of 'western' medicine, the vast numbers of drug vendors, autodidactic physicians and 'unqualified' doctors—who were often the most recognizable face of 'western' medicine for rural populations—are not seen to in any way hamper the 'systemic' claims of 'western' medicine itself. If all of these were to be seen together as constituting the social identity of 'western' medicine, it, too, would appear much less 'systemic'. It is essentially the identification of 'western' medicine with the upper end of the colonial medical bureaucracy that allows its 'systemic' image to persist. But what ultimately makes these impressions appear as the only possible historical truth is the politics of the archive.

No archive preserves traces of every single aspect of the past. Numerous technical and political limitations intersect to determine which traces shall be preserved and which not. Jacques Derrida had pointed out that each archive is defined by a guardian (archon) and a location (domicile). The archive is actually intimately connected to the archon's continuance in power. The erasure of evidence that contradicts the archon's power or its legitimacy helps to legitimize and perpetuate the archon's power. In effect, this means there is a tendency to erase traces of alternative meanings (which would by their very existence disprove the extent of the archon's power). '[L]aw and singularity [therefore] intersect in privilege'.[133] In a situation where—unlike in the case of 'indigenous' medicine—the upholders of ('western') medical orthodoxy were simultaneously also high-ranking officials of the government, it is understandable that they would be more successful than their colleagues in ayurveda, unani, etc., in erasing traces of divergence from the 'systemic' norm. It is easily understandable that lowly Compounders or Hospital Assistants, working within a strictly regimented and hierarchical service cadre, would not feel comfortable in elaborating upon areas of disagreement with the medical wisdom of those higher up. Their reports would therefore be more than likely to exhibit a degree of conformity which was inspired more by the fear of censorship than by actual practice. Even more crucially, it is highly unlikely that these lowly medical personnel would even be expected to pen their medical views in official reports. Medical reports from subordinate medical staff—especially after the 1860s—usually comprised statistical reports supplied in preprinted official forms and only minor explanations of the statistical trends. In order to get beyond this artificially imposed sense of coherence and conformity, therefore, we must engage other archives. Historians must not be satisfied by the impressions generated by the official archive. They must venture to unravel other archives that supplement the impressions of the official archive. Their critical practice must comprise not merely 'reading', but also 'finding'.

It is here that 'vernacular' language sources become important. Not only were they written outside official protocols, but, indeed, they were also relatively freer from the spectre of censorship. This however should not be presumed to make them any more 'authentic' than the English language sources. They, too, were historically contingent texts produced within specific textual economies at specific historical junctures for particular purposes. They were structured by their own textual conventions and, being written usually for a thriving medical publishing market, they were mediated by the forces of that market. The critical gaze must not seek to peer past the historically fashioned text at an anterior, 'authentic' reality, but rather, as Stephen Greenblatt has suggested, must look carefully *at* the text.[134] We cannot distinguish between the official archive and the vernacular archive on the registers of truth and falsehood, but must hope to do so at the level of different orders of information constituted within distinct textual economies. This crucial methodological clarification will be most vivid in Chapter IV. Therein we shall see how *daktars* and English doctors differed diametrically in diagnosing cases of plague. Yet, today it is impossible to claim that one was correct and the other wrong. Instead we can make sense of their diagnosis only by thoroughly contextualizing their writings. Similarly, in Chapters III and V we shall see that it was once again not a question of *right* or *wrong*, but due to the different social locations of the texts and their authors, ideas, practices and pathologies came to mean different things to *daktars* and European doctors.

The acceptance of multiple distinct registers of information might smack of postmodern relativism. In this book, however, we steer clear of any such postmodern perspective. Instead, following trends set by Greenblatt and Foucault, often referred to as new historicism, what we seek to do is to integrate the nature and context for the production of the source into our analytical framework. Sources used are therefore not mere witnesses to a lost past; their own existence—in our reading—is a part of that story of the past. The *nationalization of the body* was a process—a process that actualized the nation by vernacularizing 'western' medicine. The sources that form the basis of this book are themselves both the witnesses and the products of that process.

The process was fundamentally a political process: not merely as a liberationist project directed against the *colonization of the body* but also one to establish new hierarchies of domination. In order to unpack these subtle operations of power, we cannot limit ourselves to solely medical texts. Medical texts are not (usually) overt arenas of political debates. The power that operates within them is therefore often difficult to identify. In order to understand the subtle operations of power and the shared sentiments that constitute the affective community, we must situate the medical texts next to literary texts which are more forthright in their emotional and political affinities.

Once we reintroduce the question of power into the interpretations of medical ideas and practices, the monolithic image of a coherent *system* begins to fray at the edges. Different authors, positioned differently within a complex matrix of power, interpreted and deployed medical ideas and practices along distinctive axes. We are no longer limited to the binarism of having to clearly and absolutely distinguish between those who accepted and those who resisted 'western' medicine. Instead, we can see how a variety of actors with access to a variety of different intellectual and practical resources and with different political and emotional sensibilities could imaginatively refashion 'western' medicine. Since 'western' medicine was a crucial component of the project colonial modernity, the pluralization of 'western' medicine would also entail a parallel pluralization of modernity itself.

From around the beginning of the twenty-first century, scholars have grown suspicious of the earlier image of a monolithic, uniform 'modernity' capable of transforming large swathes of the globe into a sea of sameness. Scholars such as S. N. Eisenstadt, Nilufer Gole, Dipesh Chakrabarty, Francis Robinson, Kaviraj and others have contended that modernity was not a single homogenous entity.[135] Its chronology of introduction, the preexisting conditions it met with and its tendency to self-correct made it endlessly variable and ever different. Scholars thus proposed a theory of multiple modernities.[136] These general arguments are applicable not only to 'western' medicine in South Asia as a whole, but also in all its parts. As a whole, the contexts within which it was introduced to South Asia as part of the cultural edifice of a colonial state was very different from its origins in the 'west'. In meeting with a range of well-established medical traditions—including highly textualized ones—it differed also from other colonial contexts, such as in Africa. In continually reorganizing itself in the hands of its numerous diverse practitioners, it continued to evolve. Internally, too, it was varied and continued to vary. A number of different routes of accessing it were open to those wanting to practice it, from the multiple degrees and diplomas offered by the medical schools and colleges to a variety of contexts for apprenticeship and even self-tutoring. What emerged was not only a different *version* of 'western' medicine but also one which was internally heterogeneous. In Chapter I we shall hear more of the plurality of routes through which one became a *daktar.*

Sheldon Pollock has suggested that 'modernity' be seen as a cosmpolitan cultural form which has its own set of vernacular forms. Pollock goes further to suggest that this process of vernacularization in South Asia may draw upon much older sedimented historical experience in vernacularization of cosmopolitan Sanskrit cultural forms.[137] Pollock warns that we should avoid complicity with ethnochauvinist politics by subscribing to the view that vernaculars are autochthonous entities. Vernaculars, too, are historically produced contingent entities similar to the cosmopolitan forms. In South Asia, these two forms were produced as *Marg Sanskriti* (Culture of the Great Way) and *Desi Sanskriti* (People's Culture). The two were not always in open conflict as was often the case in the Latinate universe; instead, in South Asia a 'tactical reversal of domination—a resistance-through-appropriation' was witnessed. This did not lead to a 'mongrelization' or 'hybridization' of cosmopolitan forms—since such concepts of hybridization, etc. assume a prior purity and discreteness of the entities being hybridized—but cosmopolitan forms were recast and realigned with vernacular forms in a complex process which had issues of domination and subordination at its very heart.[138]

The concept of vernacularization has been deployed in the history of medicine by those studying early modern Europe.[139] Through their usage, they have sought to understand the process whereby Latin medical wisdom was rendered into the numerous European vernaculars such as English, German, French, etc. William Crossgrove, in reviewing such literature, pointed out that 'Vernacularization presupposes the existence of vernacular culture in opposition to something more learned, more conscious, prestigious'.[140] Crossgrove then went on to show that there was no fixed 'vernacular' identity. What was once vernacular might later become in itself a cosmpolitan form as in the case of Old Church Slavonic, which first started off as a vernacular vis-à-vis Greek before acquiring its own cosmopolitan status. Even more complicated was the case of Norman French, which was a vernacular in the English court, but was an elite language for the majority of Saxon English. Any study of vernacularization, therefore, could not avoid engaging with issues of power and social prestige. Crossgrove, therefore, went on to suggest an approach reminiscent of New Historicism, which would locate the text within its social purpose, its authorial networks and its readership. Seema Alavi's fascinating recent work, without being directly derived from this body of literature about vernacularization in the history of science, has independently evolved a very similar framework. Alavi's work brilliantly demonstrates the variety of vernaculars into which South Asian medical knowledge was rendered at different times and the multiple networks of power, 'communities of literature' and reading markets that these vernaculars tapped into. From the Mughal (Persian writings that accented health as aristocratic virtue) to, first, the Arabic medical literature of the post-Mughal era that, while accenting a more scientist notion of health also operated to hitch medicine more closely to religious identity and subsequently, then to Urdu and Hindustani, which democratised access to medical knowledge and revolutionised North Indian healing markets, Alavi presents a complex narrative of multiple vernacularizations with its own accents, markets, readers, codes, textual genres etc.[141]

The *daktari* medicine we seek to engage in this book is therefore neither a 'hybrid' nor a 'mongrel', nor indeed is it an autochthonous voice. It is, instead, a vernacularized version of 'western' medicine constituted within a specific network of authors who shared a common social identity and a particular market of readers they catered to.

About the Book

Though this book deals with Bengal, its analysis resonates with the history of a larger swathe of the erstwhile British Empire. This is not because the historically specific experience of Bengal is presented here as being typical of the rest of South Asia. Rather, since Bengal had one of the earliest medical colleges and produced a large number of medically trained personnel who often took up employment way beyond the immediate precincts of Bengal, in a sense it speaks of the somewhat atypicality of the Bengal case. Subscription lists of Bengali medical periodicals show that *daktars* who made an effort to participate in the intellectual milieu of Bengali physicians (through the subscriptions) were stationed as far afield as Lahore and Peshawar. Some Bengali *daktars* also took up appointments outside South Asia. The hero of Saratchandra Chattopadhyay's nationalist novel *Pather Dabi* (The Demands of the Road) was, for instance, a Bengali doctor in colonial Burma not unlike similar Bengali *daktars* mentioned in the subscription lists of the journal *Swasthya Samachar* in 1927. One of the *daktars* we shall meet in greater detail in Chapter I, travelled farther to Mauritius for awhile after being unsuccessful in obtaining a government appointment in Bengal.

The time frame within which this book operates stretches roughly from 1860 to 1930. Prior to 1860 the thriving world of medical publications—which we argue had a crucial influence in the development of a social identity for *daktari* medicine—was rather small. After 1930, with significant numbers of South Asians in high-ranking positions within the medical bureaucracy as well as the attempt at greater governmental control of medical commerce (especially by the Chopra Committee of 1930–31), significant changes were introduced in the intellectual milieu and politics of *daktars*. We hint at some of these oncoming changes in the decade of the 1920s throughout the book, but they have not been followed up here. Both these cut-off dates, however, are merely pointers rather than impervious walls, and much material will be found on either side of the two dates.

Another aspect that requires comment is the choice of the designation 'western' medicine, rather than biomedicine, allopathic or modern medicine. 'Biomedicine' as a category was unsuitable, because all that was practiced from 1860 to 1930 could hardly be described by that term. Moreover, it is a term which had very little currency amongst contemporaries. 'Modern' medicine in turn had wide currency amongst contemporary authors, but the sheer diversity of its deployments and its obvious political resonances with the agendas of various modernities, ruled it out. 'Allopathic' was a designation that recommended itself the most amongst all these terms. It was widely deployed by in contemporary Bengali sources and continues to be the most popular South Asian designation. The only reason for not using it is the diversity of *daktari* practice and the fact that the name *daktar* was often applied to homoeopaths as well. Eminent examples like Dr Mahendralal Sircar would be difficult to categorize as either allopath or homoeopath. Yet, they were accepted by all as being *daktars*. This brings us to 'western' medicine. The designation, of course, could be applied to homoeopaths, mesmerists and a host of other practitioners. We, however, have limited it to practitioners of medicine that claimed to be aligned with that practised by the upper echelons of the Indian Medical Service. By contrast, *daktari* medicine refers to the vernacularized forms of this recovered within the textual archives of vernacular language sources. Within the context of this book, therefore, 'western' medicine is a wider category, aligned with state medicine (but not subsumed by it) and *daktari* medicine is a narrower category designating a vernacular version of the former.

Chapter I introduces the diversity of *daktari* medicine through a number of actual *daktari* lives. Though it is seemingly descriptive in its tone, its fundamental analytical value rests in this very description. Even at the level of the biographies, the chapter points out that the politics of archive and reading shapes our understanding of who these *daktars* were. Not only are the lives of every type of *daktar* not equally well preserved, but moreover, those that are preserved are also frequently recounted within standard representational schemas. Thus, accounts of the lives of *daktars* described as 'locally entertained native doctors' are extremely rare and must be reconstructed using prosopographic techniques. Similarly, the commercial aspects of the lives of even eminent *daktars* are hard to come by in the archives, as memorial texts usually do not mention these. Representational and archival politics entangle here with the numerous entanglements in terms of pedagogy, social background and professional practice that marked the *daktars*. Any thematic survery—which may have replaced the descriptive tenor—would have risked the reification of this rich plurality, which itself marked the lives of the early *daktars*.

In Chapter II we survey the large numbers and types of medical texts that were published and the connections of these genres of medical printing to the evolution of the *daktari* label. While the chapter recognizes the existence of heterogeneity within the *daktari* texts, it challenges the received wisdom that the cheaper print markets in colonial Bengal eschewed didactic texts. It shows that the world of *Bot-tola* printing was in fact crucial to the evolution of *daktari* medicine and though its content differed from the *daktari* medicine of the more 'polite' registers, their two worlds were not cut off from each other. The chapter integrates a survey of medical publishing in the nineteenth century with an understanding of the medical market—accessible both through the numerous medical books and periodicals as well as medical advertising—into a narrative of the development of *daktari* as a descriptive category.

The Third Chapter engages the creative potential of the idea of contagion. Refusing to see the term only negatively, the chapter shows how contagion formed one of the most prolific sites for *Nationalizing the Body*. A persistent espousal of a multicausal model of disease causation—a model which itself had roots both in the 'East' and the 'West'—allowed the *daktars* to develop, constitute and reconstitute projects of somatic, cultural and spatial 'improvement' whereby contagion could be resisted. In the process they also produced the material realities of the nation.

Chapters IV through VI are three detailed case studies dealing (respectively) with an 'epidemic', i.e., Plague (Chapter IV), an 'endemic', i.e., Cholera (Chapter V) and a 'syndrome', i.e., *Dhatu Dourbalya* (Chapter VI). Each of these three case studies highlights how the combination of the professional and affective attachments entangled with specific medical crises and demands of the medical market to operationalize a vernacularization of 'western' medicine, which was marked by its distinctiveness from Anglo-Indian practice. What these three studies highlight is the process whereby *daktari* medicine acquires not only a distinctive identity as a vernacularized form of 'western' medicine but also whereby a loose affective community is given a more concrete shape as a nation. The *nationalization of the body* was therefore not an episode (such as the nationalization of a bank or an industry). It was instead a process whereby a community of affect was operationalized to frame and reframe the bodies, territories, spaces, objects and projects that were to constitute the nation as a set of material realities.

Finally, a note on transliteration would be cogent. We have tried, wherever possible to maintain more generally better-known Sanskritized transliterations of Bengali names and terms. However, where the accent has been on the specificity of the Bengali usage, we have used Bengali pronunciations as a guide to transliteration. The result, we hope, even if not always systemic, might be reader-friendly.

Chapter I

HEALERS IN CONTEXT: FORGOTTEN PIONEERS

Part of the reason that Bengali vernacular forms of 'western' medicine—more appropriately called *daktari* medicine—have largely remained absent from the historian's account of nineteenth century South Asian medical history is because the *daktars* for whom it had meaning as a distinct form of medical practice have themselves remained out of sight. Histories mainly reliant upon English language archives—both governmental and nongovernmental—have mostly tended to see this numerous group of physicians as anonymous statistics, sometimes as half-trained quacks exploiting the lacunae of medical legislation and occasionally—it must be admitted—as prominent representatives of 'native' opinion, such as Dr Madhusudhan Gupta, Dr G. C. Roy, Sir Nil Ratan Sircar or even the Congress leader Dr B. C. Roy. Little detailed account, however, has been available of the actual lives and of the numerous and varied Bengalis who came to practice 'western' medicine at various levels of the colonial establishment, ranging from the lowly hospital assistants to the grand Edinburgh- or London-trained MDs. It is through their agency and through contact with their lifeworlds that *daktari* acquired its unique identity. Any history of *daktari* medicine will therefore remain incomplete without an account of the histories of these *daktars*.

The study of individual lifeworlds, i.e., lives in context, has been popularized since the 1970s by the increasing intellectual prominence of microhistory. As one of its pioneers, Carlo Ginzburg, has clarified, for a long time microhistory was only a vague quest for a more intimate view of the past in smaller scale. Its actual ambit had remained vague and it overlapped with other emergent tendencies like local history, historical anthropology, etc.[1] A small-scale view, however, did not necessarily mean looking at individuals. It could, and often did, also mean looking at a small physical space (such as a single house), a single event (such as the 'Great Cat Massacre') or even a very small temporal span (such as a few hours preceding the Battle of Gettysburg).[2] Once the microscopic fragment to study was decided upon, there was no consensus on how to see it. Some suggested that the fragments, by revealing repetitive patterns, could eventually yield macrohistorical narratives, and others doubted the validity of the approach which sought to fit the individuality of the fragment into the repetitive structures or 'serials' demanded by macrohistorical accounts.[3] While those supporting the insertion of 'fragments' into 'serials' leaned towards 'total histories', those who 'defended the fragment' became divided, in time, into two groups. Of these two groups, one asserted the essentially 'relative' nature of the fragment to other fragments while the other propounded a 'law of levels'. According to the 'law of levels', both macro- and microhistorical narratives together constituted historical truth, though the facts of the two levels were not interchangeable.[4] This meant that the fragment, while remaining in dialogue with its context, was never wholly translatable into larger contextually determined themes. This impossibility, to writers such as Ginzburg, was related to the heterogeneity, partiality and incompleteness of the historical archive that determined access to the fragment. Put plainly, since the fragment was always recorded incompletely, from a single or a very limited number of viewpoints, and since the recording process was itself a part of the history of the fragment, it would never be possible to wholly 'contextualize' the fragment, since not all relevant 'facts' will ever be available. The best solution in such a situation was thought to be Marc Bloch's method of constant juxtaposition of macro- and microhistorical perspectives.

Though many historians interested in the fragment have adopted this general approach of combining both macro- and microhistorical perspectives, their methods and approaches have been varied. Nowhere have these questions arisen more forcefully than in the study of microhistorical biographies. In the Subaltern Studies oeuvre, for instance, historians like Gautam Bhadra and Shahid Amin have tried to de-centre the individual.[5] Amongst prosopographists, on the other hand, the tendency has been to constitute 'composite individuals' through multiple fragmentary biographies.[6] Both these tendencies fluctuate between macro and micro levels in very different ways; but both are also committed to slightly different types of projects. The first seeks to discover 'society in man' by deconstructing his identity, while the latter seeks 'man in society' by reconstructing individuals out of scattered elements which make up individual lives. They are therefore implicated in different types of archives and different types of narrative economies. The first approach shows what a particular man's identity—be it Raja Pratapchand of Burdwan or Mohandas Karamchand Gandhi—meant to others. The second approach shows how faceless individuals experienced their own lives and identities in their given societies. Both are aspects of the historical truth.

In order to reconstruct the world of *daktari* medicine through the lives of individual *daktars*, we must juxtapose both these strategies. Partly, this is to allow for comparisons, but partly, it is also determined by the nature of the archives. Since the world of the *daktars* was itself highly plural, its archives are also varied. The lives of elite college-trained surgeons, for example, are more extensively recorded in service records and memorial texts, but the lives of hospital assistants are only marginally recorded in government files. Yet both were equally crucial to the development of *daktari* medicine. Moreover, like marginal notes, memorial texts such as obituaries are formulaic narratives and give only a certain order of information while concealing much else. All of this requires a juxtaposition of different archives and different reading strategies in order to reconstitute one *daktari* life.

Jill Lepore argues that the very nature of biographical projects alongside its dominant narrative forms induces a degree of emotional attachment between the historian and the subject. This, argues Lepore, leads to the presentation of the biography as a rationalized series of facts that hints at a more 'complete' and 'essentialized' sense of the individual's life than is allowed by the inchoate historical record.[7] To guard against such implicit assumptions of wholeness, we will deliberately juxtapose not merely methods and archives, but lives themselves which are comparable. Juxtaposing distinct and comparable lives will compensate against any strong implications of atypicality and rationalization.

Khan Moulvi Tamiz Khan Bahadur (?–1882)

Tamiz Khan was one of the most successful early Bengali doctors and medical teachers, yet his legacy has been almost totally neglected by medical historians. Whereas other early Bengali doctors and teachers of Tamiz Khan's stature, such as Madhusudhan Gupta and Soorjo Coomar Goodeve Chuckerbutty, have received some attention from historians, Khan, despite being one of the most influential and highly respected early doctors, has been almost totally neglected by historians.[8]

The most detailed information on Khan's life comes from a memorial speech made at the Calcutta Medical Society by Khan's closest friend and associate and another influential figure in early Bengali history of science, Rai Kanailal Dey Bahadur.[9] Dey's speech was later reproduced in the Indian Medical Gazette in July 1882 in the form of an obituary. As might be expected from the context of its production, such a memorial text as Dey's speech provides a wealth of professional detail but very little in terms of Khan's private or social life. Dey described his friend and colleague as 'one of the most brilliant' medical minds. He went on to add that though 'a man of vast reading and very valuable professional knowledge, he was simple and unassuming as a child'.[10]

Unfortunately, not much is known of Tamiz Khan's early life. Dey merely mentioned that he was born into a family of humble means before rising to great heights in the local 'Muslim society'. Though no place of birth is mentioned, it is likely that he was born in Calcutta or somewhere nearby, as he attended the Collinga Branch School in Calcutta. He may have been born in a family of munshis, as he is occasionally referred to in later life as 'Munshi Tamiz Khan', and the title of munshi had begun to be used as a hereditary title from the beginning of the nineteenth century.[11] The munshi, under the Mughals, had been a rather numerous Persianate scribal class. It was not restricted to Muslims, and numerous Hindus acted as Mughal munshis with credit since even before the liberalization of Akbar. Their training was largely secular—and specifically secularized through educational reforms under Emperor Akbar. 'An ecumenical learning and religious pluralism' accompanied by a 'self-confident Indian claim to the use of the Persian language' had come to mark their identity.[12] Khan's early education would therefore, in all likelihood, have comprised entirely Persian and Bengali and possibly some Sanskrit, but definitely no English. The celebrated Soorjo Goodeve Chuckerbutty was said not even to have heard English before the age of thirteen.[13]

After finishing school, Khan apprenticed himself at one of the first druggist's shops to open in Calcutta. Having learnt his job at the druggist's store, he managed to then get a job as a Compounder at the Government Medical Stores. The Superintendent of the Medical Stores, Dr Grant noticed the boy's enthusiasm and talent and recommended him to Dr F. J. Mouat. It was on Dr Mouat's recommendation that Khan was admitted into the English class at the Calcutta Medical College. *The Englishman* of Calcutta mentioned in his obituary that, 'by diligence and perseverance, the young Tamiz mastered the difficult science of medicine and acquired a mastery over the English language'.[14] Sir Henry Hardinge, the improving Governor General, took an immense liking to him, and Khan obtained the Hardinge Prize for having topped his class at the Medical College. He also received the Goodeve Scholarship for midwifery for two consecutive years.

Having graduated, Dr Khan was posted first at Kumaon and then at Lahore. Hardinge had broken the back of the Sikh kingdom in the First Anglo-Sikh War of 1845–46 and by the end of the decade the Sikh kingdom had been wholly absorbed into the British Empire, but Lahore—the erstwhile capital of Maharaja Ranjit Singh—was still a hostile posting for the young Tamiz. Yet, he was remarkably successful, and *The Englishman* recounted at his death that he had done much to open a charitable dispensary in Lahore and 'made European medicine highly popular among the Sikhs'.

In 1852 he returned to Calcutta as House Physician to the Medical College Hospital. Following the death of Madhusudhan Gupta, who had taught anatomy to the vernacular classes, Khan was given charge of Gupta's anatomy classes. Soon after, the prolonged illness of Dr Shib Charan Karmakar meant that Khan had to additionally take charge of the materia medica classes as well. On the death of Prosonno Coomar Mitter, Khan was elected to the Chair of Medicine. When the vernacular classes were separated from the medical college and reconstituted as the Campbell Medical School at Sealdah, Khan was appointed First Physician.

Khan, like his friend Kanailal, looked upon himself as a member of an international scientific community and maintained an active scientific life even beyond the confines of his immediate professional life. He became a corresponding member, for instance, of the New Sydenham Society in 1867.[15] He also corresponded with the Epidemiological Society of London and the Australian Medical Journal.[16] At home, in Calcutta, when the Age of Consent Bill dispute arose over the legal age at which girls could be married off, Khan was one of the Indian doctors who gave his opinion in favour of raising the minimum legal age for marriage. He was also an active member of the National Indian Association for Social Progress in India. Moreover, he was a regular contributor on anatomical and pathological matters to the Calcutta Medical Society. Once again, like Kanailal, he was also deeply invested in building visual aids to teaching, and while Kanailal set up a number of herbaria as teaching aids, Khan set up the core collections of the Anatomical and Pathological Museums at the Campbell Medical School.

Khan's greatest legacy, however, was his tremendous influence upon his students. The eminent doctor and medical author, Dr Radhagobinda Kar—son of another famous doctor and teacher, Dr Durgadas Kar—mentioned in the preface to his immensely popular medical textbook that he had been inspired to write the book, not by his prolific father, but by his two teachers Kanailal Dey and Tamiz Khan.[17] Shortly before Khan's death, his students raised a subscription and had a portrait of him made and raised at the assembly hall of the then Campbell Medical School. Khan was also given several state honours, amongst which was the title of Khan Bahadur.

He died in June 1882 after suffering from a 'slow fever' for over two months, during which time he was treated by his student, Dr Soorjo Coomar Sarbadhikary. Khan helped fashion the role of the charismatic medical teacher who inspired generations of future doctors. While doctors of Khan's own generation had found such inspiration in a previous generation of British doctors such as Dr Goodeve—whose inspirational popularity had led one of the first Bengali doctors, Soorjo Coomar Chuckerbutty, to officially adopt his teacher's name as his own—after Khan, Bengali teachers increasingly came to fill this role. One of Khan's successors at Campbell Medical School, Dr Moulvi Zahiruddin Ahmed—professor of surgery from 1879–99 and later Honorary Assistant Surgeon to the Viceroy—went on to use this popularity amongst students to set up one of the most successful medical periodicals in Bengali.[18] Teachers like Khan and Ahmed helped to inspire future Bengali doctors and raised 'western' medicine from the level of a professional tool to that of a passion.

It is perhaps a generic constraint of the English obituaries and condolence addresses on which this short sketch of Tamiz Khan's life is based that so little can be said about Khan's nonprofessional life. Whereas Bengali obituaries give a wealth of social and personal information, and in turn are sketchy about exact professional attainments, the English obituaries tend to accent professional achievements and recognition. These generic forms lead to the selection and framing of biographical data that continue to fashion our reconstruction of these early medical lives. While in the absence of further biographic material it is difficult to go beyond such archival limitations, it is useful to be sensitive to such formulaic nature of these generic constraints even if they cannot be transcended at the present stage of research.

Annadacharan Khastagir (1830–90)

Annadacharan was born in 1830 in the village of Patiya in the Suchokrodondi Police Station Area of the district of Chittagong.[19] His family were Bengali Boidyos by caste. Though, traditionally, Boidyos were associated with the practice of ayurvedic medicine, Annadacharan's father was not a physician. Instead, Annadacharan's father, Ramchandra, possibly like Tamiz Khan's forebears had trained as a munshi. The late-seventeenth-century munshi's life and education was an embodiment of 'composite culture' in its most literal sense.[20] By the eighteenth century, the munshis were no longer merely as scribes, but had also become diplomats. Since the early colonial state had persisted in the use of Persian and needed to regularly deploy complex Persianate Mughal political etiquette in their exchanges with neighbouring post-Mughal polities, they became singularly dependent on their munshis. On the other hand, as the Mughal state crumbled, the lesser aristocracy were often forced to take up employment with the East India Company as munshis. Ghulam Hussain Tabtabi, the author of the chronicle *Siyyar ul-Mutakhkhirin*, thus sarcastically remarked that the British considered no office higher than that of munshi. The effect was that both the importance and the background of the recruits to the post of munshi rose in the eighteenth century.[21] The knowledge of Persian courtly culture, revenue systems and laws—including modes of formal legal writing—made the munshis an indispensable part of the lower courts as well. Munshi Ramchandra therefore started life as an *ukil* or *vakil* (pleader) in the Chittagong district court. He went on to become a munseff, or lower court magistrate, though it was said that 'his independent spirit was not conducive to salaried employment and [he] soon quit the munseffship to return to an independent practice'.

Annadacharan therefore had both a slightly distant tradition of medicine in his family and a more immediate tradition of government service. Though the family is said to have some lands in the region, they would more appropriately be described as middle class, service gentry rather than as landlords proper. In fact, Chittagong had been one of the last additions to the Mughal Empire in the east, and many service families had been given small land grants in the region to encourage them to settle there to form a strong loyal presence in an area known for constant attacks from the Arakanese kings.

It was during Munshi Ramchandra's stay at Chittagong town, that the government opened an English School.[22] Though most orthodox families boycotted the school, Munshi Ramchandra's more cosmopolitan outlook—almost surely a consequence of his training as a munshi—resulted in his enrolling all his wards including the young Annadacharan at the English school. This early adoption of English education ensured successful service careers for all three of Munshi Ramchandra's sons. The eldest, Umacharan, went on to become a lower court judge. The youngest, Shyamacharan, became the Head Clerk at the district court. Annadacharan, who was second amongst the brothers, went on to a successful medical career in government service. All three brothers were talented musicians as well.

However, Munshi Ramchandra had desired all his three sons to enter the legal profession. Medical service, by being a new form of governmental service perhaps, was not held in equal regard by Munshi Ramchandra. In order for them to enter the world of early-nineteenth-century legal world in Bengal successfully, he had wanted his sons to be apprenticed at court immediately after finishing junior school. Increasingly in the early nineteenth century, there was a demand for a service cadre which would combine in their person the knowledge of the old Munshi with some knowledge of English, and Ramchandra may well have thought that having given his sons a modicum of English education, giving them a 'munshi's' training would make them ideally suited for legal service or the profession. Young Annadacharan, however, was of a curious bent of mind and after having won a scholarship at junior school, he wanted to study further. His intellectual curiosity drove him eventually to rebellion. Quitting the junior school, he went to Dhaka to study at the senior school against his father's wishes. Having rebelled, he had only his scholarship to support himself. He had, however, never intended the rebellion to last long. His plan, when he arrived at Dhaka, was to finish high school and then return home and follow his father's wishes to enter legal apprenticeship.

During his stay in Dhaka he had to share lodging with two other boys. One night one of these boys suddenly fell ill. It was soon clear to the roommates that he had been struck by cholera. The third roommate refused to touch the violently ill boy, and Annadacharan was forced to care for him while the third boy went in search of a physician. Unfortunately, however, it was late at night and no physician agreed to visit. By the time the third boy returned empty-handed, the tired Annadacharan had fallen asleep and the sick roommate had died in his sleep. This experience deeply moved Annadacharan and brought home to him the need for humane physicians. It was then that he decided upon a medical career. Today, we can no longer be certain whether this story was actually wholly true, but Bengali obituaries, which are today our main sources for reconstructing several *daktari* lives, were also avowedly didactic texts. While they aimed to celebrate a life wellspent, they also equally importantly wanted to provide their readers with models worthy of emulation. The author of Khastagir's obituary in the *Chikitsha Sammilani*—from which most of the details here have been taken—avowedly seeks to provide such a didactic ethical model, and in such, text stories like the present one acted as parables. It is here that the networks of representation, narrative strategy and biography come together to constitute 'lives' for us.

After completing school, Annadacharan, having again won a scholarship of Rs 40/-, travelled to Calcutta in order to become a *daktar.* At the Calcutta Medical College, Annadacharan won another internal scholarship for Rs 20/- and successfully completed his medical education, finishing up at the top of his class. At this point, he was offered a scholarship to travel to Britain for furthering his medical education. Annadacharan, like many other Bengali boys of his age, however, had already been married and the fear of excommunication from the religious community and the attendant possible breach with his young wife made him turn the offer down. The scholarship was taken up by Dr Chandra, who had stood second in the examinations.

On entering government service, Dr Khastagir was first posted to British Burma. Thereafter, he served in several places throughout Bengal and upper India, including Vrindavan and Mathura. He was also briefly engaged in teaching at the Calcutta Medical College. After some twenty-five years of medical service, he was promoted to the position of 'Civil Surgeon' in the district of Malda. However, he soon fell out with his white superiors. Having resigned his position, he returned once more to Calcutta. It has been written by one of his biographers that 'because the government was partial towards his talents, however, it soon convinced him to accept another position'.[23] Once again, comments such as this are quite common in Bengali obituaries. They aim to legitimate the claims of the merits of the dead man by asserting that these talents had been important enough to have been noticed by 'the government'. These parables and anecdotes draw upon older Persianate canons of biographical writing, in which the genius of a man is attested by the appreciation of his superiors (human or divine) and the personal relationship he comes to hold with them. What is, in effect, an employment under a highly bureaucratized Raj, is thus rendered as a personal relationship in which 'the government' is keenly aware of the talents of the *daktar* and 'partial towards them'. Such personal contact and appreciation serve to authorize the genius and talent of Khastagir. After Malda, through the intervention of 'the government' itself, he came to be attached to the Campbell Medical School (now known as Nil Ratan Sircar Medical College). However, he was soon transferred once again, travelling to several other positions throughout Bengal before ending up eventually once more as a 'Civil Surgeon' at Shibsagar forcing him once more to resign due to the distance.

The claims of the great importance the government attached to Khastagir and the seemingly routine transfers he was subjected to, seem to be at odds. Yet the discrepancy need not necessarily be seen as an exaggeration or fabrication. The dissonance might well arise due to the different degrees of importance that the government and Bengali society respectively attached to *daktars*. To the official bureaucracy, men like Khastagir might have appeared to be relatively small cogs in a huge wheel, but to Khastagir and the Bengali society of his day—in which he played an extremely active part—his role might have appeared in an altogether different light.

Annadacharan's brief stays at Calcutta had brought him close to some intellectual stalwarts of the so-called Bengal Renaissance. Iswarchandra Vidyasagar, the noted social reformer and educator, was a close friend of his and encouraged him to develop a strong sense of criticality in both religious and professional matters. Vidyasagar—who had spent a lifetime arguing for the uplifting of women in Hindu society, also inspired in Dr Khastagir an interest in women's rights. Furthermore, it was Vidyasagar who encouraged him to study homoeopathy.[24]

Soon, however, Dr Khastagir also fell under the sway of the charismatic Brahmo leader Keshabchandra Sen. Though the Brahmos under Sen would eventually be recognized as a separate religious group altogether, initially they were considered a radical and reformist sect within Hinduism itself. When Sen emerged as the leader of the Brahmos, his radicalism had cleft the Brahmo Samaj itself, and many Brahmos under Sen had left to set up a New Dispensation (*Nobo Bidhan*). After 1870, however, Sen's grip on the radical Brahmos began to slip. A group of younger men, such as Dwarkanath Ganguly, Durgamohon Das, Shibnath Shastri and Dr Khastagir, emerged to push for more thorough and far-reaching reforms. Their main agenda revolved around a demand for equal rights for Brahmo women within the congregation. Sen at first hesitated to take so bold a step, and when the young men turned up at the congregation with the women of their households in violation of the rules of Purdah, Sen supported the old guard and asked them to leave. The rebels now set up a new meditation group at Dr Khastagir's house in Calcutta. Though this first rebellion was temporary and the radicals later returned to Sen's group, eventually, as Sen began to lean towards what the radicals considered 'superstitious strands' of Hinduism such as yoga, they split once again. Again the newly formed congregation met and prayed at the house of Annadacharan Khastagir until their new prayer hall was built.[25] However, just as Vidyasagar had urged Khastagir to take up homoeopathy, Sen urged him to work for the uplifting of ayurveda.

Though Khastagir never formally left Hinduism—as some Brahmos later did—from his student days, he developed close links with the major reformist trends within Hinduism. Ideologues such as Vidyasagar, Akshoykumar Dutta, Debendranath Tagore, Rajnarayan Basu and others sought to reform Hinduism and make it more 'rational'. Medical students became one of the most prominent supporters of this agenda for the rationalization of Hinduism. Kaliprasanna Singha's *Hutom Pnecha-r Noksha* (Sketches by a Barn Owl), which is a satirized account of the social life of mid-nineteenth-century Calcutta, cites many instances in which the eponymous 'medical student of the Bengali class' is involved in apprehending various fraudulent religious gurus and holy men through the revelation of their frauds.[26] These incidents were generally played out in front of big crowds and came to be much talked about in the city afterwards. In certain ways, this very contest between the rational medical student and the irrational guru fitted into a long tradition of performative contests which animated the urban milieu of the day. Publicly performed contests between everything, from birds like *bulbuls,* to poets (*kobi-r lorai*) and even specialists in rhymed slang (*kheur*), were the major sources of urban entertainment in early and mid-nineteenth-century Calcutta. The publicly performed contest between the rational and the irrational fitted neatly into this carnivalesque urban environment.[27] They were eagerly awaited by large crowds and both parties knew that they had to prove themselves before the crowds. On one such occasion described in detail by Singha, a member of a family of goldsmiths had fallen seriously ill. A large variety of medical and magical remedies were tried by the family—but to no avail. Finally a *Roja* or shaman was called in. The *Roja* claimed to be able to call upon malicious spirits (*bhut*) who could then be convinced through offerings to cure the patient. The *bhut*, while there, would also answer questions put to it about the future. People far and wide were informed of the *Roja*'s arrival and a big crowd began to assemble at the goldsmith's family temple on the afternoon of the appointed day. The family prepared immense offerings of the best food with a view to propitiating the *bhut*. Many 'college boys' (this was a generic term for college students in general and did not apply only to medical students) who were self-professed nonbelievers were also present. The author, however, clarified that the lines between 'belief' and 'disbelief' were not always clear and many a 'rational Brahmo' was still known to have recourse to shamans when their own near ones fell ill. Irrespective of such questions of belief, however, the performative aspects of the events at the goldsmith's house were clear. Eventually, the lights were put out and the *Roja* and his two assistants went to work, trying to invoke the *bhut*. Soon the *bhut* gave well-known signs of its presence through the apparently mysterious rain of shoes on the assembled crowd, sounds of heavy dancing and, of course, the *bhut*'s characteristic nasal voice. The first thing it did was call the 'college boys' by name, denouncing them as 'atheists and Christians'. Clearly, the shaman/spirit knew who its adversaries were. Thereafter, the spirit proceeded to threaten its usual menaces of death and destruction (a signature characteristic of its malevolent nature) on all the people assembled, and was only persuaded through the great pains of the host to partake of the offerings. As soon as the *bhut* agreed to eat the offerings, however, the crowd in the darkened temple heard sounds of vomiting. As a perplexed crowd stood around, someone brought out a light. The shaman and his assistants were vomiting. It was then that a medical student stepped forward and informed all that his medical friends and he had mixed *tartar emetic* with the ritual offerings with a view to revealing the shaman's fraud.[28] On another comparable occasion, medical students of the Bengali class apprehended a guru who claimed to have magical powers by showing that the distant flower he claimed to be able to move through magic was actually tied to his wrist by a fine hair. A Sub-Assistant Surgeon present on the occasion then proceeded to show how the guru had managed to turn alcohol to milk by pouring water into a saucer of 'American anisette'.[29] There are numerous similar stories and it is true that their comic aspect might also have a relation to Singha's satirical style of writing, but the contest between 'rationality' and 'reform' on the one side and 'superstition' and 'magic' on the other was publicly performed regularly. Moreover, the medical student and the *daktar* became an indispensable part of this urban pantomime. Irrespective of whether Singha's anecdotes are true or not, it is indisputable that religious reform and aggressive rationality came to be seen socially as very much a part of the *daktari* identity. Like Singha—but slightly later—Rudyard Kipling also noted the relish and sense of *performance* with which a spiritual healer and dealer in charms publicly engaged a 'Calcutta-taught Bengali, a voluble Dacca [sic] drug-vendor', and the way lowly hangers-on sought entertainment and possibly free treatment from these engagements rather than education and 'enlightenment'.[30] Khastagir's involvement with the 'rational' critique of popular Hinduism was thus very much a part of the social identity of mid-nineteenth-century *daktars*.

It was perhaps his immersion in the intellectual ferment of nineteenth-century Calcutta that made him turn down the posting at Shibsagar. He is said to have said that he did not want to be so far from Calcutta. Having thus quit government service, he set up one of the most successful private practices in the city. Having studied homoeopathy for nearly a decade, he started using homoeopathic medicines in his prescriptions. He did not, however, eschew allopathic medicines altogether; instead, he said that he decided on the merits of each case, what would be the best course of treatment for the patient. Under Sen's influence, he also inaugurated one of the most successful Bengali medical periodicals of the time, the *Chikitsha Sammilani*. The journal used to have three separate sections devoted to *Daktari*, *Homoeopathy* and *Kobiraji*. The objective of the periodical was to encourage dialogue between the different medical 'systems'. According to a story recounted later, on seeing the proofs of the first copy of the *Chikitsha Sammilani*, Khastagir rushed with them to Sen. On showing the copy to Sen, he is said to have said, 'Just as you have instituted a New Dispensation in spiritual life, my journal will inaugurate a New Dispensation in medicine'.

Khastagir's other major commitment remained to the cause of women's education. He was part of the group that established the *Bongiyo Mohila Mohabidyaloy*—a higher school for Bengali ladies. The school later became the Bethune School and Bethune College—the first women's college in Bengal. He also established a middle English school for girls in his native Chittagong in 1876. Later, in 1907, one of his son-in-laws transformed it into the Dr Khastagir Girl's High School, which became, in the first half of the twentieth century, one of the preeminent institutions of women's education in eastern Bengal.[31]

His authorial career was instigated both by his association with the thriving intellectual climate in which he became increasingly involved as well as his government service. During his tenure as viceroy (1872–76), Lord Northbrook announced a special award for the best book to be written by a member of the medical services on the so-called 'Burdwan Fever' in either Bengali or English. Responding to this call, Dr Khastagir wrote a small book on the subject and won the viceroy's prize. He later gave a paper at the Calcutta Medical Society, drawing upon his prize-winning treatise arguing that malaria and cholera were caused by the same germ—a position (as his biographer did not fail to point out) much later reiterated by the Malaria Commission of Egypt. His books, however, reflected both his political as well as his medical concerns. A devoted champion of women's rights and education, he published several books on women's health, such as *Sachitra Manab Janmatattwa O Dhatri Shikkhya, Stree Jatir Byadhi Samgraha O Chikitsa*, etc. In keeping with Keshab Sen's programme for organized 'nation-building' (*desh samskar*)—of which we shall hear more in Chapter III—he published books like *Shareer Rakshan* and *Ayurbardhan.*

Of his seven children, all were well-educated. Most remarkably, however, each of his four daughters received higher education in English and Bengali and went on to have prominent intellectual lives, both in their own right and through marriage to some of the most prominent men in the intellectual landscape of the day. His eldest daughter Saudamini was one of the first women to study at the Bethune College and married the Britain-educated Deputy Magistrate, Biharilal Gupta. His second daughter Manamohini, who married the late Keshab Sen's son, was also proficient in both English and Bengali and for a while edited a woman's journal known as *Paricharika.* The third, Binodini, also had a active intellectual life in association with her husband, the prominent Chittagong lawyer Jatramohon Sen. The best-known of his children however, was his youngest daughter, Kumudini. She was the first woman from Chittagong to receive a bachelor's degree and went on to become a teacher. The marriages of his daughters, which no doubt he would have helped arrange, also brings out important changes in his own outlook. Whereas in his own career he had turned down the opportunity of further education in Britain because of ritual taboos, he happily supported his daughters marrying men who had studied in Britain. Yet, whereas many radical Brahmos of the day disregarded caste restrictions and encouraged their wards to marry outside their own castes, all of Annadacharan's four daughters were married into Boidyo families in accordance with their own caste status.

Dr Annadacharan Khastagir died in 1890 after suffering from fever for few days. It was felt by his friends, however, that his health had been broken by the continuous overwork which his many interests forced him to undertake.

Annadacharan's life coincided with some of the most significant trends that shaped Bengali modernity. His birth in a Persianized service family, his taking to English education, his spiritual quest, his intellectual appetite—were all symptomatic of nineteenth-century Bengali *bhodrolok* life. In fact, through his associations with Vidyasagar, Keshab Sen and others, he was in a small way an intimate part of the far-reaching changes that led to the first de-Persianization of the Bengali service class, followed by its Anglicization, the rise of Brahmo rationalism and the eventual reabsorption of Brahmo criticality into a neo-Hindu framework. What is remarkable, however, is the convergence between his medical work and his spiritual and political commitments. It is here that Annadacharan's life begins to illustrate prominently some of the fundamental accents of *daktari* writing. The big changes that shaped Bengali modernity were not merely a backdrop to the medical history of the time, they were an integral part of it. The books Annadacharan chose to write and the highly successful periodical he founded both were fashioned as much by his political and spiritual biography as by his medical career.

Nabinchandra Datta (1852–1920)

Like Annadacharan Khastagir, Nabinchandra Datta was also born in Chittagong.[32] His family, like Khastagir's, was a Mughal service family and had travelled from Hughli with the conquering Mughal troops to Chittagong in the late 1600s. They had been settled in the village of Anwara by the conquerors. When Nabin was born in 1852, some twenty years after Annadacharan, his family were minor landholders in the region and comfortably off. Nabin's father himself, however, was not in service as Munshi Ramchandra had been. Yet, after an initial education at the hands of the family priest Juramani Bhattacharya, Nabin was sent to the Government Collegiate School at Chittagong and thereafter to Calcutta for further education. Nabin's career is symptomatic of the greater acceptability of English education in the region since the days of Annadacharan, when it was only Munshi Ramchandra's cosmopolitanism that had inspired him to break with orthodoxy and give his sons an English education. Nabin's early education shows how much more acceptable English education—and with it the possibilities of a service career—had become, even among orthodox small landed families.

Though the family were comfortably off in Chittagong, life seems to have been hard for the young Nabin in Calcutta. During his studentship at the CMC, he found employment as a resident private tutor for the son of a wealthy Calcutta family. As was then the norm, his employer's family gave him bed and board and a small stipend as well. Calcutta, however, was an expensive city and he had to work hard. He used to walk to the CMC every day from his home in Jorasanko, and walk all the way back again at the end of the day. He was physically weak and had even fainted on the way back once or twice. At home he did not have a study table and used an old box for his study. Neither did he have a proper bed, and used to sleep on a mat on the floor using his books as a pillow. His employment also meant that he had to miss classes. Often he would miss the practical classes during the day and then go back late at night, after he finished work, to dissect the remnants of already-dissected corpses by the light of a lantern all by himself.

It was during this time that he, too, like Annadacharan, fell under the spell of Keshab Sen. However, where Annadacharan was by then one of the leading members of Sen's circle and an established *daktar* himself, Datta was only a student. Enamoured by Sen, Datta tried to set up a small group of his own with friends to discuss spiritual matters. His group was called Mohan Mela and he was the main speaker at it. Sen himself, however, is said to have taken a keen interest in the doings of the youth and attended a few of his speeches. Sen is said to have referred to Datta as the 'young missionary from Chittagong'. Even this minor recognition from Sen—then arguably the most influential Bengali ideologue—gave Datta a sense of mission and a certain celebrity. On his vacations at home in Chittagong, he tried to set up his own small group for meditation and spiritual discussions in Jamalkhana. His followers were mostly his younger brothers and cousins, and once again he came to be the main speaker. Young Datta's activities might seem a little Quixotic today, but it goes to reveal how the young medical student in Calcutta came to see himself. A spiritual quest and involvement with religio-national reform were still central to the life of a young medical student like Datta.

There were other changes, however, that distinguished Datta's career from those of an earlier generation of students like Khastagir. While the latter had been wooed by the medical authorities to pursue further education in Britain even later in his career, Datta was actually turned down for government employment. As the pool available for employment increased and the priorities of medical education changed from the quest for highly qualified Indian doctors to technically qualified lower-level medical personnel, stricter selection criteria were introduced. The Medical Board, which examined students applying for government service, determined, in the case of Datta, that he was not physically strong enough for government employment. The medical examiner allegedly also told Datta, who had always been frail, that he did not have more than a few more months to live.

Demoralized, but undefeated, Datta took up employment on a coolie ship bound for Mauritius. The time spent at sea apparently had the unexpected effect of improving Datta's health and he returned from Mauritius much stronger. Taking advantage of his improved health, he reapplied to the

Medical Board. He was now accepted and posted initially at the Chittagong Jail Hospital. Subsequently, he was transferred to Dhenkanal in Orissa. During the Second Anglo-Afghan War in 1879, he served as regimental doctor to the Third Gurkha Regiment in Almora. After the war he held a string of government postings across northern India, serving in Nainital, Sitapur (in Ayodhya District), Lahore, Kanpur, Delhi, Lucknow, Moradabad, Rae Bareli, Shahbad and eventually in Tirhut as the Chief Medical Officer to the Raja of Darbhanga. Datta's service record also brings out the much wider geographic spread that Bengali *daktars* now had to cover, unlike the previous generations, where even a posting in Shibsagar or Malda could bring about a resignation.

We have already mentioned the importance of parables and anecdotes in Bengali obituaries, and some of the most interesting and revealing stories about Datta are from his time in upper India. We will cite here two such stories which bring out the apparent contradictions of the modernity Datta and others like him inhabited as well as the changes in the *daktari* culture of Datta's days since those of Khastagir.

The first story is said to have taken place during Datta's period of service in Tirhut. Having heard the news of the illness of a major landlord in the region, Datta had travelled to the landlord's home in a distant village to see him. By the time he got there, however, the *zamindar* (landlord) was dead and the family was preparing for the cremation. Datta insisted that since he had already arrived at the scene and as the Government or the Raja might later call for a report from him, he would like to examine the corpse. The family and friends of the zamindar, however, raised serious objections to this, stating that the dead man was a Brahmin, and because Datta' was of a lower caste, his touching it would defile the corpse. Refusing to give up, Datta followed the corpse to the cremation ground and having observed the body minutely from a distance, announced that the man was not dead. Once again this caused a massive furore, but Datta, now emboldened by his belief that the man was alive, together with his manservant removed the body to the veranda of the Kali Temple at the cremation ground. The door to the temple, however, was locked and none would provide the keys. Datta then decided to carry on treatment on the veranda itself. Crowds, however, continued to assemble and, tending to see him as a body-snatcher, threatened him with dire consequences. Datta held his nerve and told the villagers that if anyone interfered with his work, he would send a report to the government stating that the zamindar had been murdered. This made the villagers back down. Along with an old servant of the zamindar, whom Datta had managed to convince to help him, he continued to treat the seemingly lifeless body. Having managed to bully some villagers into providing him with meagre provisions, he set up a small tent for himself next to the temple and dug his heels in. The next day, however, there arose a massive storm. To protect his patient from the storm, Datta now sought to break open the door to the temple. This once again brought the village to its feet and their leaders, outraged at the arrogance of a low-caste man who dared to break the temple door, attacked the group on the veranda. In a dramatic scene now, Datta defended the company with a pickaxe while also splintering the temple door with it. The zamindar was now moved inside the temple and the *daktar* continued to treat him. On the fourth day, the zamindar's consciousness returned and he began to show some signs of life. Once again news spread rapidly in the village that the *daktar* was a necromancer and had managed to call down a spirit into a corpse. Now the village gathered, more determined than ever to kill the *daktar* and despatch the evil spirit that had been called down back to its lair. Mercifully, it seems the sub-divisional officer of Madhubani received news of the happenings and rushed to the village concerned with a huge police contingent just in time to prevent a massacre. The treatment continued at the temple for a few more days till the zamindar recovered his full faculties and returned home in a procession, ever thankful to Datta.

Alongside the usual rational versus irrational motif then, this narrative also shows Datta's courage and his willingness to stake everything on his beliefs. Datta comes across as a rational, courageous, principled and, above all, a talented medical practitioner.

The second story occurred during Datta's stay at Almora. Datta had loved riding horses since his childhood and bought an especially fine horse at Almora for a hefty price. The horse, however, was ill-tempered and could not be broken, despite many attempts. One day, as Datta sat alone on veranda of his government bungalow wondering what to do with the horse and about the big financial loss it had caused, a *sadhu*, or Hindu holy man, came up the hill to his veranda. As Datta rose to greet the holy man, the *sadhu* asked him if he was worried about his horse. Datta was surprised. He was even more surprised, however, when the *sadhu* assured him that he would cure the horse. The *sadhu* simply ran his hand across the back of the horse from its head to its tail, and from that moment on the untameable horse became perfectly calm and fit to ride. The overjoyed Datta used the horse for many years without further complaint until one day, while out on work, the horse suddenly refused to move a single step. It was as though the animal had stopped dead in its tracks. No amount of coaxing or beatings could make it move, until Datta heard someone calling out to him. Looking around he saw the old *sadhu* atop the next hill. The *sadhu* asked Datta not to beat the horse, for it was he who had stopped the horse with a view of discussing spiritual matters with Datta. Throughout his life Datta had many more similar experiences when *sadhus* appeared out of the blue or knew exactly what bothered him. One of them even accurately predicted his death.

His son clarified the import of these stories. Datta, said his son, 'was habitually driven by intellectual curiosity'. Having been born in a Hindu orthodox family, he had been attracted to the Brahmoism of Sen in his student days. But Brahmo rationality alone had never fully satisfied him and he thirsted for the mysterious knowledge that remained behind the veil of universal nature (*bishwo prokriti-r jobonika-r ontorale lukkayito tottworashi*). He therefore developed links in later life with such well-known *sadhus* as Bishuddhanando Swami, Basharanondo Swami, Troilongo Swami, Swami Aghorenath, Mahatma Bijoykrishna Goswami and others. He also became a member of the Theosophical Society.

The two stories occurring together bring out the changes that had affected the world of the *daktars* since Annadacharan's time. Annadacharan too, as we have seen, did not wholly sever his ties with Hindu social life, choosing to marry off his daughters within their caste. Yet, Annadacharan's generation was still committed to reforming Hinduism and ridding it off its seemingly 'irrational' elements. On the other hand, Nabinchandra's generation had been affected by the neo-Hinduism which commenced in the 1870s, but only properly came into its own in the 1890s through the works of ideologues such as Swami Vivekananda.[33] After the 1890s therefore, there was a new defensiveness of Hindu customs which sought to somehow reconcile a 'scientific rationality' with a belief in 'something more than science'. Where Annadacharan's generation, and even the younger Nabinchandra, had felt critical religiosity was an inescapable part of their medical lives, later generations would learn to keep their technical knowledge of medicine strictly demarcated from their religious practice. This generational gap is as much a matter of changing mentalities as of changing social conventions of representation. The critical rationality of Annadacharan's generation is a matter of both their personal mentalities and the way their lives were narrativized within the narrative conventions of the time. Writing in 1896, for instance, an eminent *daktar* Dr Abdul Ajed Khan Choudhury, who was briefly executive editor of the *Bhishak Darpan*, mentioned that 'science has made such progress in recent times, that most *daktars* are scared to even mention the name of religion for fear of being laughed at'.[34] Some twenty-five years later, by the time of Nabinchandra's death, however, it had become much more acceptable to speak of the religious faith of *daktars* and their firm belief in a 'realm beyond science'. One incident in particular—exact echoes of which are found also in Bengali novels of the day—showed how this reconciliation of faith and critical rationality was effected. This incident, also recounted in Nabinchandra's obituary, revolved around his wife having asked him why he had just given a hefty donation for a communal Kali worship, since she knew that he did not believe in such things. Datta allegedly replied, 'It is true that I personally do not subscribe to idol worship, but I appreciate that it is useful for some people and hence want to encourage them to worship thus'. Gyanendranarayan Bagchi's 'medical novel', *Bagher Baccha* (The Tiger Cub) narrates an almost exactly similar retort by the novel's hero when asked by a rational Brahmo as to why he, as a doctor and a man of science, supported the hook-swinging of the *Chodok* festival.[35] The most overt statement of this new marriage of medical science and religion, which eschewed the aggressive reformism of the earlier generation, came in the form of Kartikchandra Basu's *Swasthya Dharma Panjika* (Lit: Health and Religion Almanac). Beginning in the first decade of the twentieth century, Basu took to publishing almanacs with guidance on health and sanitation.[36] The almanacs, since the middle of the nineteenth century, had become an integral part of the religious life of Bengalis. By including rules of sanitation in these almanacs, Basu showed how religious life and medical science could coexist. It was a significant departure from the days of *Hutom's* satirical sketches when *daktars* were at the forefront of public 'rational' attacks on popular religiosity.

Like Annadacharan, however, Nabinchandra had been encouraged to write through his employment. During his time in charge of the Palamau Jail, he wrote a small treatise on 'jail stomatites'. The treatise was sent to Major Buchanan who had been researching the disease and had sent a letter showing his approval for the conclusions as well as his enthusiasm for such work. Where Annadacharan had become a prolific author, however, Nabinchandra did not write as much. Yet, he was honoured by the title of 'Rai Bahadur' by the government and played an important role in the public life of Chittagong where he had retired. His main rival in the town's public life was none other than Annadacharan's son-in-law, Jatramohon Sen. In part at least, this public life depended upon the social estimation of the *daktar's* career within the bureaucracy. Like Annadacharan, Nabinchandra was said to have been personally noticed for his talent and personality. On one occasion, when his application for medical leave had been adversely commented on by a superior officer requiring him to turn up for an actual medical examination by the Medical Board, he is said to have resigned saying that he 'does not wish to work for a government which does not trust him'. Later, his son said, he was made to withdraw his resignation when the Lieutenant Governor of the province personally contacted him, urging him to withdraw his resignation and offering him a promotion. Once again, such narratives establish the personal ties of the person with the ruling power, thus legitimating their social authority.

Narendranath Datta (1884–1948)

Between Annadacharan and Nabinchandra, we had seen a significant broadening of the social base from which medical students were drawn. This trend continued further, as the security of a government job along with the possibility for promising students without too many social advantages to make a successful career, inspired many more students to contemplate medical careers. Narendranath Datta was a good example of this further broadening of the social base of *daktars.*[37]

Narendranath was born in 1884 in the village of Srikail in the district of Tripura. His family was only slightly above the average landed peasantry and he was not born into the relative comfort that Annadacharan or Nabinchandra had known. His father, Krishnokumar, was a junior teacher at the Chittagong Government School and supplemented his earnings by staying at the home of a wealthy patron in town as a resident tutor to the patron's wards. His salary was not much and his remittances were infrequent. The family usually had to live off whatever little they could grow on their own patch of land. Narendranath was the third son of his parents and once his two elder brothers went to live with their father in Chittagong to further their education, Krishnakumar could no longer afford the remittances and Narendranath and the rest of the extended family became wholly dependent on the meagre income from the land. On top of this, in the autumn of 1889, when Naren's younger brother was only three or four years old, his mother died. Krishnakumar and the two older brothers left for Chittagong once the funeral was over and the two younger boys were left in the care of their aunts in Srikail. Even at this early age, the young Narendranath recognized the economic crisis his family had been plunged into. On his own initiative, he sought work as a field hand on the fields of a wealthy landowner. He used to rise early and work on the fields before going to the village school. He soon joined the Lower Primary School in the village. From the very beginning he worked at various times as a field hand or as the local greengrocer's assistant to pay his school fees. Yet, when the old greengrocer, on discovering that the boy was working so hard to go school, offered to sponsor his education, the proud Narendranath refused to accept alms.

He finished at the Lower Primary School, having won a scholarship of Rs 2/- to study further at the Middle Vernacular School in the neighbouring Dhonpotikhola village. The new school was nearly three miles from his home and he had to regularly walk to school and back. During the monsoons he had to swim across the tumultuous local river to get to school. Finally, in 1899, at the age of 13, Naren passed the provincial scholarship examinations with a first class rating and entered the Comilla District school in class VII.

Initially, he had moved into a cheap boarding house in a rundown part of Comilla town hoping to somehow find the money to pay for it. Unfortunately, he could not find the money, and once he fell into arrears, his landlord threw him out. He eventually found employment at the house of a local lawyer named Prasannakumar Chakrabarty. Prasanna was a kind-hearted man and, taking pity on the boy's plight, had offered him the position of resident tutor for his son. This social institution of staying with well-to-do acquaintances during the course of one's studentship in lieu of petty service seems to have remained unchanged throughout most of the nineteenth century. Goodeve Chuckerbutty, nearly half a century before Datta, had also stayed with a kind-hearted, well-do-to acquaintance in return for cooking for the family during his student days—incidentally, also in the town of Comilla.[38] In the meantime, he stood first in class and received both a double promotion and a 'freeship'. Though the freeship waived the need for paying school fees, he still had to find the money to support himself. Eventually, the enterprising Naren hit upon the idea of becoming a vegetable wholesaler for shops in the bazaar. After school, he would rush off to the suburbs on foot, haggle with farmers about the price, bring back the vegetables on foot and sell the vegetable to the shops in the bazaar at a very small profit. The situation the boy was in, as well as the small profit he charged, however, soon earned him a loyal band of suppliers and customers. His earnings now sufficed to support him and cultivated in him a sense of discipline and punctuality. The rigorous routine he followed, however, left little time for studies and, as the curricula of the senior classes got tougher, his studies began to suffer. His results plummeted, but he kept up his routine. Eventually, in 1906 he finished school and entered the Comilla Victoria College.

At this time, Naren's elder brother, who had become a lower court lawyer, moved to Comilla. He stayed in a cramped rented accommodation along with Naren. Soon the elder brother's wife and the two other brothers also joined them. This forced Naren to keep working in order to support the large family. His father, having remarried, did not provide any financial support for the boys. He finished college in 1908, having graduated with a second division.

Thereafter, Narendranath moved to Calcutta and got himself enrolled in the CMC. He still did not, however, know how he was going to pay for his education. He tried desperately to find employment that would sustain him through his education. His first job was when he managed to get himself a job as a laboratory assistant in the chemistry laboratory of the CMC itself. As the laboratory hours frequently clashed with his classes, however, he was soon forced to quit this job. Later, he found employment as a night-shift coolie at the Kidderpore Dock Yards. Though this was hard labour, the pay was good, since the night coolies were paid at a higher rate, and it did not clash with his class timings. This disappearance from the hostel every night raised the suspicions of his Hostel Warden, who communicated his doubts to Rev. Holland, the then principal of the CMC. Both suspected the worst and confronted Naren, who made a clean breast of it. Finding the story too fantastical, however, Holland and the warden followed him that night. On seeing that the story was indeed true, both men were suitably impressed and Holland offered to give him a stipend from his own pocket. Naren, however, refused to accept once again, asking Holland in turn why he felt being a 'charity boy' was better than honestly earning one's own living. This created a deep impression on Holland and it stood Naren to good stead throughout his career.

It was through Holland's influence that Naren stayed in college after having punched an examiner who had wrongly accused him of cheating. It was again through Holland's influence that Naren, upon graduation, was given a military commission, despite his proximity to fellow students who were known to be nationalist agitators with links to underground nationalist organizations. Part of the reason Naren so dearly wanted the military commission he got upon completion of his MB degree in 1915 was because the War Service entailed a much higher pay and, thus, the prospect of making a quick fortune. Naren was posted during the war at various places across the Middle East and West Asia, serving principally in Iraq and Iran. While there, he quickly learned Arabic and Persian and passed departmental language examinations in both languages. Each additional language known brought an increment of Rs 2,000 with the salary. Moreover, when the British troops finally occupied the Euphrates basin, Naren was the only officer who could speak the local language. This made him indispensable in the negotiations with the local population. While within the camp he was made Mess In-Charge, without he was highly commended by the local religious leaders. The ever-enterprising Narendranath now began, on the one hand, helping the local communities rebuild by using army infrastructure to train them in modern dairy farming and husbandry, while on the other hand, he solved the army's chronic supply shortages in the region by improvising upon fishing techniques he had learnt in Srikail as a boy. All this made Naren immensely popular and, after nine years in the army, his name was proposed for a permanent military commission.

Naren, however, was no longer certain he wanted to be in the army and asked for leave to come home and consider his options. Upon his return, he bought up some land and was toying with the idea of setting up a modern fruit farm. He had brought with him a young Arab boy orphaned by the war and planned to jointly work on his fruit farm. At this time he was approached by Dr Amulyaratan Chakrabarty, who had been a classmate of his at the CMC.

Amulya knew of Naren's organizational skills and enterprise and urged him to take charge of the failing Bengal Immunity Company.

The Bengal Immunity Company had been started in 1919 through the enthusiasm of a group of influential and politically active Bengali *daktars* who had sought to meet the shortage in the supply of serums due to the war by developing serum production in India. Such stalwarts like Dr Bidhan Chandra Roy, Sir Nil Ratan Sircar, Sir Kailash Chandra Basu and Dr Charu Chandra Basu had been amongst its founders. Amulya Chakrabarty and Dr Charubrata Roy were the scientists involved in the production. Since the inauguration, however, the company had been grossly mismanaged and was now on the brink of close down. It had a debt of Rs 34,000/-. Amulyaratan believed that if anyone could save the company from this position, it was Naren. This was in 1925, and Naren was still undecided about his future. Upon Amulya's request, Naren agreed to consider the option but wanted to see the accounts first. After going through everything, Naren decided to take up the challenge and turn down the permanent commission in the army. He initially proposed to work on a trial basis for eighteen months and without pay. Thereafter, he proposed, if he was indeed able to turn the company around, he would draw a salary based on a percentage of the profits he managed to generate.

Sixteen months after he took charge, Narendranath announced, at a meeting of the shareholders, that the company's debts had all been discharged and there was at this point a profit of Rs 10,000 as a reserve fund. In return for his work without pay for the past sixteen months, the company's directors decided to give Narendranath shares worth Rs 1,000/-; additionally, he was to receive a monthly salary of Rs 200/- along with incentives scaled according to the amount paid in dividends. Datta's personal supervision of every aspect of the company's work, as well as his international contacts built up during the war, led to the company's rapid expansion. By 1930 it was supplying serum to Burma, Singapore, Malaysia, Sri Lanka, Iran, Iraq and even South Africa. Despite three major schisms in which some of the technical staff left to set up rival firms, Bengal Immunity under Narendranath's supervision maintained its pre-eminence in the industry until the 'his death in 1948.

Like Annadacharan and Nabinchandra before him, Narendranath took an avid interest in promoting opportunities of education in his native Srikail and helped set up an English high secondary school there.

Narendranath's religious commitments, however, are seldom mentioned by his biographer. Though Narendranath's own writings do occasionally refer to religious matters, it is as a matter of fact and not as a spiritual quest or as something he had to personally decide upon. Religion, by the time of Narendranath, was not an active sphere of enquiry for the Bengali *daktars.*

It was a settled matter: part of their inescapable identity that did not need any further questioning. Instead, nation-building, which had remained a much vaguer, philanthropic identity in his predecessors, gained in his life a much firmer grounding in reality. Medicine, entrepreneurship and nation-building now came together, just as spiritual awakening, social reform and philanthropy had for the earlier generations. Leading *daktars* of the time sought to combine entrepreneurial zeal, medico-scientific training and nation-building. Sir Nilratan Sircar, for instance, inaugurated a host of—unfortunately wholly unsuccessful—'national' businesses based on scientific principles. These included the 'National Tannery', 'National Soap Factory', 'Eastern Tea Company', etc.[39] Closer to Narendranath's interest in 'new' business opportunities informed by science, however, was Indumadhab Mullick's venture. Mullick, a polymath *daktar* and educationist, who died in 1917, had created the immensely popular 'Ic-Mic Cooker' a rice-cooker with a timer which was supposed to have made cooked rice—the staple Bengali diet—healthier. Mullick's cooker was a huge commercial success and prefigured Narendranath's entrepreneurial zeal.[40] The amalgam of business, nation-building and entrepreneurship may even have been a model for Narendranath.

Similarly, while his predecessors sought to justify their choice of a medical career in terms of philanthropy or humanity, in Narendranath, the main reason he took to medicine was financial. It provided for him an honest and achievable goal out of the poverty of lower-middle-class life in an east Bengali village. Even later in life, his decision to join the army first, and subsequently to give it up, once again are all informed by the financial consequences. This reflects perhaps a change in the social base from which the earlier generation of *daktars* had been drawn. Whereas the men of Tamiz Khan and Annadacharan Khastagir's generation had been drawn from old service families, dating their service credential back to the days of the Mughal Empire, many men of Narendranath's generation came from lower-middle-class families that had been rising slowly during the reign of the British rather than the Mughals.

Gohur Khan

Unlike the more eminently 'qualified' *daktars*, whose lives were often commemorated in memorials, obituaries and biographies, the numerous *daktars* who did not have any fixed qualifications—though they played a very important part in the history of *daktari* medicine—were not always recorded in as much detail. These *daktars* were initially described simply as 'native doctors' and later, once college-educated Indian doctors became increasingly available for appointment in the Subordinate Medical Service from the 1850s, as 'locally entertained native doctors' or, indeed, as 'local native doctors'.[41] They were not, strictly speaking, 'unqualified', though they were often referred to as such. Their education was distinct from the more 'elite' *daktars* in that, instead of attending a college, they had trained through a system of apprenticeship, either in the army or in the numerous dispensaries that had sprung up throughout the provinces. The lives of these apprenticed *daktars* are difficult to reconstruct, for very little specific information about individual 'Native Doctors' is available. Yet numerous references to various individuals are to be found fleetingly in the files of the medical department, and prosopography is the only way to combine these various individual references into a single composite life.

Gohur Khan's name props up briefly in the dispensary records of Bengal in the early 1840s. He is described as a Native Doctor from the Chittagong region who enjoys considerable local support.[42] There are no other details about him that can be ascertained with certainty. Yet, using such fragmentary details gathered from a host of different records, we can try to gain some understanding of what Gohur Khan's life may have been like.

'Native doctor' was a notoriously ambiguous term used throughout the eighteenth and nineteenth centuries to a variety of Indian medical personnel employed in the lower rungs of the medical service. By the end of the eighteenth century there were already a hundred 'Native Doctors' serving with the various 'native' regiments of the East India Company's armies. These doctors were generally employed after a period of apprenticeship with the white doctors. Once various classes of college-educated medical graduates started becoming available from the 1850s, the designation for doctors who came through the apprentice system changed and they were, as stated previously, described as 'locally entertained native doctors'. In the early years, the white doctors themselves, too, had had a variety of different educational backgrounds and very few in the eighteenth and very early nineteenth century had any comprehensive medical training. Graduates of the short-lived Native Medical Institution set up in the 1820s, following a mixed curricula of 'indigenous' and 'western' medicines, were also called 'native 'doctors'. Much later, graduates of the vernacular medical classes would also come to be called 'Native Doctors'. Civil dispensaries, too, had been proliferating since the last decades of the eighteenth century and here, too, the doctors or Sub-Assistant Surgeons placed there recruited their own apprentices and assistants, who, in time, qualified for independent postings. These men were chosen due to local considerations and there were no standard eligibility criteria or necessary subsequent education—each being educated according to his prior knowledge, aptitude and the interest taken by the particular Sub-Assistant Surgeon.[43] All this made the training that 'Native Doctors' received highly uneven.

Those who came to be locally attached at the various early dispensaries, especially through the apprentice system, tended to come from locally prominent loyalist families. All of the three new apprentices employed at the Kanpur dispensary the year after the first reference to Gohur Khan in Chittagong, for instance, were of 'good caste and good family' and two of them were sons of non-commissioned native officers. After two years of apprenticeship in 1842, three men—Najaf Ali, Mohammed Baksh and Sheikh Jahangir Baksh—were certified as been eligible for independent appointment.[44] The following year, the Kanpur dispensary mentioned taking on another apprentice, Kishenprasad, who was the son of a 'native 'doctor'.[45] Similarly, at the Mathura dispensary, of the three apprentices taken on, one, Seo Gobind, was the son of the local *Dak Munshi* (Postmaster); another, Swaroop Singh Rajput, was the son of an invalided cavalry trooper; and the third, Sukhanand, was the son of the local Shroff (moneylender).[46] Gohur Khan, therefore, is quite likely to have been from a locally prominent family with some familial ties to the regime.

He may also have been a scion of a locally important family of indigenous physicians. There are some examples where members of very prominent 'indigenous' physicians' families applied for apprenticeship in order to learn the new mode of healing. The best example of this is Neemchand Dasgupta, who was an apprentice to T. A. Wise at the Dhaka dispensary. Dasgupta came from one of the oldest and best-respected Boidyo families in the region. He had travelled from his home in eastern Orissa to Dhaka in order to learn medicine under Wise.[47] Much before him in the 1840s, Sub-Assistant Surgeon of the Dhaka dispensary, E. J. Lazarus had also mentioned the employment of a local 'Cabrauz' (Kobiraj) as an apprentice.[48] In fact, Lazarus himself was a Native Doctor of Jewish extraction who had risen through the ranks to become Sub-Assistant Surgeon, but had an abiding interest in high Sanskrit literature and quite likely knew the ancient ayurvedic texts. He later converted to Christianity and became a noted orientalist scholar based in Benares.

The terms of Khan's employment, however, were uncertain. Unlike those who qualified from the CMC, men like Khan were seen largely as filling a gap and, hence, often felt to be dispensable. When Rajkrishna Chatterjee, the Sub-Assistant Surgeon appointed to Chittagong, finally arrived in Chittagong to take charge, he found that his arrival had resulted in the summary dismissal of the man who had till that time—since the very inception of the dispensary—been in charge. Chatterjee, wrote in his annual report that 'Gohur Khan, Native Doctor, who has been officiating as Executive Medical Officer since its Establishment, has been discharged. I am given to understand that he performed the duty in a very efficient manner, and so well has he gained the confidence of the people, that [sic] I beg to recommend him for appointment to the situation of vaccinator in the Dispensary'.[49] Later, when in 1845 the dispensary is once again without a Sub-Assistant Surgeon, we hear the Civil Surgeon J. Duncan saying once again that, 'Since December last, in the absence of a Sub-Assistant Surgeon, the duties have been carried on by Gohur Khan, Native Doctor, in a very creditable manner…'.[50]

The fact that dispensaries depended significantly, for both financial reasons and for patients, upon the goodwill of the locals, made them very sensitive to local opinion. Local support was thus crucial to the careers of *daktars* in dispensary practice. Thirty years after the first references to Khan, we still find numerous petitions from the local people in support or opposition to the appointment, continuance or dismissal of *daktars* at the local dispensaries. In one case in 1874, when one Dr Harinarayan Banerjee of the Jamoakandi dispensary had been involved in a dispute between the local peasants and the landlord, the local eminences petitioned the government for his removal. The Civil Surgeon, after finding Banerjee innocent of any wrongdoing upon enquiry, still recommended his transfer on the grounds that keeping him on might bring the dispensary itself to a standstill.[51] By contrast, when an anonymous petition brought to light that Beharilal Paul of the Bogra dispensary was selling medicines from the government stores to his private patients at a premium rate, the investigating Surgeon, Sandiford, despite finding the charges valid, could not proceed against Paul, as the entire local population declined to testify against him and the locally constituted managing committee said Paul had acted with their permission.[52] This crucial element of local support was even more critical for 'local native doctors' like Khan, who did not have any fixed qualifications and were therefore unlikely to be transferred elsewhere in the way that Banerjee was. That the local support was a consideration in Khan's career is borne out by a comment by Khan's superior officer. Writing at the end of 1845, when Khan had once again been put in charge of the dispensary, his superior, Duncan wrote (much in the same vein as Chatterjee had), 'Gohur Khan who at present carries on the executive duties of the Dispensary, possesses and appears to me to be deserving the confidence of the natives who resort to the Dispensary, and I have every reason to be pleased with the manner in which he conducts himself'.[53]

From 1876 to 1877, however, the government began to have an excess of graduates from the vernacular classes applying for appointments. Even allowing for a 20 per cent reserve, the government still had a surplus of medical graduates applying for jobs in the Subordinate Medical Service who could not be employed. A decision was therefore taken at the behest of Surgeon General J. F. Beatson to not employ 'local native doctors' whenever more-qualified candidates were available.[54]

The policy, however, failed to totally abolish the role of the 'local native doctor'. Two important factors kept up their recruitments. First, the qualified candidates were often unwilling to travel to the backwaters of the country. Thus, when the Assam government, which had a shortfall of medically qualified personnel, asked the Bengal government for volunteers at the very time that there was a surplus in Bengal, Beatson replied to the Bengal government that he had been unable to find a single volunteer who would be willing to work in Assam unless some greater inducements were offered.[55] Second, the chronic outbreaks of many endemics, in epidemic form at various distant stations, created a chronic shortfall of college-educated *daktars* at hand. At most times, such outbreaks required urgent action, and the men at hand were employed by local authorities and ratified later. Compounders, Hospital Assistants and others who had received some medical training were thus transformed into 'local native doctors' during such outbreaks. In 1876 in Tirhut, an epidemic outbreak of cholera, for example, led to the appointment of Hospital Assistants Syed Luteef Hossein and Abdul Gafoor, to cholera duty.[56] The Compounder Sanatan was appointed in the same year for cholera duty in the interior of Dinajpur.[57] While Dinabandhu Mohanto and Sheikh Misser were appointed 'Acting Native Doctors' in Pabna,[58] Chintamoni Das was appointed on a comparable basis to treat cholera in Medinipur.[59] Local Native Doctor Wazullah was appointed to treat cholera in Baruipur in 24 pergunnahs.[60] Some idea of the extent of the divergence of the priorities of local appointment practices at times of epidemic outbreaks and Medical Department policy can be gauged from an appointment made in Arrah during a cholera outbreak in the mid-1890s. In 1896 the Arrah municipality had appointed a self-professed homoeopathic practitioner on cholera duty. The Lieutenant Governor took severe objection to this and wrote to the municipality referring to the appointment as 'unjustifiable'. Since ratification was ex post facto, the government paid the homoeopath's salary as per agreement with the municipality, but advised them to terminate the employment forthwith.[61]

It is difficult to gauge what sort of medicine Khan or those like him may have practiced. Coming from diverse social and educational backgrounds and existing at the very margins of state medicine, their actual medical practice remains a tantalizing enigma. Some general idea, however, of the nature of their practice might be had through some anonymous manuscripts preserved in Dhaka University's manuscript collections. Most of these are handwritten texts written in either Urdu or Persian. Texts such as the *Nizamat Tibb*, written in 1836; the *Risala Qanuncha*, written c. 1848; the *Kitab-i-Daktari*, written c. 1869 and the *Nushkhajat*, written between years 1224 and 1237 of the Maghi (Arakanese) Era (AD 1862–75) all show considerable knowledge of 'western' medicine but are always accompanied by indigenous ideas.[62] The *Kitab-i-Daktari*, for instance, even while using English names for some diseases, continues to cite *djinns*, or evil spirits, as one of the causes for them. The *Nushkhajat*, which is basically a collection of prescriptions, also advocates prayers for some diseases. However, books such as the *Risala*, which give a brief and incomplete summary of the 'western' ideas of anatomy as well as the aetiological sections of the *Kitab*, clearly prove that the knowledge of 'western' medicine these authors possessed was not wholly superficial. That the authors had close connections to the government is suggested by the fact that two of the books are written on foreign paper usually only used by the government departments. The pages of the *Risala*, for instance, are watermarked 'Bordeaux & London'. The *Kitab* is similarly written on paper with the watermarks 'Pro Bono Publico' and 'Universal Foolscap'.

The existence of such mixed regimes of treatment can also be inferred from the existence of numerous accounts for the purchase of 'country' or 'bazaar' medicines by Native Doctors. The Commissioner of Bardhaman, for instance, forwarded bills for Rs. 83-1-1 for 'country medicines' from Native Doctors deputed on cholera and smallpox duty in Hughli in 1875–76.[63] A mere three months later, another bill was sanctioned from the Hughli Native Doctors for Rs. 46-9-3.[64] Earlier in the year, Bharatcharan Das, another Local Native Doctor, was paid Rs. 6-5-6 for 'bazaar medicines and travel' into the interior of Cuttack to treat cholera.[65]

Numerous marginal scribbles in other hands further prove that, though the books remained unprinted, they did indeed circulate and have a wider readership. The texts possibly circulated along the lines of the preprint manuscript economies which overlapped with the institution of apprenticeship. The *Nushkhajat*, for one, clearly shows formal similarities to the *Bayaaz* (unani prescription collections) or the lists of *Taliqa Kobirajes* (physicians who treated by consulting a small list of remedies they had learnt).[66] Such texts also suggest that people like Gohur may have in turn become further agents of dissemination of their version of *daktari* medicine. Tarashankar Bandopadhyay's critically acclaimed novel *Arogya Niketan* (The House of Healing) describes one such *daktar* and his role in disseminating 'allopathic' medicine in the interiors of Bengal:

> From the north of the village used to come Rangalal *daktar*—he wore pantaloons made of *tussar* and a coat buttoned upto his neck. Around his neck used to hang a pocket-watch on a black chord. He used to travel in a palanquin. He used to live some four miles from the village. It was he who introduced allopathy into this region. He was an amazing physician. A talented man. He had never studied at a medical college or school.

> He had studied medicine at home. He would scour the cremation grounds and the riversides for abandoned corpses and bring them back home. Dissecting these according to the guidance of his books, he had learnt anatomy. Astounding was his dedication and so was his success. His home had originally been in the Hughli district. He had come here to the banks of the Mayurakshi in the capacity of an English teacher at the Raj High School. His grasp of the English language was said to be unparalleled… after his long medical education, one day he declared that he would practice medicine. Within a few years he gained an immense reputation as a physician. It was not Rangalal alone who was firmly established through his fame, allopathic treatment itself came to be firmly established due to his fame.[67]

Herein lies the crucial importance of men like Khan: they may feature only marginally in the government archives, but for the majority of the people living in ill-connected, way-out Bengali villages in the nineteenth century, they were the living face of *daktari* medicine. It was they and not the stalwarts of the medical colleges who established *daktari* medicine in rural Bengal, and until their legacies are recognized, 'western' medicine in India will continue to be spoken of as being cocooned in 'enclaves'.[68]

Daktars like Gohur, though increasingly disliked by the more professionalized graduates of the government colleges, continued to have some, albeit limited, medical standing in *daktari* and social circles until the beginnings of the 1920s. The humorist and essayist Rajshekhar Basu, for instance, wrote a short story in the early 1920s based on the character of an ageing *daktar* very much in the mould of Gohur Khan. Basu's Dr Jodunondon Gorgori, is presented as the last of a dying breed of *daktars*. His methods combined a practical/technical experience of 'western' medicine, particularly in surgery, with a belief in ghosts, devils and other hobgoblins. Basu, who was known for his accurate characterizations, paints a vivid picture of Jodu *daktar*, which could well double up for Gohur's had he lived till the 1920s. Basu wrote:

> His age at present is ninety, but he is still firm in body. He is slightly short of hearing, however, and occasionally babbles on nonsensically. No one is quite sure as to exactly where he learnt his *daktari*—perhaps in Calcutta, perhaps Bombay or maybe even Rangoon. Some say he is one of those old VLMS *daktars*. Others disagree, asserting that he is a pure and simple quack. Whatever detractors might say, there is no denying that at one time he had innumerable patients, the common people thought of him as being a big surgeon. He has given up his

> practice some twenty five years ago and spends his days now in prayer and discussing religious matters. He had donated the building for the [Calcutta Physi-Surgic] Club. As a mark of respect therefore, he has been made life-time President of the Club. All [the members] respect him, but behind his back all of them crack jokes about him as well.[69]

For Gohur Khan to have been put in charge of a dispensary in 1840, when Annadacharan was a mere boy of ten, would have meant that he was in all likelihood born sometime in the 1820s, if not earlier. For a period of nearly a hundred years. then, from the 1820s to the late 1910s, there had continued to be *daktars* like Gohur Khan and Jodunondon. While the many changes had dramatically affected that level of medical service that was inhabited by Annadacharan, Nabinchandra and Narendranath, a relatively lesser known, but possibly more populous stream of *daktari* practice had flowed at a completely different rhythm at Gohur's level, where the impact of major changes was always blunted by its filtration through a more ad hoc system of pedagogy. While one of the significant motors of change at the level of Narendranath and others was changes in educational opportunities and terms of service, at Gohur's level things changed more slowly, since the educational structures for this level were based on older structures of apprenticeship and manuscript texts. At the last instance, men like Gohur Khan continued to be employed because there continued to be a chronic shortfall in the state's—however major or minor—acknowledged commitments to public health.

Pran Horon Nondon

Where Gohur Khan's class of *daktars* had some limited hands-on training in 'western' medicine and received a limited official recognition through short-term government service, the class of *daktars* represented by Pran Horon Nondon was utterly devoid of any significant training or recognition. They were mostly autodidacts and, hence, came into being only in the second half of the nineteenth century. Whereas there had always been a wide variety of 'indigenous' practitioners of various kinds of healing, it was only in the second half of the nineteenth century that *daktari* came to enjoy sufficient popularity and legitimacy to whelp its own stock of quacks. At the same time, cheap books and periodicals on *daktari* became fairly widely available, allowing enterprising men to acquire a smattering of medical knowledge without any real training. Dr Jadunath Mukherji, a licentiate from the Medical College and a prolific *daktari* author, when publishing a collection of articles from his defunct periodical titled *Chikitsa Darpan*, for example, quoted a letter he claimed to have received from just such a quack. The letter ran thus: 'Dear Sir, Before the publication of your *Chikitsa Darpan,* we used to be inwardly ashamed to call ourselves physicians, but now we can hold our own against any physician'.[70] Twenty-four years later, another letter from one *daktar,* Purnananda Chattopadhyay, was published in the *Chikitsa Kalpataru,* once again repeating how rural quacks (*hathurey*) had received 'enlightenment' through the publication of the *Kalpataru.*[71] A few years later, Durgacharan Ray described how old and useless medicines from leading pharmaceutical firms in Calcutta such as Bathgate & Co were bought up by rank quacks who then peddled these useless drugs in distant villages posing to be *daktars.*[72] It is not important to decide whether any of these stories were little more than clever ruses. What their frequent publication does prove, indubitably, is that quackery was believed to be a fairly widespread problem—particularly in the rural hinterlands. So grave was the problem of quackery that at one point in the 1870s, the tax-payers of Rajkristopur and Howrah submitted a petition to the Government, 'representing that they are infested with a host of quacks, who kill more than they cure', and praying for instructions to the Civil Surgeon to institute some kind of scrutiny to control the menace.[73]

Understandably, this class of *daktars* left even lesser documentary evidence than the Gohur Khans and the Rangalal Daktars. Having never been in government employment, they did not usually enter the government medical records—unless as the subject of criticism. Neither were their lives grand enough or public enough to be celebrated by memorial texts. Their lives must therefore be reconstructed from the critiques and lampoons of their adversaries. The name Pran Horon Nondon (Lit: one who delights in appropriating the life of others) appears in a now forgotten but once popular Bengali farce called *Thengapathic Bhnuiphor Daktar* by Kunjabihari Deb. The drama was published in 1887. The term 'bhruiphod' means an upstart and 'thengapathic' is a mocking reference to the variety of 'new systems of medicine' (all of which used the suffix '-pathy') that *daktars* of this class claimed to practice. Describing Nondon's origins, a song mouthed by a rural singer in the drama states:

> Leaving his own home, the son of a poor man goes to another land; Putting on a pantaloon and a chapkan there, the quack opens a dispensary there, Pretending to be man of substance.[74]

Nondon, therefore, is nearly always an outsider to the place he practices in, thus allowing him to invent tall claims; he is also usually a man of very humble origins. His attire, however, is a conscious attempt to mimic the styles of the anglicized college educated *daktars.* In fact he makes further attempts to pass himself off as a college-educated *daktar* by prominently displaying and showing off a few fat medical books. In an exchange with another character in the play, Nondon mentions:

> **Upstart:** The proof of the pudding is in the eating thereof, whether my 'treatment' (English word in original) is effective or not you can see with your own eyes. Look at these three fat English books on the table. I always consult them.
> **Chalak Das:** Sir! Please read something from them.
> **Upstart:** Will you understand anything? You won't understand a thing, its full of 'technical' (English word) words. One is for Sarjari, another for Midifari (Midwifery) and the biggest one is a tainer (trainer).[75]

Sarah Pinto, studying the dynamics of medical authority in a postcolonial village in north India, has identified many of these characteristics in people she calls 'ersatz doctors'. Pinto's 'ersatz doctors' are people who exist on the fringes of medical legitimacy, but are not wholly illegitimate. They manage to tap into a diffused aura of legitimate authority or 'Sarkar' (which is not wholly reducible to the institutions of the state) by performing certain rituals of power. These rituals, Pinto points out, are performed through forms of dress, address, speech, etc.[76] Nondon exhibits each of these characteristics. His deliberate use of English words, his 'westernized' attire, etc., can be seen as the performance of the rituals of power, which he hopes will allow him to partake of the aura of legitimacy. Yet, crucially, Pinto points out that the pre-existing social authority of the person concerned is as important in the successful articulation of ersatz medical authority as is the ritual performance. Therefore, not all who perform the rituals are accepted into the folds of legitimacy.

The 'trainer' referred to by Nondon is an artefact that shows the permeability of the boundaries between 'legitimate' and 'ersatz' medical authority. The 'trainer' usually referred to a simple compendium of treatments and prescriptions, with the aid of which, it was alleged, one could successfully practice medicine without any further training. It was a book such as Nafarchandra Datta's immensely popular *Sahaj Daktari Shikkhya* which went into several editions.[77] This small but highly popular book that went into at least ten editions, though claiming to teach the reader *daktari* treatment, in fact included sections on ayurveda, hekimi (unani), homoeopathy, mushtijog (herbal simples) and even patent medicines. The section on *daktari*, or allopathic treatment, comprised mainly actual prescriptions for different common maladies and some hints on how to compound the necessary medicines.

Publishing collections of prescriptions of renowned doctors was another important and lucrative genre of medical publishing, and these, too, would have acted like 'trainers'. Despite this seemingly dubious credentials of the 'trainer' genre, some of the best respected *daktars* of the day also produced 'trainers'. *Daktars* such as the erudite Dr Radhagobindo Kar, a professor at the Bengali class, himself published a collection of his father Durgadas Kar's prescriptions in 1879.[78] Kar was a teacher at the medical school in Calcutta and his having written a 'trainer' therefore clearly blurred the lines between college-taught, degree-carrying, 'legitimate' *daktars* and autodidact, 'ersatz' *daktars.* Even the highly respected Bengali medical periodical *Bhisak Darpan,* known for its proximity to the government, later in its career took to publishing prescriptions of renowned doctors. Bandopadhyay mentioned a dispensary Compounder blindly prescribing 'penicillin' for everything, since he had learnt of the drug.[79] Orwell also mentioned 'half-trained Assistant Surgeons' who kept stacks of pre-written prescriptions to be dealt out after the most cursory queries.[80] His practice was bolstered by clever commercial ploys. He had gathered around him a band of loyal 'agents', recruited from amongst the unemployed middle-class youth of the area. Deb describes these agents in his drama:

They are all agents of The Upstart. Whenever someone in the village falls ill, their brains start ticking. It is not Bokku alone, but every locality in the village has one of them roaming the streets.[81]

Advertising is another prominent feature of this class of *daktars.* As entrepreneurs, they make full use of the opportunities opened up by the thriving mid-century medical market and the booming print culture. They combine every conceivable source of authority in these advertisements in a bid to sell their medicines. Nondon, for example, does not even hesitate to claim that some of his medicines were revealed in a dream by the god Shib. Such advertisements, which combined both claims to 'western' medical wisdom and older sources of divine legitimization, can easily be seen in plenty in the publications of the day. The *Edwards' Moondie-Essence,* for instance, claimed, despite its name, to be an 'old and established remedy used by native physicians for the last Ten Centuries…'. The *Non-Mercurial Pills for Syphilis,* similarly, claimed both to be a 4,000-year-old Vedic remedy and to have been given to the present seller's father by a 'Mohammadan Fakir in the jungles of Nepal during the Indian Mutiny'.[82]

Sale of medicines, in fact, formed one of the most lucrative sources of income for this class of *daktars.* The substances sold, however, were not always sold merely as medicines. Several farces on *daktars* written in the late nineteenth century and at least one cartoon printed in a popular satirical periodical of the day spoke of the sale of liquor to known local drunks as medicines (to avoid the usually high *abkari* taxes) as constituting a major source of income for these *daktars*. The shops of unscrupulous *daktars* were also resorted to by those who wanted to consume alcohol after the grog shops had been closed for the evening. Later, when the government sought to sell quinine—a drug widely used by both *kobirajes* and *daktars*—through the local postmasters at a fixed rate, quinine black-marketeering became another source of income for these *daktars*.[83] In a context where dispensing still largely formed part of the *daktar*'s profession, such abuses were symptomatic of the lack of common standards of medical ethics or capabilities of regulation. Such examples, however, also show how these marginal *daktars* utilised new commercial opportunities created by legal changes in dynamic ways.

From the 1880s, particularly, a new source of legitimation emerged to cash in on this growing market for private *daktari* practice. Private colleges now sprang up claiming to provide *daktari* education for those who could not make it into the handful of medical schools and colleges established by the government. The quality and standard of education provided by these colleges were extremely variable and some were said to be mere fronts where one could simply 'buy' a degree.[84] In 1882 the government first made an attempt to regulate these privately qualified *daktars*, but did not succeed. It was discussed again in 1908. Finally, the Medical Registration Acts introduced in 1913 and 1914 in each of the three British Indian presidencies succeeded in introducing legislative safeguards. One especially perceptive *daktar*, Dr Kulachandra Guha, LMS, however, writing in 1913, blamed colonialism itself for the variable standards of *daktars*. Instead of seeing it as a legal lacuna, Guha argued that the only way a common standard for medical training and practice could be established was through common socially validated norms. Such common norms, wrote Guha, were to be seen amongst the 'Europeans and other ancient nations'. In India, however, its colonized status (*poradhinota*) had fractured society and long-established social norms had been displaced. In their place had arisen numerous partially expressed, partially understood and infinitely varied norms.[85] Not all, however, agreed on the causes or the consequences of the rise of this class of *daktars*. Writing in 1888, Dr Jadunath Mukhopadhyay pointed out that these *hathurey* (the word is usually used to refer to quacks, but possibly arose originally from physicians who practised at weekly *haths* or village markets) *daktars* should not be seen merely as a problem. They provided a much needed service for the majority of the population who could afford neither the high fees of the qualified *daktars* or that of the established *kobirajes*.[86] Writing a few years later in 1891, Sir Nilratan Sircar, pointed out that the demand for medical help was so great that it far outstripped what the handful of government medical colleges and an almost equal number of well-trained *kobirajes* could hope to meet. Unless, Sircar argued, opportunities of medical education were expanded dramatically and immediately, the problem of *hathurey daktars* could not be solved.[87] Guha, on the other hand, felt that any immediate expansion of medical education would prove self-defeating since it would force a parallel dilution of the standards of medical students and their education in any case.

Several factors combined to produce this particular class of *daktari* practitioner: A sudden rise in the popularity of 'western' medicine creating a rise in the demand for this mode of treatment, a related but not identical expansion of the medical and print markets, a lack of regulatory mechanisms, a lack of common social standards of medical practice, the numerous commercial opportunities not directly related to medicine but capable of medical exploitation—all these together produced the phenomenon identified with Pran Horon Nondon. It is little surprise, then, that characters like him frequently crop up in literary sources and more occasionally in police and judicial records. The most concerted discussions on the subject were occasioned by Medical Registration Acts. Until the state agreed to a far greater involvement in public health or some forms of social regulation emerged in time, *daktars* like Pran Horon Nondon, remained a socio-historical fact.

It is cogent to remember that the particularly negative portrayal of this class of *daktars* may not have been wholly justified. Many extramedical considerations framed the texts which recorded their lives. The farces, for example, remained tinged with socially conservative anxieties about the 'upstart' status of the *daktar* who came usually from humble backgrounds. In at least one case of prosecution for selling dangerous quinine, it was argued by the defence that the local functionaries of the government were trying to protect a purely commercial monopoly they enjoyed. Positive comments such as those of Dr Mukhopadhyay, who highlighted the necessary service these much-maligned *daktars* provided, though rare, cannot be ignored.

Nibaranchandra Sengupta

Nibaranchandra Sengupta is a character in Gyanendranarayan Bagchi's novel *Bagher Baccha* (The Tiger Cub). Bagchi himself was a *daktar* and wrote the novel confessedly using autobiographical elements. Though a work of fiction, it is grounded in the real experiences of a *daktar*. The work is particularly useful in giving an insight into the commercial world of established medicine. As we have seen in these biographies, there was a tendency to represent the cruder aspects of medical commerce only in relation to the *hathurey daktars*. Even in the case of Narendranath Datta, whose biographer was relatively more forthright

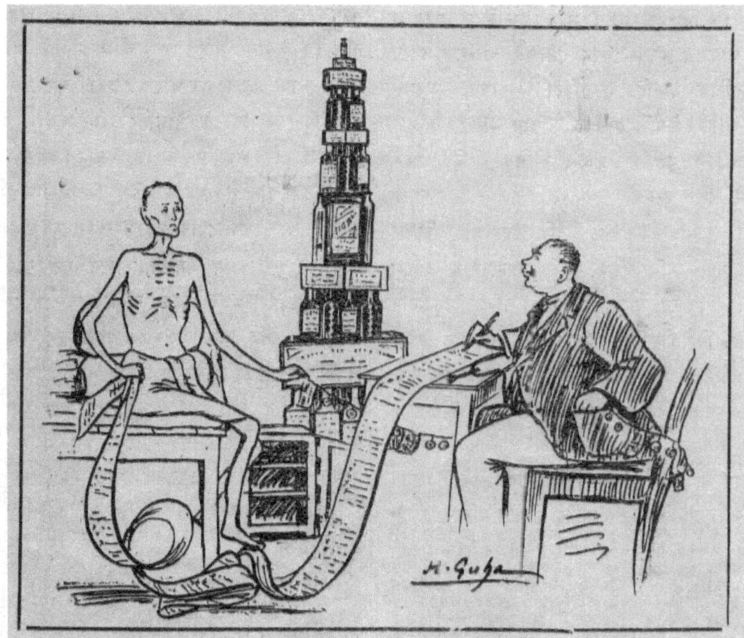

Fig. I. Caricature of exploitation of patients by reputed *daktars* by H. Guha in Sri Nripendrakumar Basu, "*Parasparik Haran*" (The Mutual Robbery), *Swasthya Samachar* 16, no. 1 (1927): 30.

about his financial motivations, the commercial aspects of Naren's life remained entangled with narratives of nation-building and professionalism. Bagchi's novel and his characterisation of Dr Sengupta, a wealthy and highly successful city *daktar*, is therefore a useful corrective. By the 1920s, this literary trope of the renowned but exploitative *daktar* had become fairly popular. H. Guha's caricature, which accompanied Nripendrakumar Basu's poem on the subject in the journal *Swasthya Samachar*, provides a potent visual representation of the trope. (Fig. I.)

Nibaranchandra lived around the turn of the twentieth century. Since by 1920 he was already one of the leading *daktars* in the city, it is safe to assume that he had begun practice some time in the late 1890s. Chronologically, this would place him between Nabinchandra and Narendranath and a decade or so after the death of Annadacharan. He is presented to us as living in a large house in Calcutta within a huge walled compound, having many household servants and owning a car. He is, in short, the picture of wealth in the Calcutta of his day. He is usually always clad in 'western' clothes, choosing to wear a formal suit, waist court, silk tie, hat and shoes, even when the tropical heat makes these extremely uncomfortable.[88]

He owns several city dispensaries which are accompanied by dispensing services. He himself no longer attends patients at all his practices. Every morning he sees patients at home. This is apparently a philanthropic gesture and Dr Sengupta accepts no fees from these poor patients he attends to. However, he makes it a point of making them buy the medicines he prescribes from his own Compounder. Through this subterfuge he manages to both earn a name for himself as a philanthropist and a friend of the poor and continue to make a profit from these poor souls.

His other dispensaries in both the city and the suburbs are run by young medical students such as the novel's idealistic hero—Dr Deen Choudhury. Young *daktars* like Deen, who—somewhat like Narendranath—are hard-working and bright but come from lower-middle-class backgrounds and do not have the capital to set themselves up in practice, are forced to work for established *daktars* such as Dr Sengupta. These *daktars* are employed by Sengupta on a purely commercial basis and made to sign a legal contract. According to the contract, a young *daktar* is meant to turn over the majority of his earnings everyday to the senior *daktar* who in turn provides him with a chamber, the necessary medicines to treat and a small allowance based on his takings at the practice. To Sengupta, this practice is a purely commercial enterprise and everything must be done to maximise profits. Thus, medicines are prescribed for everything, whether the patient needs them or not, and often these medicines are little more than coloured water. Deen also soon finds out that Sengupta is not very scrupulous about exactly who he employs. One day he bumps into an old friend from the medical college, who also now works for Sengputa, but who, significantly, had failed to graduate from the college.

During his treatment, Sengupta was said to show no interest in the particularities of his patient. Though he treated both his rich and his poor patients alike, he treated all with equal callousness. He had neither the time nor the interest in getting to know his patient or in exploring ways of treating him without medicines merely by encouraging him to alter his daily diet or routine as Deen was often keen to do. The author further lamented, that if there were one or two such heartless and unprincipled *daktars* in the city, it might be all right, 'but alas! The majority of the *daktars* in the city today are like Sengupta'.

Dr Sengupta's prototypes continue to crop up in other literary texts in the 1930s. Col Banerjee in Kamakhyaprasad Roy's drama entitled *Mayapuri* and Dr Bikramadityo Roy in Sachindranath Sengupta's drama entitled *Narsin Hom*, published respectively in 1937 and 1940, both share their greed and unprincipled exploitation of medical authority with Bagchi's Sengupta.[89]

Though each of these texts tries to redeem the profession of *daktari* as a whole by positing an young idealistic *daktar* like Deen, who is the very counterfoil of the greed seen in the senior, established *daktars*, in actuality these trends may well have existed in varying degrees within the same person. Texts, as we have repeatedly drawn attention to previously, tend to frame lives in keeping with specific narrative conventions. Biographies and other hagiographic texts, therefore, seldom mention those incidents which may have brought out the commercial motives—leave alone greed—in the more successful *daktars*. Rereading some of these hagiographic texts in the light of literary creations like Sengupta, however, can reveal hints, even within celebratory texts. Nabinchandra's obituary, for instance, mentions that he was popular among his juniors in government service because he often recommended them to private patients so that they could earn some extra money. He himself, it is said, earned so much from private visits as it is, that he could afford to be generous with some of his 'calls'. Read in the light of the literary representations, this comment brings out the importance of 'private calls' for government *daktars*, the keen competition caused by these and the importance of the support of senior *daktars* for the success of juniors. All this, while wholly legitimate, may well have been subject to abuse, as is suggested by the literary depictions.

Texts such as *Mayapuri* also reveal new sources of medical corruption. Whereas older tropes like the sale of alcohol now disappear, new occasions of corruption arise in writing medical certificates (a privilege given exclusively to *daktars* by virtue of the Medical Registration Acts), the illegal confinement of wealthy heiresses, the testing of pharmaceuticals on hapless poor patients thus endangering their lives and knowing that given their poverty they would never be in a position to challenge the *daktar's* treatment—all emerge as new sites of corruption.

Previously, physicians, of whichever system, had been individuals. But with the growing popularity of *daktari* medicine people came into contact with physicians who did not practice in isolation but worked within larger institutional structures like hospitals, asylums, medical cadres, etc. While there is ample evidence to suggest that medical exploitation and corruption had long existed and that there was no golden age, when sagely Kavirajes and Hakeems were, as a rule, above exploitation, the new institutional frameworks made medical corruption more virulent. As is seen in both *Mayapuri* and to a lesser extent in *Bagher Baccha*, the sheer extent of the corruption makes it well-near impossible for a single individual to fight it. That such institutionalized corruption was not merely the stuff of fiction can be seen in the several cases of medical corruption that came to light in the late nineteenth century. In a case reminiscent of *Mayapuri*, several doctors and employees of the Dhaka lunatic asylum, for example, were apprehended as being party to a well-organized embezzlement racket in the 1870s.[90] The head clerks of the office of the Civil Surgeons of Malda and Shahbad were both apprehended on corruption and embezzlement charges.[91] The aforementioned case of Dr Beharilal Paul, who was found to be selling government medicines to private patients allegedly with the connivance of the managing committee, is perhaps the most striking in terms of actual instances of institutionalised medical corruption in the nineteenth century.[92] Surprisingly, Paul went on to have a very successful medical career and even temporarily became Civil Surgeon of Rangpur during the plague epidemic years.[93] It was this new institutionalised clout that corruption came to wield that was depicted in the dramas *Bagher Baccha, Mayapuri and Nasin Hom.* Whereas earlier farces and dramas about corrupt *daktars* such as *Daktarbabu* or even *Thengapathic Bhnuiphod Daktar* could have been resolved happily with the errant *daktar* being beaten up by the irate locals, this new species of organized medical corruption did not have a dramatic happy ending and the conclusion was often bleak.

'Fictional' characters like Col Banerjee and Dr Sengupta reveal those aspects of successful medical careers which are not recorded in the more 'factual' archives. Memorial texts consciously silence these aspects of medical lives, while the very success of the people concerned, as is depicted in *Mayapuri,* is due to the fact that they can evade detection or punishment by the government by using their clout. As minor medical figures of the day, people like Bagchi, could not have sustained such allegations against successful *daktars* of their days, fiction, therefore, gave them an opportunity to present, in the guise of 'fiction', what was in fact a social reality.

Conclusion

These many and varied lives give a brief glimpse into the lives of the real people who animated the world of *daktari* medicine in the nineteenth and early twentieth centuries. The many juxtaposed archives and the few contrasted lives, allow us to glimpse, albeit briefly, that anxious space between the formulaic recordings of men's lives and actions and the chaotic irreducible logic of lived lives. In the next chapter we shall interrogate the books these men read and wrote.

Chapter II

DAKTARI PRINTS: THE WORLD OF BENGALI PRINTING AND THE MULTIPLE INSCRIPTIONS OF *DAKTARI* MEDICINE

The major debates in the history of printing in Bengal until recently have revolved around the early typefaces and the contribution of Bengalis in making these.[1] The actual impact of printing on Bengali life and culture, by contrast, was assumed to be fairly straightforward. The impact of printing in this straightforward narrative was assumed to have been formative of the wide-ranging cultural phenomena commonly dubbed as the 'Bengal Renaissance'—a cultural ferment usually framed as one that sought to replace the traditional Bengali cultural milieu based on orality by a textually grounded and rationalized set of cultural practices. Anindita Ghosh's fascinating recent study, however, has challenged this linear account of the relationship between print and cultural transformation.[2] Ghosh argues that the impact of print was much more pluralised and multivalent than has hitherto been acknowledged. Its relationship with precolonial worlds of oral culture was not necessarily one of opposition, and the high literary texts of the Bengal Renaissance were not necessarily the only new cultural trend which took advantage of the new printing technology. Ghosh's work has provided a long-awaited critical framework within which to approach the vibrant plurality of Bengali printing that had already been noticed by a previous generation of historians, such as Tapti Roy and Ramakanta Chakrabarty, and some amateur enthusiasts such as Nikhil Sarkar (better known as 'Sripantha').[3] The reformist high literature was only a small component of the entire print output. A more voluminous corpus—often described as Bot-tola prints, named after the locality where the majority of the presses were located—eschewed any reformism as such and gave voice to a variety of tastes and genres that did not always sit well with the high-reformism of the Renaissance.[4] Bot-tola texts regurgitated numerous precolonial oral narratives, thus giving them a new lease on life in print, as well as tapped into a rich seam of low Victorian literature and reformatted it into Bengali Considering this totality of Bengali printing reveals that the world of Bengali print was not dominated by the small group of *bhodrolok* authors who are identified as the ideologues of the Renaissance or by any clear-cut reformist tenor. Instead, Ghosh has shown that there existed a far more diverse range of authors and publishers—many of whom were drawn from relatively marginal sections of society. Similarly, in terms of consumption, too, Ghosh argues that such practices as the use of pages from printed tracts to wrap medicines ensured a much larger circulation of fragments of printed works. Ghosh's work raises interesting questions for the historian of medicine.

Given the complicated and multivalent nature of the world of publishing, how did it affect individual areas of cultural practice such as medicine? Since we can no longer carry on seeing printing as a straightforward agent of massive cultural displacement, how, in the field of medicine, do we map the complex processes of renegotiation that printing may have introduced? How far were books on medicine shaped by the politics of the print industry? What impact did these texts have on ideas about health and healing—both amongst the laity as well as the physicians?

The historiography of medicine has only recently begun to engage seriously with the history of printing. Kavita Sivaramkrishnan's work on Punjabi indigenous medicine has drawn attention to the fiercely political nature of the project of printing indigenous medical texts and especially the classics in colonial Punjab.[5] Seema Alavi has noted how printing helped to create new forms of authority for a new class of unani physicians in Awadh who did not have access to the traditional sources of authority.[6] Guy Attewell's work, too, has highlighted the new forms of authority and power that became entangled with the domain of unani printing.[7] All of these fascinating works, however, deal with 'indigenous' medicines and printing; none look at the impact vernacular printing had on western medicine in South Asia. Partly, this oversight is the consequence of the continuing propensity to see western medicine simply as state medicine which was foisted on an unwilling South Asian people and remained—to varying degree—until after the First World War, an alien affair. On the other hand, this tendency is also the result of seeing western medicine in India as a relatively 'closed system' of medicine discussed in the Introduction. The identity of *daktari* medicine is thereby thought to be a given matter not open to historical negotiations in South Asia.

The term *daktari* as a self-descriptive category, however, only emerged in Bengali print used by those seeking to affiliate with a 'western' medical tradition from around the 1860s. Though books on 'western' medicine as such had been printed well before that, they did not use '*daktari*' as a self-descriptive term and continued to use a common medical vocabulary with the 'indigenous medicines' to refer to their medicine. Even after the first emergence of *daktari* in the 1860s, many eminent authors such as Radhagobinda Kar continued to write books such as *Bhisak Suhrid* and *Kar Samhita,* which drew upon older vocabularies and genres and thus positioned 'western' medicine as *the* medicine, the heir to past medical traditions rather than a competing medical alternative.[8] For the early authors, the world of medicine was not divided into multiple different 'systems'. Instead, there were different competing ways of treating specific ailments and *daktari* was one of these. Despite their efforts, however, after 1860 the term *daktari* increasingly caught on and gained currency as denoting a separate 'system' of medicine distinct from the variety of 'indigenous systems'. In effect, then, this term came to denote the 'provincialization' of western medicine. It challenged the universalized notions of 'one' medicine and replaced it with the idea of various competing 'systems' of medicine. At length this provincialization went hand-in-hand with the vernacularization of 'western' medicine as well. It came to acquire a very specific regional identity as a special form of medicine and many of its proponents, however grudgingly, accepted that they existed in competition with other forms of medicine. This process of provincialization, vernacularization and the subsequent 'inter-systemic dialogue' cannot be understood without reference to the emergent markets for printed books on medicine.

The First Phase: 1818–1851

Seema Alavi has suggested that once lithographic printing had arrived in India, it was the contestation between the 'native' elite and John Company to style themselves as medical patrons in a bid to further legitimize their political authority that by the late 1820s produced an efflorescence of vernacular medical printing.[9] Alavi also draws attention to the crucial role played in this period by British doctor-authors such as John Tytler, Peter Breton and others.[10] Some of these early English doctor-authors carved out a hugely lucrative niche for themselves by combining their government salaries with prolific vernacular writing.[11]

While these trends held true as much in the case of the Bengali print sphere as in the other vernaculars investigated by Alavi, there was one crucial way in which the Bengali vernacular print sphere was beginning to diverge. Already, from the second decade of the nineteenth century, printed medical books in Bengali had began to appear whose authors or contents were not directly shaped by either a declining 'native' elite or the company's medical establishment.[12] The first known printed book on a subject related to medicine appeared in 1818. Ironically, this small, anonymous book was meant to ridicule physicians irrespective of disciplinary or national affiliations. The *Boidya Ninda* drew upon an old adage that 'the destruction of 100 lives makes a physician (and that of) 1,000 makes a doctor'.[13] The text clearly functioned outside the economies of elite power. Indeed, it manifested a degree of oppositional consciousness to the power of the elite physician groups. As William Ward and, much later, Tarashankar Bandopadhyay had pointed out, physicians' fees—at least in the case of the better-established ones—had been steep, and it was possibly in response to this that there had grown a culture of aggressive self-medication which denied the professional wisdom of physicians.[14] As a result, some came to argue that it was unnecessary to have recourse to physicians to cure illness. A song by the famous Bengali mystic and songwriter, Dabiruddin Mondol—better known as Duddu Shah—stated, for instance, that:

> Life and Death are in your own hands
> Who says Khuda (God) has anything to do with it?
> If you preserve your virile juices, you live
> If you waste it, you die
> Ayurbed describes, and I conclude.[15]

Since indigenous medicine was also tied up with issues of ritual and caste status in rural Bengali society, such assertions challenged the social and ritual power of the indigenous physicians. It is perhaps not insignificant that Duddu Shah himself was born in a peasant family in Harishpur in Jessore district—the district known to be the bastion of the Vaidya caste who were preeminently associated with the practice of 'indigenous' medicine.

It was perhaps because of the lack of elite patronage dependence in Bengali medical publishing that the degree of homogeneity that Alavi observes in the case of the north Indian vernaculars, cannot be found in the case of Bengali. Instead of standardisation of medical knowledge being the only observable trend, in Bengali printing, standardisation competed with a continuous thrust towards pluralization and multiplication of medical knowledge. Prankrishna Biswas' *Ratnavali* published in 1833, for instance, was a compendium of numerous 'rational' and 'supernatural' cures. It was more in line with the 'gnostic' encyclopaedias of the Mughal era that Alavi mentions than the standardizing texts of the early nineteenth century. Biswas, a resident of the small town of Khardaha just outside of Calcutta, was not a Vaidya and confessedly drew upon a wide range of medical 'opinions' (*moth*) ranging from the 'English' to that of the 'hakims' and even lesser known 'opinions', such as those of the 'people of the hills' and that of the divine bird, *Garuda*! Texts such as Biswas' did not fit into any of the three major medical 'systems' that are usually observed by the medical historians. They drew significantly upon mutually contradictory ideas about health and healing in circulation in the region without always seeking to organize them into a homogenous system.[16] The eclecticism, however, was not limited to the nonmedical men alone. The Calcutta grandee Ramkamal Sen, one of the leading Vaidyas of his day, published the *Aushadh Sar Samgraha* in 1819 in very similar vein. In this 95-page publication, Sen drew eclectically upon a range of locally held ideas and traditions about the uses of medicines such as *jalap*, *rhubarb*, *castor oil*, *mercury*, etc. Sen was a corresponding member of the Medical and Physical Society of Calcutta, and English extracts of his writings also made it into the *Transactions* of the society and, therefore, could have possibly entered the usage of Anglo-Indian doctors as well.[17] Another book appearing in the same year, however, attested to the reverse flow of medical knowledge. Ramgopal Sanyal's *Aushadh Sar Samgraha* was a collection of remedies from the British Pharmacopeia. The most voluminous Bengali work on a medical subject in the period, however, was not authored by a medical man Instead, *Vaidya Haravali*, published in 1820 (and running into over 600 pages) by Felix Carey—son of the Serampore missionary and pioneer of Bengali printing, Rev. William Carey—was originally written with the intention of forming a part of a general Bengali encyclopaedia. In its published version, it outlined the basic 'western' understandings of the human anatomy in Bengali for the first time, but did not make any explicit disciplinary claims.[18]

Though Peter Breton, the charismatic head of the short-lived Native Medical Institution (NMI) in Calcutta, had a firmer standing as a medical man, his *Olautha-r Vivaran*, a slim, 26-page tract describing cholera, still seemed largely unaware of disciplinary boundaries that divided ayurveda and 'western' medicine.[19] In fact, Breton's tract, which was published and freely distributed by the School Book Society in 1826—as will be discussed later in this book—drew upon the experiences of the numerous indigenous healers who had been employed to treat victims of the cholera epidemic. This early eclecticism in print mirrored the more open world of medicine that had persisted in the early colonial years. Until the end of the decade of the 1820s, there had been remarkably little by way of 'systemic' rivalries. 'Western' medical authors such as James Johnson had often sought to learn from 'native' ideas about health, and a good many so-called 'Black Doctors'—numbering up to a hundred by the end of the eighteenth century—had apprenticed under British doctors in the army.[20] Until the end of the second decade of the nineteenth century, the colonial government's medical policy had itself been largely unencumbered by systemic prejudice and much more open to local medical knowledge. The Native Medical Institution, founded in 1821, gave an institutional shape to this spirit of openness.[21] A mixed syllabus drawing upon both elite Indian medical traditions such as ayurveda and unani tibb and 'western' medicine was taught at classes held at the Sanskrit College and the Calcutta Madrasa respectively. At the same time, numerous reports from Anglo-Indian doctors in journals such as the *Transactions of the Medical and Physical Society* showed their curiosity and interest in learning from indigenous medical tradition and practice.[22]

In the 1830s this openness began to change. In its place emerged stricter disciplinary prejudices signalled by such widely discussed gestures as the abolition of the NMI and the founding of the Calcutta Medical College (CMC). The first generation of medical graduates from the CMC, however, were woefully inadequate to either meet the country's health needs or, indeed, to form the basis of an emergent vernacular identity. Having said that, it must also be added that the effects of the changes instituted in the 1830s has too often been overstated in the existent historical scholarship on the subject.[23] While the abolition of the NMI and the setting up of the CMC unquestionably marked a significant shift in the colonial government's policy, in actual practice, the collaboration did not stop immediately. While the CMC remained an elite institution, the ever-growing numbers of government dispensaries became the real interface for medical eclecticism and collaboration.[24]

The government charitable dispensaries (CDs) had been in existence since the eighteenth century, but their numbers grew rapidly in the nineteenth century. By the end of the nineteenth century, Sir Henry Burdett described 'the dispensary system' as the truly original institutional innovation of British India.[25] The increasing numbers of these dispensaries allowed a degree of autonomy to the Bengali Sub-Assistant Surgeons, who often held de facto charge of these dispensaries. The nature of this collaboration, as we have argued elsewhere, became in turn much more complex and structured by the identities of the Bengali Sub-Assistant Surgeons. Instead of the days of the NMI where pluralism usually implied only collaboration with elite—usually textual—strands of 'indigenous medicine', the 1830s and 1840s saw a much more variegated pattern of plural medical practice at the level of the CDs. What was considered worthy of acceptance and use and what was considered ineffective depended largely upon the identity and background of early doctors like Drs Ishwarchandra Ganguly, Rameshwar Awasthi, E. J. Lazarus, etc.

Another, related reason behind the nonemergence of a separate *daktari* identity at this time was undoubtedly the fact that these early Sub-Assistant Surgeons had a sense of participating within the larger homogenous edifice of 'western' medicine in India. These doctors were encouraged to investigate and innovate at the local level and to write reports about their findings. This obviously generated a sense of importance for the experimentation and collaboration being practised on the ground by these early doctors. Their enthusiasm and sense of participation is clearly evident in the lengthy and detailed reports they annually wrote on various new drugs or diseases they encountered in their practice and of their enquiries about these from local people or physicians. Their British superiors often commented on the zeal and interest of these early doctors. There was a clear sense in their writings that they thought that their work and writings were being taken seriously by their seniors in the medical establishment. Men like Rameshwar Awasthi or Iswarchandra Ganguly clearly did not feel excluded or unimportant within the IMS and, hence, it would be meaningless to speak of their work as a 'vernacular' form of 'western' medicine.[26] A 'popular' form (truly so-called), can only exist in relation to a 'cosmopolitan' form. As Andrew Wear has pointed out while discussing a very different medical context in early modern England, it does not make sense to speak of 'popular' medicine before a split has even occurred between 'popular' and 'high' traditions.[27] Categories of analysis must emerge from the historical archive itself and should not be imposed anachronistically.

So while a sense of a distinct 'western' medical tradition was beginning to emerge by the 1830s and 40s, this tradition was still sufficiently open-ended and did not seem to alienate its Bengali participants. This is reflected in the domain of medical publishing. Whereas the books up to 1835 (when the CMC was opened) did not overtly connect to a single medical tradition, those after 1835 sought to affiliate directly with any one tradition while continuing to be open to collaborations. The first book to appear in the period after 1835 was Udaychandra Adhya's 99-page 1836 translation of Dr Bramley's discourse on the 'nature, cause of diseases and the European mode of treating them', delivered on the occasion of the opening of the CMC. The text entitled *Bramley-r Boktrita* significantly also acknowledged the contribution of the local *Boidyo* writers on medicine. Iswarchandra Bhattacharya's *Dravya Guna* also appeared in 1835. Though Bhattacharya, too, clearly affiliated with the ayurvedic tradition by copiously quoting from the 'shastras', his text was clearly based upon an open-ended, flexible idea of the tradition of his choosing.[28] The 'shastras', after all, were a relatively open-ended category in themselves, and any locally available Sanskrit text (most frequently late-medieval Bengali compositions) could pass as such. It was an easy way of giving a corpus a recognizably 'classical' Sanskritic identity without necessarily narrowing its scope in any way.[29] Madhusudan Gupta's pharmacopoeia entitled *Aushadh Kalpavali*, which appeared in the following year in 1836, also affiliated putatively with the 'western' medical tradition while being open to indigenous influence.[30] Gupta thus included Bengali and English names for his medicines. A little later, in 1849, Rajkrishna Mukharji authored a very similar book entitled *Atmarakshya*. Though Mukharji also quoted the 'shastras', his text drew upon Madhab Kar's *Nidan*—a medieval Sanskrit text from Bengal. He also used very broad, popularly held ideas about the preservation of health.[31] These texts, printed in the 1830s and the 1840s, thus clearly show the emergence of a loose sense of distinct medical traditions, yet the scope of these traditions are left vaguely defined. When the Rev. James Long compiled his *Descriptive Catalogue* of Bengali books in the mid 1850s, therefore, he continued to use the term 'doctor' to refer to both practitioners of 'western' and 'indigenous' medicines.

The 1830s and 1840s was also the period when the idea of a 'Hindu system' of medicine equated with ayurveda was gaining popularity as a powerful intellectual resource amongst Anglo-Indian writers. The two most significant authors in this regard were J. F. Royle, whose *Essay on the Antiquity of Hindu Medicine* appeared in 1837, and T. A. Wise, whose *Commentary on the Hindu System of Medicine* appeared in 1845.[32] F. J. Mouat's 1847 essay on 'Hindu Medicine' in the *Calcutta Review* was also an important text that popularised the idea of a 'Hindu medical system'.[33] The idea that 'Hindu medicine', or ayurveda, formed a 'system' had already emerged in the writings of the orientalist H. H. Wilson in the 1820s.[34] The emergence of the *daktari* texts in the second half of the nineteenth century owed much to the emergence of the idea of a 'Hindu' or 'Ayurvedic System'. By insisting on a clearer definition of ayurveda, authors like Wise, Royle and Mouat also paved the way for the emergence of the *daktari* system. Despite their best intentions—particularly Wise—by clearly defining medical inheritance in terms of 'national' identities (Wise spoke of, apart from the Hindus, of the 'medical systems' of 'Asiatic Nations', such as the 'Buddhist' and 'Chinese systems of Medicine'), they succeeded not merely in Hinduizing and Indianizing ayurveda, but also 'provincializing' the medicine he and others such as Rameshwar Awasthi or Ishwarchandra Ganguly were practising at the time.[35] To define ayurveda as the historical inheritance of South Asia alone was to imply at the same time that the medicine being practised by Wise, Ganguly and others was the inheritance of some other place, i.e., the 'west'. To accent the nationality of ayurveda was thus to also challenge the universality of 'western' medicine.

In terms of imperial ideology, too, there was a growing ascendance—though not as linear as previously thought—of Anglicist insistence on the adoption of 'British style of life', instead of the previous openendedness of the orientalists.[36] This ideology, in its own turn, would have been instrumental in framing the question as one of adopting alien, but superior, 'western medicine'.

Arnold has rightly pointed out that the purpose of the NMI was never to support 'indigenous medicine'; it was simply to provide cheap medical care for the company's servants. He also points out that the NMI did not intend to place 'western' and 'indigenous' medicines at par and always presumed the superiority of 'western' medicine.[37] The framing of the NMI, however, had been such as to avoid the portrayal of 'indigenous' and 'western' medicines as conflicting 'national' medicines. Driven as it was, by pragmatic considerations, it was a characteristic institution of an epoch in which 'western' was presented in texts such as *Olauthar Vivaran* or *Bramley-r Bakrita* as 'updated' (and therefore superior) versions of a shared medical practice.

This provincialization of medicine was not immediately visible in the world of English printing on South Asian medical subjects. Partly, this was because there was still no significant number of South Asian medical authors writing on 'indigenous medicine' in English, but partly, it was also because English authors wrote for a readership—Anglo-Indian or continental—for whom the supposed antiquity and achievements of ayurveda was a thing of the distant past and not an actual treatment option. Most of those who wrote on ayurveda, i.e.,Wilson, Wise, Royle, intended their works to be read by a continental readership. Wise and Royle both published editions of their books in London. This automatically meant that they were writing for a readership which would be very unlikely to ever come across ayurveda as an actual treatment option. Thus, authors like Royle could create a global genealogy of medicine where Europe had borrowed from the Arabs who had supposedly in turn borrowed from the 'Hindus'. This reconciliation of present-day conflict and competition through an acknowledgement of distant historical debt could only work in a situation where there were no actual physicians competing for patient custom. Bengali texts, however, were predictably printed only for circulation in South Asia. Here the readers encountered proponents of several different medical traditions. These texts, therefore, did not have the luxury of resolving contemporary conflict through positing a historical debt. They had to position themselves and their authors vis-à-vis the other competing physicians and their (the latter's) texts. Once ayurvedic texts had been given a clear systemic and national identity and they continued to exist as actually available medical alternatives, 'western' medicine in Bengali had to adopt a self-description which implicitly acknowledged its own 'provinciality' by merely acknowledging the contemporary existence of other 'systems'.

While the need thus arose in the world of Bengali print to distinguish between ayurveda (and, to a lesser extent, unani tibb) and its 'state-backed Other, the provincialization of 'western' medicine also implicitly challenged the claims of the increasing number of Bengali 'doctors' like Awasthi or

Ganguly, who had energetically participated, in what had, for a while, seemed to be an ecumenical medical world, as equal participants (in their view) and contributors to that world. The Annual Dispensary Reports which had arguably been the main forum for the original writings of lower-level Bengali doctors were stopped in March 1852. The government simply decided that it had neither the need nor the interest to collect or read what these doctors had to contribute to the 'universal corpus of medical knowledge'. Though these reports were revived after 1865, the government now supplied pre-fixed formats in which the reports were to be written. Interested principally in statistical data, the government forms specified, in red letters on top, that the reports were 'Not to Exceed 25 Pages'. Not only was the only scope of original medical work for the doctors therefore abolished, but they were further told in no uncertain terms that as far as the higher levels of the medical establishment were concerned, their intellectual innovations or experiments were immaterial. They were reduced to the level of mere technicians manning the lower rungs of a system from which they were increasingly intellectually alienated. Whereas in the 1830s and 1840s, the Assistant Surgeons in-charge of the many dispensaries had been seen as valuable 'native' pioneers of 'western' medicine, after the 1860s they came to be seen increasingly as unreliable, half-trained subordinates. In 1868, the Inspector General of Civil Hospitals of Bengal wrote:

> The inspections of the dispensaries have, on the whole, been satisfactory; yet I cannot but feel that, over the minor ones especially, more supervision is necessary. Native Doctors, and even Sub-Assistant Surgeons, left to themselves too long, are apt to get into the habit of performing their duties in a perfunctory manner… As dispensaries in out of the way districts go on increasing year by year, the present difficulty of inspecting them will have to be met, for no institution can be left un-inspected to itself, without being productive of more harm than good to the people, and to the name of these benevolent institutions all over the country.[38]

Thus, while the numbers of 'native' staff required continued to grow, their image changed radically in the eyes of the IMS superiors after the 1860s. Some idea of how extreme the mistrust between Bengali surgeons and their immediate superiors was can be gained from the especially tragic case of Dr Pulinchandra Dey. Dey, a graduate of the Bengali medical class and placed in charge of the Purulia dispensary, kept on writing to his immediate superior, Dr Wilson, asking for sick leave in the early 1870s, only to be repeatedly refused. Dr Wilson was convinced that Dey was not telling the truth about his own health.

Ultimately, the Bengali doctor fell dead of extreme exhaustion. The government rebuked Wilson and withheld the increased pay he was entitled to for six months.[39] But what is revealing about Dey's death is the extent to which the relationship between Bengali surgeons and their British superiors had changed since the days of the Awasthis and Gangulys. The personalized, encouraging and intimate contact that Dr Butter shared with his Bengali subordinate Dr Ganguly, or that Dr Davies shared with Dr Awasthi, had, by the 1870s, been replaced by so much distance and suspicion as to make Dey's death possible.[40]

On the other hand, in response to the growing demand for technically qualified manpower, the Medical College had been forced to introduce vernacular medical classes as early as in 1839. These classes were taught in Hindustani. In 1851 classes were also introduced in Bengali. This shorter course produced a growing number of medical men whose linguistic skills were mostly confined to Bengali. These new doctors who became the *Vernacular Licentiates in Medicine and Surgery* (VLMC), created a further motor for the vernacularization of 'western' medicine. While their increasing numbers created a growing demand for Bengali books and periodicals, their lack of knowledge of English made their own location within the 'western' medical tradition uneven and inchoate. One such Bengali class graduate who went on to later write a treatise on 'malarious fevers', for instance, confessed that his knowledge of the 'western' medical tradition on fevers was derived solely from running class notes taken during the lectures of Professor D. B. Smith.[41] It was hardly surprising, then, that the system he described in his small treatise, though bearing a superficial resemblance to the 'western' medical ideas about fevers, also bore a strong resemblance to certain indigenous ideas about fevers, their causes and types.

The idea of 'national medical systems', the alienation of the Bengali Sub-Assistant Surgeons within the medical establishment and the establishment of the Bengali medical class—all contributed towards the Bengali medical publishing industry's production of texts on vernacularized 'western' medicine. It is crucial, however, to remember that *daktari* was, at least in its early decades, a relational term. It was used principally to distinguish the medicine practiced by Bengali physicians practising 'western' medicine from those practicing ayurveda, unani tibb, etc.

Neshat Quaiser is perhaps the first historian of South Asian medicine to have drawn attention to the role of the label of 'doctory' or *daktari* in the reform and revival of 'indigenous' medicines.[42] Others since have also highlighted the constitutive role that *daktari* medicine and its dialogue with 'indigenous' medicines had in shaping 'modern indigenous medical systems'.[43] Little account however has been taken of how far the 'doctory' or *daktari* itself was shaped by such dialogue.

Second Phase: 1851–1918

The second half of the nineteenth century witnessed an enormous explosion of Bengali medical publishing. As per Long's catalogue, while merely 14 Bengali books had been published in the thirty-two years from 1818 to 1850, ten Bengali medical books were published in the mere six years between 1850 and 1856. Even allowing for the characteristic underreporting of Long's catalogue, it does point towards a massive expansion of the market for Bengali medical literature. From the second half of the nineteenth century the print industry in Bengal in general witnessed massive growth. By 1891, 26,347 people were being employed in various capacities by the printing industry.[44] By 1901, 35,917 depended upon the print industry as either employees or their dependants.[45]

Along with this massive expansion of Bengali medical publishing, there arose an unprecedented variety in the texts themselves. A general idea of this vibrant plurality of Bengali medical publishing is essential to any appreciation of the context within which *daktari* became a meaningful category of self-description. For the sake of convenience and comparison, we will therefore try to organize the numerous medical texts of the second half of the nineteenth century into generic groups.

The first of these genres was undoubtedly the Bengali texts produced as a direct result of the establishment of the Bengali medical class and sought to fulfil the demand for Bengali medical text books by the students. P. Kumar's 280-page *Oushodobyaboharok* published in 1854 was an early example of this genre. Kumar was a lecturer at the Bengali class and presented his book as a translation of the latest European medical authors. His book was also clearly against any inter-disciplinary borrowings. He claimed that by translating the European authors he hoped to save his countrymen from the 'clutches of native quacks'.[46] This trend of Bengali class lecturers producing Bengali text books was continued later to great success by the prolific Dr Durgadas Kar, and to a lesser extent by his son, Dr Radha Gobinda (R. G.) Kar. As already hinted at in the foregoing section, texts such as these which overtly eschewed 'inter systemic' dialogue, borrowed vocabularies and formal traits from the 'indigenous' traditions. They were therefore conspicuous in refusing to explicitly agree to the provincialization of *daktari* medicine, positioning it instead as the heir to the accumulated medical history of the region.

A strand within this genre of Bengali medical textbooks also comprised the numerous homoeopathic textbooks. In the absence of prominent institutional structures for the instruction of homoeopathic medicine in the early days of the second half of the nineteenth century, these textbooks were far more important to the dissemination of homoeopathy amongst practitioners than their 'allopathic' counterparts. While in the case of allopathic medicine, the textbooks were usually supplemented by a variety of structures of personal instruction ranging from apprenticeships to the more formal enrolment in Bengali medical class and even enrolment in numerous private medical colleges; in the case of homoeopathy, many practitioners were autodidacts for whom the textbooks were the main source of knowledge. Though Kalikrishna Mitra's small treatise on the treatment of dysentery, entitled *Homiopathic Chikitsa*, was one of the earliest homoeopathic texts, Hariprasad Chakrabarty's later *Homiopathic Bhaisajyatattwa*, published in 1880, was much more comprehensive as a textbook.[47]

These textbooks were also closely related to another genre of books which had commenced way back in the 1820s with Peter Breton's efforts, i.e., that of Bengali medical vocabularies. These vocabularies tried to provide Bengali alternatives to English technical terms. The subsumption of this genre briefly in the 1860s and 1870s by authors such as Durgadas Kar provided these authors with one of their most fertile sites for vernacularization.[48] Like the textbooks, vocabularies eschewed provincialization by deploying terms drawn from 'indigenous' traditions within a uniform 'western' medical framework. Thus, any typical statement from an author like Kar was composed of a Bengali term followed by the English term it sought to replace (but written in Bengali) and finally the English term that appeared parenthetically in English. Thus, a typical example from Kar reads: '*Bhoutik Shakti, Ingraji, Mekanikal Influens* (Mechanical Influence)'.[49] The original concept thus introduced was presented first as an 'indigenous' term, and subsequently the English terms were introduced as synonyms. The order of reading the sentence automatically presented the Bengali term first and therefore implicated it in already-available associations before introducing the later English term as a synonym. At every level of explanation, therefore, the English terms were being grafted onto existing ideas rather than displacing them. Like the textbooks, implicitly by setting up correspondences between 'indigenous' and 'western' categories, vocabularies refracted 'western' concepts through 'indigenous' concepts with older genealogies. The choice of words used in the texts were by no means obvious choices and it allowed the authors to map the European concepts they claimed to be translating onto preexisting indigenous ideas and concepts, despite their assertions of the disciplinary difference and distance between indigenous and European medical traditions. The 'active principles' of drugs such as *quina* in cinchona is described as being its '*virya*'—a highly loaded term within the locally popular Tantric vocabulary, in which it is related to 'sperm'; the *gallbladder* becomes the '*pittwakosh*'; the tube connecting the *gallbladder* and the *kidneys* become the *Kaishik Shira*—both, once again, terms with powerful Tantric resonances.[50] Partly, this mode of translation was dictated by the demands of the medical market. The books were written not to implement colonial (or any other policy) but as commercial ventures and they would only sell if they were understood by the people who comprised the market. As one *daktar* writing in 1896 pointed out, irrespective of what popular ayurvedic terms like *bayu, pittwa* or *kaaph* may mean in technical terms, they had a great popularity amongst the lay people. 'Until a patient hears one of these terms already known to him from his *daktar*', wrote Dr Lalibhamohan Chattopadhyay, 'no matter what the *daktar* says, the patient will not comprehend his affliction'. The *daktars* therefore, Dr Chattopadhyay pointed out, were often forced to use such terminology to explain their 'western' pathological categories.[51]

By the late 1880s and 1890s, however, the growing use of some 'western' medical terminology—especially some anatomical designations such as "nerves" and some pathological categories such as "malaria"—by those outside the 'western' medical tradition once again caused an independent genre of vocabularies to reemerge from the shadow of the textbooks. So great was the demand for books markedly on 'western' medicine—which would obviously deploy a fair amount of 'westernised' terminology—that one Jadu Mandal petitioned the Bengal government, asking for books on 'how to treat diseases' according to the 'western' system, which Mandal claimed he could easily sell at a profit and therefore make the government a lot of money.[52] Prasadkumar Mukhopadhyay's *Chikitsakosh*, published in 1894, was a good example of this reemergence, as was Hariprasad Chakrabarty's *Daktari Abhidhan,* published from Dhaka in 1890.[53] The most remarkable in this regard, however, were the efforts of the prolific and charismatic Bengali scientist and essayist, Ramendrasundar Tribedi. Tribedi, incidentally, took Breton's earlier work as his starting point, though the changes he made were very significant as well. We will discuss Tribedi's translations further in Chapter V.

The second half of the nineteenth century also saw the publication of a significant number of smaller treatises by Bengali *daktars* on specific areas of specialization within the larger 'European' tradition. Four areas of specialization were particularly productive of such smaller treatises: sexual diseases, disorders of the spleen or liver (these often concentrated mainly of 'malarious fevers'), children's diseases and women's diseases (including tracts on midwifery). These texts were more often than not produced by *daktars* working with relative autonomy in CDs. Hur Chunder Sen's manual of venereal diseases published in 1882, while he was working as the medical officer in charge of the Sherpur dispensary, and Annadacharan Khastagir's *Manabjanmatattwa* are both good examples of this genre.[54] Sometimes textbook writers, too, would try their hands at this genre, hinting perhaps at the fact that this was a large and lucrative market. Jadunath Mukhopadhyay, one of the most prolific textbook and manual writers, also tried his hand at writing specific disease-focussed books on fever and cholera.[55]

Apart from these three *daktari* genres, there were also three significant genres of 'indigenous' medical publications. Primarily, of course, there were the numerous new printed editions of Bengali translations of Sanskrit ayurvedic texts. The works of Charak, Madhab Kar, Gobinda Das, etc., appeared in easily accessible Bengali translations in multiple editions by a host of different redactors.[56] This prolific genre marked the process of ayurveda's classicisation and its attendant process of canon formation. Alongside these classics, there also appeared a set of ayuvedic 'lists'—comprising both texts listing names (vocabularies) and those listing qualities of substances (*dravya gunas*). The renowned Kaviraj Binodlal Sen's *Ayurvediya Dravyabhidhan* (An Ayurvedic Encyclopaedia of the Qualities of Substances), published in 1876, was one of the first of this genre, and Haralal Gupta's *Ayurbed Bhashabhidhan* (A Linguistic Encyclopaedia of Ayurvedic Terms), which went into at least five editions, was one of the most successful.[57] Finally, there was a set of texts on 'indigenous' medicine that could not strictly be located within the evolving canon of ayurveda's classical heritage. They drew, instead, on a welter of localised 'smaller' traditions. Prankrishna Biswas' *Ratnavali*, published in 1833, had already inaugurated this genre and flourished, especially in the voluminous productions of the cheap presses of the Bot-tola area in Calcutta.[58] In fact, Bishwas' legacy was directly invoked in a number of these later texts, such as in Jadunath Datta's *Prankrishna Aushadhavali* (Prankrishna's Medicines), published in 1877, or Moulvi Abdus Sobhan's *Sahi Elaj-e-Lokmani* (The Authentic Treatment of Lokman), published as late as in 1921.[59] Pramathanath Ghosh's *Sarpaghater Chikitsa* (The Treatment of Snakebites), published in 1868, was another good example of this trend.[60] The trend was most conspicuous, however, in genres known as '*garhasthya chikitsa*' (home remedies) and '*mushtiyoga*' or '*totka*' (simples).[61] These texts played an important part in institutionalizing numerous marginalized medical ideas and practices as, for instance, in the case of the *Malboidyo* treatment of snakebites.

Alongside these lower-brow 'indigenous' medical texts, there also appeared a wide variety of 'low-brow' Bengali texts that claimed to be translating marginalised 'western' traditions. Premchand Chaudry's 1850 book on *Jal Chikitsa* (Water Treatment), which claimed to be translating European texts on hydropathy, was perhaps the earliest example of this genre.[62] Later similar texts on treatments like mesmerism or chromopathy also appeared.[63] There was, however, a crucial change in the publication structure of the early books such as Chaudry's, drawing upon 'alternate' strands of 'western' medicine. It is also worth pointing out that these books were often published by some of the most respectable presses of the day. Chaudry's work on hydropathy, for example, was published by Rozario & Co., the same company that published Madhusudhan Gupta's translation of the British Pharmacopoeia, proving that the trend had not changed in the second phase of publishing. The Bengal Medical Library, which had published such Bengali literary giants as Tagore and Saratchandra Chatterjee, also published Surendramohan Bhattacharya's work on mesmerism in 1911. Another point of interest regarding these 'western' heterodox texts was their attempt to doubly code their treatments by laying claim to both elements of the 'western' tradition as well as strands within the South Asian traditions. Surendramohan Bhattacharya's book on mesmerism entitled *Dakini Vidya* and published in 1911, for instance, sought to equate mesmerism with the knowledge possessed by mythic Assamese witches (*dakinis*).[64]

It was this vibrant plurality and market for cheap textbook-like compilations that may have inspired the production of a certain genre of cheap Bengali texts aimed at the market for the autodidacts but claiming to teach *daktari* medicine. This peculiar genre, which propagated a certain bowdlerized version of 'western' medicine in Bengali, cannot be understood simply by reference to the erudite textbooks of medical scholars such as Durgadas Kar, or through the institution of the Bengali medical class alone. It becomes meaningful only within the unique, polyvalent and voluminous market for Bengali medical manuals. Thus, whereas the textbooks of Kar and others usually avoid using the term *daktari* and often use vocabulary reminiscent of preexisting healing cultures (though they do not openly embrace any conceptual links with 'indigenous' medical traditions), the cheap *daktari* texts prominently display the word *daktari* to designate their contents. The names given to the books amply bring out this contrast. For instance, in Durgadas Kar's arguably best-known work, *Bhaisajya Ratnavali*, though the text avoided positing any direct conceptual connections with ayurveda, the name itself was identical to the vastly influential eighteenth-century ayurvedic classic by Gobindo Das. Similarly, his compilation of 'western' prescriptions was called *Bhisak Suhrid*. As already suggested, these books, while avoiding any direct inter-borrowings, used a vocabulary that subtly displaced 'western' medicine onto older registers of medical signification, which resonated with older 'indigenous' medical traditions. In this, however, texts such as those of Kar preserved the universalist claims of medicine to some extent. By seeking to establish these interconnections and equivalences between traditions, they avoided having to frame different traditions as being distinct from each other. For the more plebeian authors of the *daktari* manuals, however, such universalism was impossible. In a market already jostling with medical manuals ranging from texts on chromopathy to those inspired by local faith-healing traditions, these authors were forced to present their medicine as belonging to yet another discrete and distinct medical tradition. The most conspicuous provincialization of the 'western' medicine in Bengali, therefore, occurs in texts such as Nafarchandra Datta's hugely successful *Sachitra Sahaj Daktari Shikkhya*.[65]

It is cogent to point out that the existence and immense popularity of cheap didactic medical texts qualify—at least in the case of medicine—the assertion by some scholars that the *Bot-tola* publications 'were markedly disassociated from…educational publications'.[66] Datta's book was published from No. 117 Upper Chitpur Road (at the very heart of what is known as the Bot-tola area) and the use of the word '*shikhya*' (education) in the title leaves little doubt about its advertised 'educational' character. Advertisements of Datta's book also advertises many similar didactic medical titles such as *Sahaj Kaviraji Shikhya, Patent Aushadh Shikhya Boro, Nadigyan Shikhya*, etc., offered by the same publisher.[67] The difference between the higher-end publications and the cheaper ones lay in their format and structure rather than in their subjects.

It is by attention to the actual layout and format of the text that we can clearly distinguish Datta's *daktari* texts from those by scholars like Kar. Whereas Kar had deployed a complex translation format linking indigenous words and concepts to English terms, thereby avoiding any overt reference to 'other' or 'indigenous' medicines, Datta's book, after prominently using the word '*daktari*' in the title, includes named sections on each of the other available medical traditions in the region. *Daktari Shikkhya* is divided into distinct sections devoted respectively to *Ayurvediya Mote Chikitsa* (Treatment according to Ayurveda), *Oushodh Prostuth Pronali* (Preparation of [ayurvedic] Medicines), *Materia Medica Arthat Bhaisajyatattwa* (European Medicines and Prescription), *Homiopathic Mote Chikitsa* (Treatment according to Homoeopathy), *Hekimi, Mushtiyoga ebong Abadhouta Mote Chikitsa* (Treatment according to Unani, by Simples and Faith-Cure), *Dhatri Shikkhya* (Midwifery) and, finally, *Pliha o Jokkrit Sangkranto Jwor Chikitsa* (Treatment of Fevers of the Liver and Spleen). The sections seem absurd at first. Why should a book claiming to teach *daktari* medicine be comprised of sections on ayurveda, unani, homoeopathy, etc.? The structure only becomes meaningful once we realise that each of the sections resonates with one of the important genres of publication mentioned above.

In effect, *daktari* becomes a universal category within which all else that is known by the name of medicine can be accommodated. Thus, whereas Kar and authors like him had eschewed openly professing 'western' medicine's universalism by using an elaborate system of conceptual correspondences, authors like Datta deliberately frame their texts in terms of 'western' medicine's universalist claims. However, what that 'universalism' comes to stand for in Datta's register of meaning is itself very different from the polite understandings of the concept. For Datta, the universalism of 'western' medicine lies not in its superiority to other systems, but in precisely its ability to assimilate and use all other systems of medicine. Not only do we see here the idea of 'medical systems' being made explicit, but, indeed, the universal claims of the 'western' system is expressed as a power to subsume and absorb, rather than as an innate difference and superiority.

The second point of distinction between 'polite' and 'rude' forms of *daktari* lay in the specific identities their authors sought to project. The title pages of the books amply clarify this difference. While the 'polite' *daktari* authors prominently displayed their 'medical' qualifications and expertise, the authors of the 'rude' texts prominently advertised their previous publications—be they medical or not. Thus, while the polite authors showed themselves to their readers as good doctors, the rude authors projected themselves as established authors. The author of *Karyasadhok Aushadhgyan*, Fakirchandra Basu Barman, for example, introduced himself as the author of two racy historical romances 'Shivaji' and 'Ujir Putra'.[68] Nafarchandra Datta introduced himself as the author of *Patent Aushadh Shikhya, Chikitsa Kalpataru*, etc.[69] By contrast, Kar was introduced as Sub-Assistant Surgeon and Jadunath Mukherji was introduced as 'Jadunath Mukherji, LMS'.[70] This format of presenting a generalised intellectual authorial identity shows that in certain sections of the thriving medical market, preprofessional notions of medical legitimacy continued to persist into the twentieth century. Prior to the professionalization of medical authority in the second half of the nineteenth century through the insistence on 'properly qualified' medical personnel, physicians were expected to be wise men and intellectuals, and the type of authority projected by authors like Datta show that such paradigms of medical legitimacy had not been totally displaced, even within those claiming to work within the *daktari* tradition.[71]

Though poor preservation makes the ruder forms of *daktari* medicine more difficult to access today, their existence clearly proves that *daktari* medicine itself was not a homogenised praxis.

Periodicals

Numerous Bengali medical periodicals were floated in the second half of the nineteenth century. Most of these tended to be very short-lived and disappeared after a few early issues. Apart from a very few, such as *Bhisak Darpan, Chikitsa Sammilani* and the *Swasthya*, most did not live beyond the first two years of their inception. Lack of preservation, however, makes it impossible to say with certainty how many such periodicals were launched or exactly how many issues each published. Those issues that have survived provide a fascinating, albeit inchoate, glimpse into the rich intellectual culture of the Bengali *daktars* working at the lower end of the medical bureaucracy.

The greatest boom of Bengali medical periodical publishing came in the period after 1875 right up to the 1930s and 1940s. In the case of Britain, W. F. Bynum and Janice Wilson have pointed out that, after the 1860s, the medical journals industry became more stable. The rate of growth slowed down significantly, but the longevity of the journals published increased and there was an increasing trend towards specialization. Much of this, suggest Bynum and Wilson, may have been due to the consolidation of the profession itself after the Medical Registration Act of 1858.[72] In Bengal, on the basis of the very limited evidence that has survived, this was not the case. Short-lived journals continued to appear and disappear with great regularity. The kind and degree of specialisation observed in Britain was totally absent. Indeed, there was constant pressure to expand the ambit and be more general. Bengali journals, however, were unique in allowing a robust dialogue between different 'systems' of medicine. Even those such as the *Bhisak Darpan,* which was virtually a demi-official publication, included occasional pieces where a dialogue with ayurveda was visible.

That the periodicals were not primarily commercial ventures can be inferred by the chronic indebtedness of the ventures. Those starting a medical periodical could hardly have done so in the hopes of making money through it. Even the best-run and longest-running ones remained chronically in debt. Of the three periodicals known to have run with the greatest success, the *Bhisak Darpan* (BD), which is known to have been published more or less regularly for at least twenty-three years since 1890, the *Chikitsa Sammilani* (CS), which appeared for at least twelve years since 1887 and the *Swasthya,* which appeared for at least seven years from 1897, none ever made a profit.

Usually the periodicals were run by one or more editor-proprietors who invested their own money in starting the journal. Dr Binodbihari Roy of Talanda, Rajshahi, who briefly published a journal called *Chikitsak* in 1889, mentioned that he had had to incur a personal debt of Rs 600—a very considerable sum of money at the time—to set up a press from which to publish his journal.[73] Numerous other periodicals, too, repeatedly hinted at the personal financial difficulties of the editor-proprietors due to irregularity of subscriptions. Since advertising—though voluminous in the general periodicals of the day—was scanty in the medical periodicals, the bulk of the periodical's earnings were dependent on subscriptions. Irregular subscriptions forced editor-proprietors like Dr Roy to invest their own money not only in setting up the journal, but also in trying to keep it going. Even successful journals such as the BD and the CS repeatedly urged recalcitrant readers to send in their overdue subscriptions. A wide range of strategies were deployed by the editor-proprietors to try to ensure the payment of outstanding subscriptions. Apart from regularly publishing appeals about the straightened finances of the journal and its editors, some editors, such as those of the CS, threatened to socially embarrass the recalcitrant subscribers by sending subsequent issues by 'Value Payable post'.[74] Other editors went even further and took to publishing the names of the defaulters in their journal as another way of socially embarrassing them.[75] Another variation on this strategy was for editors to publish the names of those who *had* paid their dues—both as a mark of acknowledgement, but more to castigate those who did not pay up.[76] However, apart from such varieties of social embarrassment, there seemed to be little that editors could do to recover bad debts and unpaid subscriptions.[77] The most successful periodicals, therefore, managed to identify individual patrons who subsidised their costs regularly. The benevolence of these patrons, in turn, was prominently acknowledged in every issue of the periodical alongside the names of the editors. The CS was regularly subsidised by Rai Jatindranath Choudhury, the zamindar of Taki. The BD received financial subsidy from the Bengal government itself.[78] Though there is little direct evidence to suggest that the patrons directly interfered with every aspect of editorial policy, the patron's support was crucial to the editor's continuance in office. That the patron's support was ultimately crucial for the editor becomes particularly evident in the case of the BD. The BD had been started by Dr Moulvi Zahiruddin Ahmed, a charismatic professor of surgery at the Campbell Medical School. Dr Girishchandra Bagchi joined the editorial team from the middle of the sixth year in the capacity of working editor, having replaced the previous incumbent, Dr Abdul Ajed Khan Choudhury. The circumstances of this replacement were not clarified for the readers. Chances of the replacement having been anything but amicable, however, are slim, since Dr Khan Choudhury continued to contribute articles to the journal frequently even after his departure from the editorial team.[79] On the departure of Dr Ahmed in 1899, however, Dr Bagchi was involved in a bitter struggle for control of the journal. The dispute even led to the temporary suspension of publication for four months. Eventually, Dr Bagchi and Dr Kalimohan Sen emerged as joint editors of the periodicals. By a public announcement made in the delayed issues of the year 1900, the editors clarified the reason for the delay and further stated that they had eventually been given control of the journal through the intervention of the government.

This close association of the government of Bengal with the BD also assured the journal's closer implication within the professional life of the Bengali *daktars*. The journal came to regularly publish lengthy monthly lists of inter-hospital and inter-regional transfers of lower level medical personnel, results of intra-departmental examinations for promotion, examination papers for various medical examinations and drafts of proposed legislative bills that had any bearing on the Subordinate Medical Services. All this helped to consolidate a professional identity for the Bengali *daktars*. It also helped formulate opinions and develop a common stand on controversial topics such as the Medical Registration Act of 1914. The various publications and discussions related to different medical examinations also made the journal attractive to medical students at all levels, and the journal consistently offered special subscription rates for medical students, hinting perhaps at the continued importance of student subscribers to their overall subscription lists. Its importance to Bengali medical staff and its proximity to the government also inspired many British authors such as Dr William Henry Porter, Dr R. E. Rafdhar, Dr William Sedgewick, Dr Palmer Vadley and others to contribute articles to it.[80] The editors also regularly published extracts and summaries of the latest research from Europe and America. For many of the Bengali *daktars* of the Bengali class working at the lower end of the medical bureaucracy, these pieces in the BD were the only contact they had with the intellectual milieu of the upper end of Anglo-Indian medicine. The BD, however, also accepted a large number of contributions from Bengali VLMS *daktars*. The journal's guidelines for submission stated: 'Any physician can contribute to the *Bhisak Darpan*. For articles to be accepted, however, they must posses a degree of individuality (*bisheshottwo thaka dorkar*)'.[81] Unlike in the case of medical textbooks, therefore, this was not merely a forum for the presentation of Anglo-Indian medical knowledge in simplified form for the *daktars*. It was also a forum for the active intellectual engagement of these *daktars* with higher-end medical writings.

The closer proximity of the BD to the Bengal government made it in many ways atypical of the general trends seen in Bengali medical periodicals of the day. The CS was possibly more typical in this sense. While its founder-editor Dr Annadacharan Khastagir was a well-known Bengali *daktari* author and had long served in the IMS as a Sub-Assistant Surgeon, the journal had encouraged writing on *daktari*, homoeopathy and ayurvedic medicine. For most of its career, the journal was clearly demarcated into a '*daktari*' (within which section it included both 'allopathic' and 'homoeopathic' articles clearly distinguished by a subheading) and a '*Kaviraji*' sections. Apart from the obvious commercial interest in broadening the appeal of the journal, such cosmopolitanism of the

Bengali journals also arose from a genuine interest of Bengali *daktars* in intellectually engaging with the indigenous medical traditions. Protracted and often bitter debates between exponents of the two systems attested to the fact that the journals were not merely a forum for commercially driven eclecticism. Dr Pulinchandra Sanyal, MB and one-time editor of the CS, for instance, was engaged in a bitter and long-drawn-out debate in print with Kaviraj Prasannachandra Maitreya on the issue of whether the contemporary practice of ayurveda was based upon fallacious fundamental principles. At the same time, however, the very fact that Sanyal had edited the CS for a few years proved that his commitment to intellectually engage with ayurveda was not limited to mere superficial debunks.[82] In fact, Dr Roy, the editor of the *Chikitsak* of Rajshahi, clearly stated in the first issue of his journal that the reason for launching it was his belief that since ayurveda was the 'national' medicine, the *daktars* had a duty to ensure its improvement as well as learn from it.

This intellectual dialogue based upon a commitment to 'improve' ayurveda, but also equally upon a belief that as the older and 'national' medicine of the region it could enrich 'western' medicine, helped to shape *daktari's* own identity. *Daktari* writings were marked increasingly by a concern to 'nationalize' (or more accurately perhaps, 'de-alienate', i.e., make less alien) their medicine. Their active intellectual dialogue with ayurvedic medicine helped them not only to popularise their distinct—if provincialized—identity, but it also helped them to actively align their own medical repertoire with what they saw to be local cultural mores and traditions. Since medical traditions had already been reimagined along 'national' lines and *daktari* medicine was clearly framed as being non-Bengali, Bengali *daktars* increasingly came to resist the idea that they were mere 'mimic men' blindly following a 'western' tradition. *Daktars* like Jadunath Gangopadhyay wrote with passionate sarcasm: 'We are becoming like children, just as children do exactly what their teachers tell them, so, too, do we blindly follow the lead of our English teachers. We do not have our own independent way of thinking, we do not have novel opinions, we don't even aspire to such originality or in seeking to teach others as such. We have become like a mass of dead flesh, enlightened by the light of English wisdom but unable to reflect that light.'[83] Gangopadhyay argued that it was not enough to merely translate 'western' knowledge and texts. What was needed, asserted Gangopadhyay, was that authors translating 'western' medical texts had to give more importance to their own local experience and incorporate these into the texts they translated. Among the few people who Gangopadhyay thought had done this successfully were Madhusudhan Gupta, Durgadas Kar, Mir Ashraf Ali, Gunga Persaud Mookerjee, Bholanath Basu, Udaychandra Dutt and Annadacharan Khastagir.[84]

It was this search for originality and a unique identity that instigated the Bengali medical periodicals to progressively engage with local medical ideas and traditions. Even journals such as *Bhisak Darpan*, which eschewed open dialogue with the indigenous system, actively tried to vernacularize 'western' medicine by realigning it with local cultural beliefs. Even the editor of the BD, Dr Girishchandra Bagchi—who had by then also been honoured by the title of Rai Bahadur, presented to him at the Coronation Durbar in Delhi—wrote to align *daktari* understandings with ayurvedic disease categories.[85] This process of realignment, which was so amply visible in authors associated with the BD—arguably the journal most committed to 'official' (state-sponsored) 'western' medicine—was even more central to *daktari* authors writing in journals such as the CS, the *Chikitsak* (both the Rajshahi and Calcutta journals of that name) and the *Swasthya*.

The quest for a unique identity that contextualized and situated 'western' medicine within local needs and traditions also led to several periodical editors writing textbooks which engaged vigorously with local concerns. Annadacharan Khastagir's work in this regard was mentioned by Gangopadhyay. Others like Dr Devendranath Ray, sometime assistant editor of the BD, Pulinchandra Sanyal, sometime assistant editor of the CS and Jadunath Mukherjee, editor of the *Chikitsa Darpan* all authored popular Bengali medical books in which they engaged with local traditions and requirements. Editorial work in medical periodicals, therefore, came to inspire further medical writing, and the broader exchanges characteristic of the medical periodicals may well have influenced the search for a unique local identity in the medical textbooks the editors came to author.

This pressure to make *daktari* medicine relevant to local contexts was also generated in part due to the particular readership profile that these periodicals came to have. Though readership data is fragmentary and by no means exhaustive, it is clear from the available data that the readership of these journals was usually not restricted narrowly to *daktars* alone, or even to just physicians for that matter. From a subscription list published in the CS in 1887, we find that one subscriber, Mr Brajendrakumar Sheel, was a judge in the district of Bankura; similarly, Dr Gurudas Bhattacharjya was a lawyer in the Calcutta High Court, Mr Amritanarayan Acharjya Choudhury was a zamindar at Muktagachha, Mr Radhagobinda Roy was a manager at the zamindari estate of Tada, etc.[86] A survey of the next year's lists shows a further expansion of the nonmedical readership. Apart from the many from 1887 who renewed their subscriptions, others such as Mr Bhagabaticharan De, station master, Ayudh, Rohilkhand; Mr Ramjoy De Biswas, lawyer, Sunamganj, Sylhet; Nimaicharan Ghosh, employee, engineering office, Dhaka, etc., also appear on the list for 1888.[87] By the ninth year of the CS, the editors published an announcement in which they clarified that: 'The *Chikitsa Sammilani* is a medical periodical, therefore, whenever in recent times we have commented on non-medical matters, critics have not failed to criticise us for speaking out of turn. However, it is important to clarify that though the CS is a medical periodical, the majority of our readers now are non-medical people, so what option do we have, as editors, but to pay heed to the interests of place, time and person? Would it be fair to write solely about obscure medical topics and thus ruin the periodical or rather to occasionally "speak out of turn" in order to ensure its continued popularity?'[88] Dr Roy, of the *Chikitsak* of Rajshahi, who also had a number of nonmedical subscribers for his short-lived periodical, even sought to actively cultivate this nonmedical readership. In a bid to solicit more nonmedical readers, he wrote in the fifth issue of his journal: 'Many might think this is a medical periodical, why should I as a layman subscribe to it. To them we say, all of us have a body and all of us need to be acquainted with that body'.[89] One short-lived journal, the *Chikitsak O Samalochak* (Physician and Critic) even tried to base its appeal upon this combination of lay and medical interests by publishing a mixture of medical and literary pieces. The editor, Dr Satyakrishna Roy, announced in the inaugural issue that, apart from discussions of *Daktari, Homiopathi and Kaviraji* medicine, it would also include 'serialised novels, dramas, short stories and poetry'. Such nonmedical readership—as is amply brought out by the comments of the editors of the CS—forced the editors of these journals to actively seek to align their discussions to popular sensibilities.[90] Discussions in such journals could not become arcane and always needed to keep track of the opinions of the average intelligent layman. While a core of vigilant medical readers, such as those whose criticisms evoked the response from the editors of the CS, ensured that discussion of medical topics were not too far diluted, the need to appeal to a broader nonmedical petty-intellectual class composed of clerical employees, small landholders, lawyers, stationmasters and the like, meant that the medical discussions could never become as alienated and abstruse as purely professional discussions might. What the editors of the CS called paying heed to the interests/ circumstances of 'place, time and person' (*desh, kal, patro bichar*) was therefore a pressure to ensure further alignment of *daktari* medicine to local ideas and sensibilities.[91]

Some of the central features of *daktari* medicine, such as its abiding interest in 'Predisposing Causes' of disease and its insistence on the capacity of the individual to be able to resist contagion through conscious choices—which we shall deal with in greater detail in the following chapter—very likely arose partly from the material need to appeal to a nonmedical readership. As Dr Roy mentioned in his advertisement, the subscription to the journal by nonmedical readers was based upon the idea that laymen could benefit from knowing about their bodies. The journals, therefore, prevented professional isolation of the authors which is to some extent visible in the writings of an earlier generation of textbooks authors such as Durgadas Kar.

Finally, the widespread dispersal of Bengali professionals throughout the British Raj in various capacities meant that these periodicals reached way beyond the political and geographic boundaries of Bengal proper. Apart from subscribers in various parts of Bengal, the more successful journals often had subscribers spread out across northern India. The 1888 issue of the CS, for instance, mentioned a Dr Gopalchandra Bandopadhyay subscribing from Lahore; a certain Mr Bhaironprasad Khetri from Colonelganj, Patna; Mr Bhagabaticharan De from Rohilkhand; Pundit Nabinchandra Roy from Ratlam State; the Maharaja of Manipur; Mr Ashutoshnath Roy of Munger, etc. The subscription of some of these Bengali medical periodicals by the Medical Department itself also led to further dissemination of the periodicals. In 1876, for instance, the government approved a subscription of 30 copies of the *Chikitsa Kalpadruma* in place of the *Chikitsa Darpan* which had ceased publication.[92] Whether or not these distant readers beyond Bengal proper in turn became agents for the further dissemination of *daktari* writings amongst non-Bengali colleagues cannot be ascertained with certainty without further research, but this much can definitely be concluded: that the impact of *daktari* medicine as espoused in the journals of the late nineteenth and early twentieth centuries was not wholly limited to Bengal proper.

Notwithstanding its broad appeal and fairly widespread reach, there was one area in which the Bengali medical periodicals remained limited. Despite the existence of several Bengali Muslim authors, the readership remained overwhelmingly Hindu. Very few Muslim names appear on the subscription lists. Moreover, whereas there was, as already outlined, a rich intellectual engagement with Kaviraji and ayurvedic medicine, unani tibb or hakimi medicine was almost totally ignored. Nor were there any hakims who contributed to these periodicals, whereas there were several kaviraj contributors. The only periodical which had a significant engagement with hakimi medicine was Hakim Majibar Rahman's short-lived periodical titled *Hakim* which appeared in 1910.[93] Rahman was also the only Bengali Muslim to hold editorial responsibilities of a Bengali medical periodical after the departure of Dr Ahmed from BD in 1899. Given the poor state of preservation of this genre of texts, it is impossible to say with certainty whether other smaller, lesser-known publications might have sought to fill this gap. However, the fact that such periodicals, if they existed, were not as well known proves that among the more well-established journals, at least there was clearly a progressive marginalization of what was thought of as 'Islamic' medicine and Bengali Muslim culture. The cultural realignment of 'western' that we have mentioned previously, therefore, increasingly took on a strong Hindu flavour. Even later articles in the demi-official BD had a distinct alignment with Hindu cultural traditions.[94] How much of this was driven by the fact that the majority of the subscribers were Hindus and how much by the fact that most of the more learned literature of unani tibb existed in Arabic and Persian is difficult to ascertain. The end result of this marginalization, however, was clearly to make the nationalization of *daktari* medicine a markedly Hindu project.

Advertisements

Medical advertisements, though one of the most conspicuous genres of medical texts, have only recently been taken up for serious study. Madhuri Sharma has explored its role in creating medical 'consumers' (as opposed to 'users'). She cogently points out that advertising has helped to sustain certain patterns of 'flows of goods' (and we may add 'services') and to 'extend the space occupied by the commodity' through texts and images.[95] Working with similar Hindi advertisements, Rachel Berger has proposed a threefold categorization of medical advertisements of the time. Berger has divided them on the basis of the nature of the commodity being advertised into first, those concerned with 'products targeting the power (or lack thereof) of Indian men'; second, those aimed at 'information about babies and families'; and finally, those selling 'indigenous food products'.[96] Unfortunately, our interest in medical advertising within the context of the present chapter, does not allow us to explore these typologies within the fascinating world of Bengali advertising. Instead, we will interrogate what Berger terms the 'education of desire' with regard to the development of a systemic identity for *daktari* medicine, i.e., why did people choose to buy *daktari* medicines and how did these reasons shape the identity of *daktari*. Instead of looking directly at the actual commodity being sold, we will explore how the advertisements contributed to a popular understanding of the identity of the *daktari* 'system' of medicine. As Sharma rightly points out, the constitution of a 'medical consumer' is a historically specific event and this consumer's 'desire' for certain commodities must also be historically fashioned ('educated'). Thus, implicit in this process of constitution and education are the codes that define and frame medical objects ('medical systems', medicines and diseases). Before we decide to buy (or ignore) a certain advertised commodity, we must figure out what the commodity means and what its consumption might do for us. The advertisements codify these meanings. Advertisements after all aim to sell goods, but, as Jean Baudrillard points out, the exchange, sale and circulation of goods also constitute a 'language' or a 'code'.[97] It is a code that invests the transaction engendered by the advertisement with a specific meaning. Buying, or even merely reading the advertisements everyday in the morning, entails certain kinds of transactions, even if it does not eventually result in the purchase of the medicine concerned. Stefan Ecks has pointed out that many contemporary pharmaceutical companies selling antidepressants in Calcutta do not aim to inspire an immediate purchase, but only endeavour to 'grow the market' by slowly replacing traditional categories of mental states like *mon kharap* ('bad mind') with medicalized, pharmaceutical-consumption-oriented categories like 'depression'.[98] It is this code we wish to decode in a bid to find out how the social identity of *daktari* medicine was expressed in these.

Gautam Bhadra's fascinating recent work on book advertising has raised a crucial question about what precisely constitute the vernacular categories for 'advertising' and how they are distinct from the English word 'advertisement'. Bhadra points out that by the late nineteenth century, the prefaces of printed books had come to be called '*bigyapan*'—the word commonly used for 'advertisement' in Bengali.[99] Clearly, then, the function that a '*bigyapan*' was supposed to perform was broader than that connoted by the English word. It is perhaps due to this mismatch in the English and vernacular meanings that we find a large number of advertisements which look very different from what one tutored in the English meaning of the word would expect. Instead of a layout limited to a single page, for instance, we come across a large number of advertisements—inserted into popular almanacs, for example—which run like small independent texts.[100] These texts have their own page numbers and can sometimes run for twenty pages or more. In some cases, the pages of advertisement are smaller in size than the text they are inserted into or of a different colour, thus further accenting the autonomy of the text.[101] The uniformity of the visual space of the page where advertisements and nonadvertising texts coexist—which have been described by scholars like Charu Gupta—is hence fractured in many Bengali *bigyapans*.[102] These texts, moreover, did not advertise a single commodity, but rather an entire assemblage. In some cases, it was limited to a single type of commodity, i.e., a variety of medicines or books, but at other times, even the nature of the commodities sold were different. Too often, the editors of periodicals advertised books they had written, medicines they sold and the periodicals themselves together. Furthermore, there would often be substantial pecuniary incentives to buy the commodities together.

This peculiarity of Bengali *bigyapans* meant that the desire they sought to cultivate was not directed at a single commodity, but oriented towards a particular framework which encompassed a range of different commodities and products. For instance, the tenth edition of Nafarchandra Datta's immensely successful *Sahaj Daktari Shikhya* discussed earlier, was advertised in the *Gupta Press Dairektari Panjika* (Bengali almanac) of 1915 by Bharat Pustakalay alongside a list of over five hundred other titles sold by them. Significantly, *Daktari Shikkhya* was one of the few that had an entire page dedicated to it (Fig. II). On the page facing it, appeared books such as the *Chikitsa Darshan* (The Philosophy of Medicine), the *Dravya Guna Parichay* (Encyclopaedia of the Qualities of Substances), *Pashu Chikitsa* (Veterinary Medicine), *Sachitra Grihasthya Jeevan* (Illustrated Domestic Life) and *Brahman Itihas* (History of the Brahmins), all advertised by the same Bharat Pustakalay. The *Chikitsa Darshan*, which was allegedly compiled from ayurvedic sources, was said to be useful to '*daktars*, kavirajes and householders in general'. Further down the long list of titles, we find texts like the *Sahaj Kaviraji Shikhya* (Easy *Kaviraji* Primer) and *Sahaj Hekimi Shikhya* (Easy *Hakimi* Primer).[103]

While Bharat Pustakalay sold books, S. K. Roy & Co. sold medicines. They, too, had inserted a multi-page *bigyapan* in the same almanac that Bharat Pustakalay had advertised in. Their text, however, was organized into different clearly defined sections devoted to 'homoeopathy', 'patent medicine' and 'allopathy' or '*daktari*'.[104]

Aimed as these *bigyapans* were at a broad lay-consumer market, the main function of these lengthy *bigyapans* was to create a visibility for an entire range of products, i.e., the books of Bharat Pustakalay or the medicines of S. K. Roy & Co.; they did not intend to sell any specific type of medicines or any specific type of medical books. Though advertisements selling commodities belonging to 'specific systems' can also be seen, in the vast majority of cases, real (as opposed to alleged) differences between the systems becomes hard to sustain in the face of the *bigyapan* texts. What these *bigyapans* promoted, therefore, was a nonspecific surface identity for different medicines and medical books. Medicine was, in these texts, an ecumenical world in which numerous different approaches coexisted. Thus *daktari* as a 'label' became well known in contradistinction to other labels like *kaviraji* or *hakimi*, without necessarily clarifying anything about how these 'labels' differed from each other. The *bigyapan* texts, therefore, educated the medical consumer to recognise *daktari* as a distinct type of medicine, but did not base this distinction upon any conceptual elaboration.

The surface distinction between the systems, therefore, became a matter of names. Nomenclature became an important mode of conveying distinct systemic identities of commodities. Dr S. K. Roy, proprietor of S. K. Roy & Co., advertised homoeopathic, patent and allopathic medicines. However, what distinguished his 'allopathic' medicines were their English names. His list of *daktari* medicines comprised such medicaments as *Roy's Head Cure*,

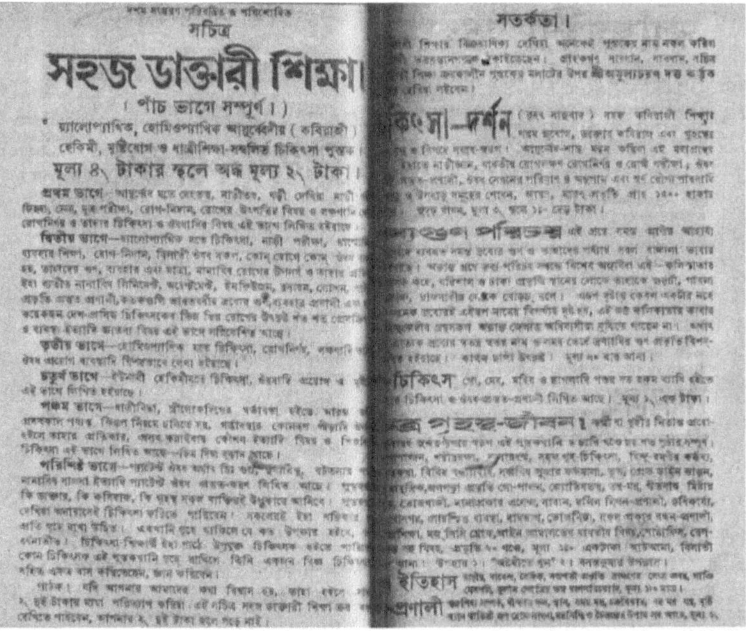

Fig. II. Advertisement for *Sahaj Daktari Shikhya, Gupta Press Dairektari Panjika for 1322 BS.*

Nervine Tonic, Magic Ointment, Dental Powder, Pain Balm, etc., appearing once again next to numerous ayurvedic medicines with names like *Madananda Modak, Mahashakti Salsa, Omlo-Shul Nashak Churna, Ratiranjan Batika,* etc. The *kaviraji* and *daktari* medicines thus came to be distinguished primarily on the basis of English and vernacular names.

Medical advertising also sought to explicitly operationalize the touted proximity of the 'allopathic' medicines to the colonial establishment by naming drugs after symbols of colonial authority. The early Bengali pharmaceutical wholesaler, Butto Kristo Paul & Co., for example, named drugs after the Emperor of India, Edward VII.[105] An earlier advertiser had called his medicine after Edward's father, Albert.[106] Another eminent 'western' pharmaceutical firm in Calcutta, D. Gupta & Co., even named an ointment after the much-resented Lord Lytton.[107] This overt proximity to the colonial state was increasingly erased in the years following the Swadeshi Movement of 1905. Hardly any medicines sold after 1905 were named after colonial administrators. The prefix 'Imperial', however, continued to be used in numerous medical advertisements.[108] The 'exotic' or 'foreign' character of *daktari* also continued to be promoted.

'Exoticism', as a popular framework for operationalizing a surface identity for *daktari* medicine, did not remain limited merely to alleged links to Britain and the colonial power. One Motilal Basu advertised, for example, a Napoleonic Tooth Powder for disorders of the mouth.[109] The advertisements of one Dr Syed Abul Hossain, MD, who used to advertise his medicines in the *Mohammadiya Panjika* (Bengali Islamic Almnac), drew an even more diverse map of medical provenance and authority.[110] Yet, amongst his medicines were such exotic substances as the *Chin-Chuasi* (which was allegedly made with herbs from 'China, Japan, Darjeeling and Bengal') and the *Herambari* (which was made by mixing herbs from 'Egypt, Arabia and Unan [Ionia, Greece]', according to a certain 'Indopathic system'). One drug, called *Sinkuasa,* was said to be made from herbs obtained from Australia and Tasmania.[111] Advertisements such as those of Dr Hossain, amply demonstrate the incomplete hegemony of 'western' medical authority amongst many *daktars.* Plural cartographies of medical authority continued to be transacted by *daktars* in popular social registers. Medical authority in these cartographies was not always seen to derive from centres in the 'west'. Instead other centres of medical authority were seen to be located in Egypt, Arabia, China, Japan, Greece and perhaps somewhat unexpectedly, Tasmania. The hegemonic, 'universalist' aspirations of 'western' state medicine came undone and were recoded in the world of *bigyapans* within a framework of exoticism. Berger's revealing study of ayurvedic medical advertisements, refers to the 'consumption of indigeneity'. In *daktari* advertising we have a complementary example of the 'consumption of exoticism'. The angst of the lower-middle-class *keranis* (those in clerical or semiclerical jobs)—the prime consumers of the surface modernity of *bigyapans,* undoubtedly influenced the popularity of such exoticism. Chained as the *keranis* thought they were to the soul-killing urban rhythms of clerical work, they came to crave the imaginary escape offered by the exotic.[112]

This exoticization of the surface identity of *daktari* medicine also draws attention to the essentially self-prescriptive nature of the Bengali medical market of the day. The fact that a vast amount of medical advertising appeared in nonmedical forums like the almanacs also reaffirms the existence of this do-it-yourself (DIY) ethos in medicine. The first step in this ethics of self-treatment was deciding which mode of treatment was best suited for a particular ailment. Humorist and essayist Rajsekhar Basu, writing in the early 1920s, pointed out in an essay on 'scientific medicine' that though, as a nonmedical man, he had no right to write on medicine, what gave him the right was that as the head of an average middle class family, every time someone fell ill in the family, he was called upon to decide what course of treatment would be best and he had to decide from amongst the various available modes of treatment ranging from *daktari* and *kaviraji* to amulets and the saying of propitiatory prayers.[113]

This DIY ethos of medical advertising also led to the progressive medicalization of everyday complaints and anxieties associated with lower-middle-class urban lifestyles. Markus Daeschel identified in this DIY ethos a reformatting of the selfhood itself. This ethos projected by the advertising and such, like ephemeral texts, argues Daeschel, reconstituted the ways in which South Asian societies experienced and expressed their most intimate selfhood.[114] Indigestion, constipation, lassitude, weakness, problems of anxieties about the adulteration of cheap foodstuff, etc., came to take on significant medical dimensions which eventually even forced the more 'polite' forms of *daktari* practice to discuss these issues.[115]

Literature and Medicine

Advertisements were obviously not the only form of print that constituted the social meanings of *daktari* medicine. A variety of literary texts also contributed towards the social identity of *daktari* medicine.

The immense popularity of late nineteenth century Bengali theatre and the heterogeneity of the audience made dramatic texts arguably the best indices to social meanings.[116] There were, in fact, a number of dramatic texts ranging from serious drama to satires and farces that dealt with *daktari* medicine. So important were these dramatic texts in shaping public perceptions, that in the 1890s the Calcutta municipal authorities, embattled by the public resentment of their sanitary policies, funded one of its own *daktars*, Dr Sundarimohan Das, to write a drama in the traditional *darpan* genre to popularise its sanitary policies and win public approval.[117] However, several dramatic texts appeared before Das' *Munisipal Darpan*, which undoubtedly shaped the social image of *daktari* medicine.[118]

Whereas Das' text followed the *darpan* or 'mirror' format which claimed to 'reveal' the true nature of things, the more popular texts followed a *prahasan* or 'satire' format.[119] The *prahasans* were more ribald in their tone and satirical in flavour. Possibly the earliest *daktari prahasan* was Bhubanmohan Sarkar's 1874 text titled *Daktarbabu*.[120] Kunjabihari Deb's *Thengapathic Bhnuiphod Daktar* appeared in 1886.[121] Another *prahasan*, also called *Daktarbabu*, appeared in 1889, authored by Rajkrishna Roy.[122] All three of these texts painted a largely similar picture of the *daktar*. All three *daktars* were presented in dress and character as being utterly alienated from their society. Even when practising in the rural backwaters, they were shown to be wearing European dress, smoking cigars and sprinkling their dialogues with English words. Sarkar, the author of the very first text, who himself was a practising *daktar*, mentioned, in the foreword to his text, 'As far as I have seen, I feel that doctors, at least a significant number amongst them, consider themselves somewhat at a distance and at a higher title than their fellowmen. Society, too, seems to see them thus and respect them for such'.[123]

Other dominant concerns expressed in the texts revolved around the excessive commercialization and pecuniary greed of *daktars*, their being social upstarts and usually outsiders to the local milieu, as well as their lack of moral probity, especially with regards to the treatment of female patients. Sarkar's Manmatha Daktar, Roy's Joy Daktar and Deb's Pranharan Daktar—all conformed to this image of alienation, moral corruption and sexual predation.

All this was often contrasted with the more familiar and sexually reliable, if less erudite, image of the village *kaviraj*. Rajkrishna Roy's *Daktarbabu*, for instance, drew a clear parallel between the much-better-trained, but alienated and sexually predatory, Joy Daktar on the one hand, and the half-literate Bhajahari Kaviraj on the other. The contrast once again helped to cement the image of different, discrete medical systems with their own practitioners and their unique styles. This idea of each discrete but comparable system with its own practitioners and their signature social and medical styles including forms of speech, dress and ways of relating to patients was caricatured in the 1920s in one of Rajsekhar Basu's best-known short stories entitled *Chikitsa Sankat*. In it, Basu painted pen-pictures of four different physicians—a homoeopath, a kaviraj, a *daktar* and a hakim. While Basu's short story evidenced the further institutionalization of distinct characteristics used by different types of physicians, it continued to depict the *daktar* as being distant and alienated from his patients. Using a comic-metaphoric ruse, the author represented this alienation through the different ways in which different physicians felt the pulse. While the intimate but 'unscientific' *kaviraj* pretended to divine the life history of his patient while feeling his pulse, the *daktar*, whose speech was littered with alien English words, used a contraption made from a car's spark plugs to monitor the pulse, thereby avoiding all physical contact/intimacy with the patient.[124]

These popular images, developed originally in popular drama, began to migrate to other registers of print. For instance, a song describing the corruption of the early *daktars* in Sarkar's *Daktarbabu* was reproduced alongside a cartoon sketch of the character in the short-lived early Bengali comic periodical, *Harbola Bhnar*.[125] (Fig. III) That the cartoon appeared in the same year as the play was released might also hint at the play's popularity.

By the 1930s and 1940s, this image of alienation, commercial greed and unreliability, particularly in the care of female patients, had crosshatched

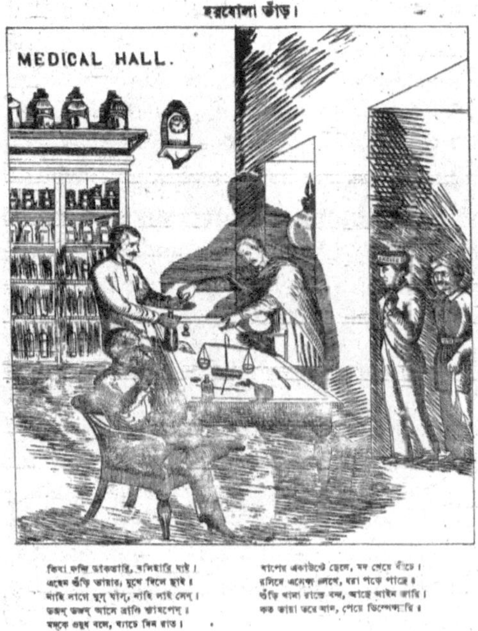

Fig. III. Plate 6, *Harbola Bhnar* (The Ventriloquizing Jester: Journal of Cartoons and Caricatures) 1, no.1 (1874).

with Victorian tropes of 'wrongful confinement' to produce new fears and anxieties about the doctor.[126] Kamakhyaprasad Roy's 1937 play *Mayapuri* and Sachindranath Sengupta's 1940 dramatic text *Narsin Hom* both depicted corrupt, alienated doctors using their power and authority to wrongfully confine young heiresses to make money through bribes from rival claimants to the legacy.[127] Social anxieties, however, did not always bear a direct chronological correspondence with historical facts. The implication of corrupt doctors in property disputes that ended up in the deprivation of hapless heirs was nearly a century old as a social occurrence before it appeared as a popular literary plot. One Dr J. R. Crawford had, for instance, been convicted by a Grand Jury in Calcutta as early as August 1859, after it was discovered that he had connived with an eminent Calcuttan, Sibkrishna Banerjee, in a plot by the latter to defraud his late brother's family of their share in the family fortune. It was a widely publicised case and Crawford got eight years of rigorous imprisonment for his part in the affair.[128] Yet none of the nineteenth-century depictions of corrupt *daktars* introduce this dimension of medical corruption. It is only in the late 1930s that it becomes a popular literary ploy.

By the 1920s, however, another more positive image of the *daktar* had also been evolving. In most cases, this image of the 'good doctor' came to replace the old image of the rustic but intimate *kaviraj* as the counterpoint to organised medical corruption. According to this image, which was best represented in Dr Gyanendranarayan Bagchi's *daktari* novel, as he called it, a young idealistic medical graduate, Deen Choudhury, takes on the corruption of the medical world in an individual crusade to reorient medicine within a framework of '*desh seva*', or service to the nation.[129] Similarly in *Mayapuri*, despite the ultimate cynical triumph of the corrupt forces, the plot revolves around the personal crusade of the young eponymous medical student, Sebabrata Das. The most powerful and best known version of this image of a highly principled, incorruptible and nationalistic Bengali *daktar* was produced by another *daktar*-author like Dr Bagchi—Dr Balaichand Mukhopadhyay, who was better known by his nom de plume *Banaphool.*[130] Banaphool's novel *Agni*—which was later made into a hugely successful Bengali film in 1975 starring the matinee idol Uttam Kumar, depicted a brilliant Bengali doctor working in the IMS in the closing years of the Raj. The fictional Dr Agniswar Mukharji maintained his seemingly alienating 'westernized' attire and lifestyle in continuity with the Joy Daktars and Manmatha Daktars of the nineteenth century. He is also seen to always insist upon his exact fees. However, further on in the novel, the readers are shown that this insistence on an alienating attire and apparently heartless insistence on fees is not borne out of moral corruption, but rather out of a principled belief in following the right professional norms. The fees obtained from hard-pressed poor patients are therefore secretly returned to the patients as anonymous donations by Dr Mukharji. Underneath his seemingly anglicized exterior, there is also seen to hide a deeply patriotic heart. He jeopardises his career to help injured freedom fighters escape from the jail hospital and writes successful Bengali poetry under a nom de plume. The fact that both Mukhopadhyay and Bagchi were themselves *daktars* suggests that a new generation of *daktars* were seeking to actively combat the medical corruption as well as the negative social image of the profession.

Another similarly positive *daktari* image that emerges from the 1920s is that of the *Ledi Daktar.* The image is one of a loving woman whose medical skill is subverted in the plot by the personal ties that she either discovers or enters into with her patient. Basu's *Chikitsa Sankat*, for example, ends with the marriage of the hapless but wealthy patient who has been duped by all other types of physicians to the loving but slightly bossy Dr Vipula Mitra. In Kaliprasanna Dasgupta's 1921 drama *Ledi Daktar*, on the other hand, it turns out that the immensely caring and morally upright lady doctor Gangadasi caring for Dheereshbabu's pregnant wife, is none other than Dheeresh's first wife Maya, who had been kidnapped and sold into prostitution before being rescued by an old lady doctor and trained as a doctor.[131] It is perhaps significant that though this image of the lady doctor is very positive, it is depicted essentially within a framework of familial rather than national duty and service. This framework of 'familialization' of medical care in the context of *ledi daktars* may have actually reflected different modes of practice. Tapan Raychaudhuri in the preface to his translation of the only published autobiography of a Bengali *ledi daktari*—Dr Haimabati Sen—mentions 'her habit of forming putative relationships and referring to sundry people in terms of the minutae of Bengali kinship terminology'.[132]

On the whole, however, there is a clear renegotiation of the image of the *daktar* in literary texts in the period between the 1880s and the beginning of the 1940s. In these sixty years, the image of an alienated, immoral, highly commercialized and predatory *daktar* is replaced by two parallel images in the social consciousness. The first of these is of the good *daktar*, a man of strict principles and deep philanthropic commitment like Dr Agniswar Mukherjee. The second image—of the bad *daktar*—is more redolent of the older images of corruption, predation, greed, etc., but in keeping with the times, these base qualities are now expressed through new tropes which reflect the new power that *daktars* possess.

Conclusion

The impact of print on the emergence of a vernacular identity of 'western' medicine is vast and multidimensional. It is neither homogenous nor uniform. There are numerous different worlds of vernacular printing ranging from medical periodicals, to textbooks and advertising, to dramatic texts. All of them produce different significations of the *daktari* label. These significations often resonate with each other, such as in the case of the erudite *daktari* discussions of 'weakness' or constipation through its contact with the world of advertising. Yet these different significations cannot and should not be reduced to a single social meaning of *daktari*. While *daktari* did acquire a certain social recognizability as a distinct and foreign 'medical system', the range of meanings ascribed to it often varied widely, depending upon the particular section of the vibrant and plural world of Bengali print culture that it inhabited. Importantly, its valence was always as a relational reality, i.e., its identity as a 'medical system' derived from its competition within the medical market with the images of other 'medical systems' such as ayurveda. It represented, therefore, a partly commercially motivated provincialization of the universalist claims of 'western' medicine and partly a response by Bengali practitioners to the charge of the alienation of 'western' medicine owing to the close proximity of this medical tradition to the colonial state.

The diversity of the influence of print technology and market upon the evolution of *daktari* serves to underline two crucial points: First, it cannot be understood as being an internally homogenous domain of knowledge and practice. Second, its evolution and character cannot be adequately understood simply with reference to its own internal logic. Its meanings and identities must be situated in its dialogue with the forces of the market and dialogues that were instigated by that market. This must then further be read with regard to the meanings ascribed to it by lay members of society, such as average consumers and theatre-goers. Indeed, the production of the identity must be juxtaposed with its consumption to get some idea of the range of significations *daktari* acquired at the time.

Chapter III

CONTAGIOUS NATIONALISM: CONTAGION AND THE ACTUALIZATION OF THE NATION

The idea of contagion, i.e., the transfer of disease from one who is afflicted to one who is not, though seemingly obvious to most contemporary readers, has had a complicated and chequered history within the medical traditions of the world. In the premodern era, as in the modern era—and some have suggested even in postmodern contexts—the idea of contagion has been a powerful and polysemic idea. The only extant studies of the idea in South Asia, however, pertain to premodern societies. The discussion of the idea in the history of medicine in colonial India remains merely incidental to concerns about epidemic diseases. This has led to a rather simplistic understanding of the concept with regard to its usage by colonial Indian doctors. In stark contrast to this, studies based in other colonial contexts, such as Australia, have suggested that the relationship between contagion and colonial modernity was anything but simple and straightforward. Alison Bashford and Claire Hooker have suggested that the 'geographies, policies and identities' that emerged under colonial modernity through the entanglement of 'metaphor and public policy…intertwin[ing] personal conduct with the management of populations, nations and economies' within the idea of contagion, were rich, polyvalent and had even an almost fantastic dreamlike character to them.[1]

The study of the history of contagion amongst Indian doctors in the late nineteenth century raises some interesting methodological as well as conceptual problems. Unlike colonial Australia or modern Europe, there was in India not one, but several contending, competing and collaborating medical modernities. As we have discussed in the Introduction, the Indian doctors, though working within a seemingly homogenous colonial modernity, had access to several distinct and overlapping modernities—each with a slightly different ideational and practical conception of contagion. Moreover, each of these modernities was, in turn, differently implicated in various premodern legacies. Conrad and Wujastyk further argue that premodern societies, including South Asian ones, were 'prepared to accommodate the subject in multiple contradictory registers'.[2] The methodological and conceptual challenge for the historian, then, is to evolve a framework capable of engaging and explaining this vibrant plurality without being reductive or anecdotal.

The plurality also highlights another aspect of contagion that, though implicitly present in the accounts of Bashford and Hooker, are not developed therein, i.e., the productive and creative aspects of contagion. Bashford and Hooker focus on the state's 'dream of hygienic containment', its use of contagion to develop 'strategies and technologies of isolation, containment, barriers and policing of spaces'.[3] However, dreams are also occasions for the most prolific production—of images, spaces and narratives; every technology of isolation and containment is also a mode of producing new territories. Every 'containment' and 'bounding off' also produces two new spaces on each side of the boundaries: spaces and contexts with their own semantic and connotative investments. This productive aspect of contagion that produces new geographies, new identities and new solidarities does not conform to the demands of the state. Instead, they are the fructification of the already present 'excess' contained in statist notions of contagion noted by Bashford and Hooker. It is this creative multiplication of the excess into nonstatist registers that we will need to engage within the new analytical model of contagion.

Following Christopher Hamlin's fascinating work in the case of Victorian England, we will argue that seeing disease causation merely in terms of an either/or binarism between contagionism and anticontagionism is unhelpful.[4] The rich history of notions about disease causation and transmission in the nineteenth century cannot be understood in terms of these simple binaries. A more comprehensive appreciation of how Bengali *daktars* came to talk, write and think about disease causation and transmission will require, first, an appreciation of the actual terms of their discourse, which does not usually fit into a contagion/anticontagion binary, and second, a parallel appreciation of the productive nature of this discourse, wherein it went beyond the regulatory mechanisms of control and limiting off, and also created new ideational contexts which incited new ways of acting on bodies, beings and spaces.

National Bodies

The conception of contagion in the late nineteenth and early twentieth centuries had come to intersect with two other powerful concepts in the writings of the Bengali doctors—those of racial immunity and racial predisposition.

And it was precisely at this intersection that a specifically Bengali national body was medically produced.

Jean-Paul Gaudilliere and Ilana Lowy have argued that the attempts to distinguish between 'vertical transmission' (heredity) and 'horizontal transmission' (infection) had remained inchoate and episodic in the same period in 'western' medical discourses.[5] Such overlaps are clearly visible in the *daktari* writings as well. In the case of madness, for instance, the word *sankraman* (contagion) is often used to designate heredity. In these writings, however, the overlaps between vertical and horizontal contagion acquires a very specific valence through their entanglements with other discourses. Discourses such as those of 'predisposition' to diseases and unique 'national constitutions' overlapped and entangled with the discourse on contagion to give it a very specific identity, even whilst it did have elements of continuity with the 'western' medical discourses. In the instance cited earlier, for example, though the report in the *Swasthya* had mentioned it only while summarizing the annual governmental Report on Lunatic Asylums of Bengal, it introduced a very specifically Bengali inflection into the idea. It said that it had been found that 13 insane patients had had the contagion passed on to them (*sankramita*) 'due to reasons of lineage' (*kulaja karan-e*).[6] Its preference for the term *kulaja*, connoting a particular culturally specific and ritually loaded notion of lineage, rather than the more frequently used *vamshaja*, which connotes 'familial', is revealing. While *vamsha* is limited to an individual family, *kul* could refer to a wider kin/hereditary group such as a clan.[7] This indeterminacy between individual familial heredity and larger clan/caste/national heredity was one of those fruitful excesses that gave Bengali *daktari* writings on contagion their characteristic identity. The concept of *kul* was, moreover, not a purely 'biological' notion. It also resonated on registers of morality. Thus, the moral qualities of an individual's actions are often described as either bringing glory or infamy to the *kul*. The notion of 'blood' that forms one of the crucial axes of the notion of *kul* has prominent ritual, moral and biological valences.[8] Gunga Persaud Mookerjee's hugely successful *daktari* textbook in the 1870s, while classifying hereditary forms of predisposition to contagions as '*Kaulik Dehaswabhav*' (The Habits of the Body Caused by Lineage), clearly stated that 'this [factor] is not limited in its effects to mere disease causation'. Mookerjee went on to describe how some people such as the royals of ancient Rome had proven to be excessively cruel in every generation.[9]

Though the discourse on 'national constitutions' has been observed to be developing within the emergent ayurvedic and unani public spheres from the 1860s and 70s by scholars like Alavi and Berger, it can also be observed in the Bengali *daktari* texts.[10] It was asserted forcefully in the *daktari* periodicals of the time that 'Bengalis were not Englishmen' (*Bangali Shaheb nohey*), Bengali constitutions were different from British constitutions and this difference, in turn, made them differentially susceptible to contagions.[11] Though most *daktars* accepted germs as being at the root of contagions, almost all insisted on a multicausal model of disease. The body's power to resist disease was, therefore, considered as important as contagions in causing anyone to be afflicted by a contagious disease. This constitutional susceptibility was designated as 'predisposition'. Mookerjee's textbook, *The Principles and Practice of Medicine in Bengali*, in describing the 'aetiology *ba karantattwa* (the theory of causes)' stated that disease occurs due to both 'intrinsic' and 'extrinsic' causes.[12] The 'intrinsic causes' were described as 'predisposing causes' (*purvavarti*) while 'extrinsic' causes were described as 'exciting causes' (*uddipok*). Nearly twenty years later, another highly influential textbook writer, Devendranath Ray, while deeply invested in the Germ Theory of disease, continued to divide the causes of disease into *uddipok* (exciting) and *purvavartak* (predisposing) causes.[13] Some later authors even tried to establish an anatomical basis for such predisposition. Dr Satyasaran Chakrabarty, for instance, argued that each cell had within it three types of vital or life force (*jeevanishakti*).[14] These were: first, self-defence (*atmarakshya*); second, towards growth (*vriddhi-r dikey*) and third, determination of favourableness or unfavourableness of its immediate environment (*bahir jagater anukul-pratikul nirupane niyajita*). Dr Chakrabarty argued that the predisposition to being affected by infectious diseases arose due to the weakness of the third type of *jeevanishakti*.[15] Dr Chakrabarty further explained that an infection acquired by a pregnant mother could structurally hamper the cellular structure of the child and thereby make the child predisposed to disease. Dr Kulachandra Guha, writing on infantile tuberculosis, also accepted the theory of inherited predisposition.[16] Since there remained a fundamental indeterminacy about individual/particular familial heredity and broader 'national' heredity, such ideas about inherited predisposition easily and often got entangled with the discourse on national constitutions.

The idea of 'national constitutions', however, did not designate a strictly biological inheritance of predisposition to disease. It often combined both biological and cultural inheritance. Thus, inherited cultural practices such as types of diet, dress, lifestyle, etc., could create 'predisposition'. While presenting a paper on *sankramak shoth* (which was translated both as 'Epidemic Dropsy' and 'Beriberi' by contemporaries) on the 25 November 1907 at the Medical Club of Calcutta, Dr Satyasaran Mitra pointed out that the disease affected 'only the rice-eating people. No Marwari is therefore affected…'.[17] Srirupa Prasad has pointed out that, as the *bhodrolok* increasingly lost economic power in late colonial Calcutta to Marwaris, rice emerged as a potent tool for *othering* for the former.[18] Dr Lakshmikanta Ali, also discussing *sankramak shoth*, observed that '...poor Muslims who live in huts with earthen roof tiles have been observed to have up to four or five in every home suffering from the disease'.[19] Similarly Dr Lalmohan Ghoshal drew upon his experience at the Rajshahi Government Hospital to write that Bengal fever (*Banglar Jwor*)—which according to him was 'mostly malaria'—affected Bengalis more than Europeans, men more than women, villagers more than townsmen and the poor more than the genteel (*bhadralok*).[20] The most extensive early statement of this notion of a biocultural inheritance that shaped one's predisposition to contagion can be found in Mookerjee's *Medicine in Bengali*. Among the various predisposing causes that Mookerjee investigated, one of the most elaborate is 'weakness' (*durbalata*). Under this heading, he proposed to discuss all that made people of 'this country' (*etoddeshiya*) more susceptible to diseases. The discussion is then divided into nine separate heads and includes numerous 'cultural' factors, such as the diet (including both the nature of the food and the way it is cooked), the type of occupations, etc.[21] The underlying assumption was that cultural traits such as food and lifestyle—when persisted with over a long time—could lead to subtle anatomical and physiological changes which in turn affected the susceptibility to diseases.

This insistence in itself was not unprecedented or unique. Indeed, the great British doctor William Cullen himself had stressed the importance of 'debility' as a predisposing cause.[22] Its roots possibly went back through the eighteenth-century doctor Boerhaave all the way to Galen, Hippocrates and Aristotle. Later writers like James Copland, Sir Thomas Watson and others had developed the idea as late as in the 1840s and 1850s.[23] What is remarkable about the Bengali *daktari* situation, therefore, is not the originality of the ideas about 'predisposing causes', nor should it be assumed that it came to the *daktars* directly or exclusively from neighbouring 'indigenous' practitioners who used similar notions. What is noteworthy in *daktari* writings, however, is their selective appropriation from a heterogeneous 'western' tradition and the consistency that these ideas came to acquire. The *daktars* were not inert and absorptive sponges soaking up a clearly defined 'western' tradition. Instead, they were exposed to a heterogeneous 'western' tradition, from which they selectively picked and chose what to develop. What they did choose, however, came to acquire some canonical value amongst later *daktari* writers who developed the notions chosen by their forebears. Mookerjee, for example, in describing and discussing the role of the four different temperaments, i.e., sanguine, phlegmatic, bilious and nervous, went on to say that multiple distinct temperaments might coexist in the same person, thereby making any clear understanding of the subject difficult.

The example he used is even more telling. He stated that light-skinned, blue-eyed, thick-haired, thin-lipped men actually had 'diastheses', i.e., multiple contradictory temperaments, which made them exceedingly susceptible to diseases like scrofula and tuberculosis.[24] Similarly, Ray, while discussing the older notion that the same contagion might give rise to different diseases in different people, stated that Dr Liebermeister had asserted that the same contagion must always cause the same disease in every country and in every patient.[25] Yet, he gives the example of 'chill', which might cause 'cough' in some, 'indigestion' in others and 'toothache' in still others. Ray accepted Leibermeister's rule, but only for diseases like smallpox, while also accepting the 'Chill Theory' as well as the theory that the same cause could produce different diseases in different people owing to the existence of predisposing causes. Neither of the latter two theories had universal acceptance amongst the Anglo-Indian doctors of the mid-1890s.[26] Ray's adoption of them, even while being aware of the force of contrary opinion, thus constituted a conscious selection which was in line with that of his predecessors like Mookerjee.

The point is not to argue that such assertions were either right or wrong. They were indeed based upon factual observations. Dr Mitra's lecture at the Medical Club was based upon the observation of 137 different patients in 33 households, while Dr Ghoshal's assertions were based on his long experience of working at a busy government hospital, and Dr Ali, too, wrote from personal observations. Moreover, *sankramak shoth* (whichever translation is accepted) is indeed (according to contemporary understanding) a dietary disorder that affects certain groups with specific dietary patterns. Malarial fever, too, might well affect —in the light of contemporary understandings of the disease—certain groups with specific nutritional and habitual patterns more than others. What is interesting for us is not the accuracy of these observations as such, but the explanatory framework within which contagion was understood. None of the connections *necessarily* needed to be framed in terms of religious or ethnic communities. Dr Ali's 'poor Muslims' were presumably not the only ones in Bengal who lived in 'huts with earthen roofs', nor need Dr Mitra's Bengalis have been the only rice eaters. The implicit assumption in these medical formulations was that certain 'communities' had fixed lifestyles that affected their physiological predisposition to contagion. That many Marwaris—a community which had been in Bengal since precolonial times—may have also been rice eaters or that many poor Hindus may also have lived in earthen huts very similar to those of the 'poor Muslims', were not considered. Individual lifestyle choices were therefore thought to be almost nonexistent and subsumed within community lifestyles. Moreover, disease transmission was framed within a multicausal model of pathogenesis which belied the strict dichotomy between contagionism and anticontagionism, while also drawing upon older ideas about constitutions and temperaments which could slip with ease between strictly biological, biomoral and biocultural registers of meaning. Dr Harimohan Sen, for instance, wrote that 'A person who has a predominance of *sattwa-guna*, one who is healthy and in internal harmony [*samabhavapanna*], one whose life has no artificiality, one whose life is in accordance with nature' had a much lower predisposition to disease.[27] The conceptual vocabulary Sen used drew explicitly upon older conceptions of *gunas*, primordial qualities that defined people's characters and temperaments, as well as forming a dynamic mechanism of constant exchange between the individual subject and his/her environments.

While contagion often cut across conceptions of vertical and horizontal disease transfer, there did emerge, in certain discussions, a separate, specific and distinct idea about the role of biological heredity (*abhijattya*).[28] Though such usages are not very frequent, the existence of such distinct words is significant in conclusively establishing that despite the importance of constitutions and temperaments, a notion of contagion was indeed clearly understood and used by the Bengali *daktars*. Vivian Nutton, in his study of the idea of contagion amongst ancient Greeks, has suggested that one way of settling the issue of whether a particular corpus of writing recognizes the concept of contagion or not is to see if there is a specific technical word for it and to see how precise that word is. The development of two distinct words *abhijattya* and *sankraman* therefore clarifies that a conception of contagion was understood by the *daktari* authors. Eschewing a body-independent notion of abstract contagion, however, *daktari* writings developed a formulation where the afflicted body and the afflicting contagion were equally important for the development of disease. The metaphor that was repeatedly used was that of a seed germinating and growing to an adult plant on a receptive surface. Dr W. J. Buchanan, the Inspector General of Jails in Bengal, who often contributed articles to the *Bhisak Darpan*, developed this plant metaphor elaborately in one of his most influential serialized essays on *Sankramak Rog*.[29] The onus here was as much on the 'surface' as on the 'seed' of disease.

It was this accent on the body that led to the forceful articulation of ideas about 'vital force'. This 'vital force' or *jeevanishakti* was said to reside in the individual cells of the human body. It was this vital force which was said to give life to the foetus at conception and it was this vital force in the cells that resisted contagion.[30] Writers such as Dr Taraknath Roy confessedly drew upon ayurvedic texts in order to further develop these ideas.[31] It was because of this force that, even when all other circumstances were identical, some people developed a disease and others did not. Every effort thus had to be made to further invigorate this vital force and desist from anything that might attenuate it. Hence, crucially, this accent on the body's predisposition, instead of validating physical weakness, became a positive potential in the hands of the *daktari* authors—a potential for building fitter bodies better capable of resisting disease. Instead of framing disease transmission by fantasies of controlling bodies and spaces, it became a trope that returned power to the afflicted patients by insisting on their own capacities to resist and fight contagion through personal lifestyle choices. In Foucaultian terms, this shift in accent might be described as a shift from governmentality, which fashions docile subjects pliable to the ends of power, to an 'ethics of care of the self', wherein caring and developing a more active and articulate self becomes a 'practice of freedom'.[32]

It was these two ideas of a culturally fashioned bodily difference and the existence of a vital force that could ward off illness that together inspired the project of national bodily development. By implicating contagion within a framework that implied bodily difference and, thereafter, the imagination of that bodily difference as cultural—and hence perfectible—rather than biological qua immutable, the *daktari* authors created the intellectual space to articulate a project of national physical development.

Strength/Weakness

One of the central axes along which this project of national physical development was articulated was that of the binary of strength and weakness or debility. In her recent fascinating study, Julie Livingstone has pointed out that notions of 'debility' develop in the 'intersections of cultural and somatic life', where the relationship between the 'body' and 'personhood' is worked out through a 'moral imagination'. There are, therefore, no pregiven criteria for the determination of 'debility'. Notions about 'strength' and 'weaknesses' are imaginatively developed in response to changes in the social, cultural and somatic histories of bodies.[33]

Particularly in Bengal, but generally in South Asia as well, colonial hegemony came to be based upon a constant assertion of the hypermasculinity of the colonizers. The nationalist project consequently often came to be articulated as a quest for the recovery of lost manhood.[34] Hence, the national constitutions came to be defined in terms of a lack of strength and the need to regain such strength. The predisposition to contagion was said to be greatly increased by this ubiquitous lack of strength, and in order to prevent contagious diseases, every effort had to be made to reverse this debilitating weakness. As already stated, the insistence on 'debility' itself was not novel to the *daktari* writings. But whereas eminent British doctors like Cullen and Watson had used it to describe individual constitutions, in the hands of the Bengali *daktars* it became a 'national' predicament.[35] Sir Thomas Watson, in a lecture given in 1845 at King's College, for instance, mentioned that, '…as the body is weakened and exhausted, it yields more readily to the pernicious influence of contagion, or of malaria; but by obviating all causes of debility, and fortifying the system, we walk with comparative security amidst surrounding pestilence'.[36] While Watson was clearly articulating an 'ethic of self-care', nowhere did he speak of nationally specific bodies. By contrast, Mookerjee, commenced his discussion on 'weakness'/'debility' (*durbalata*) by specifying that he was speaking of people of 'this country' (*etaddeshiya*). The national character of the debility that plagued Bengalis/Indians was further accentuated by the mention of dietary habits, prolonged exposure to heat, etc. Moreover, this dangerous debility was not merely physical weakness. It encompassed both the body and the mind. Mookerjee therefore clarified that: just as soldiers in battle are exhausted and hence predisposed to contagion, so, too, are students before examinations due to their mental fatigue.[37]

Christopher E. Forth has shown how ideas about contagion, through their accent on willpower, came to articulate the anxieties of nineteenth-century French masculinity. In Bengal, the crisis of Bengali masculinity had, under colonial ideological hegemony, become almost a verity. The discourse on vital force therefore quickly blossomed into a full-blown project for the development of masculine, virile strength. *Daktari* authors wrote passionately about the role of *vyam*, or cultivation of the body in the invigoration of the vital force and, consequently, in preventing disease. Dr Kulachandra Guha, writing in 1910, warned that 'We need to attend to the cultivation of the body [*vyam*] with as much urgency as we do these days to our diet [*ahar*]—possibly even more urgently—this has become our solemn duty now, or else, our nation [*jati*] shall soon fall prey to a variety of Contagious Diseases and disappear from the face of this earth'.[38] Thus, to ensure the survival of a healthy nation, the twin axes of *vyam* and *ahar* had to be manipulated. New national bodies more capable of fighting contagion had to be built. Dr Harimohan Sen clarified that what later *daktars*—like Mookerjee before them—meant by *vyam* was not limited to physical exercise. It included also *manasik vyam*, or mental exercises. *Manasik vyam* was aimed at the improvement of '*vivek* (conscience), *buddhi* (intellect), *smriti* (memory) and *kalpona* (imagination).[39]

Vyam was not mere unstructured exercise. Instead, different types of exercise were said to suit different nations. *Vyam* was often equated with formal sport and an attempt was made to codify the various effects different games had on different people and their health. Dr Sen, for example, argued that while tennis was good for almost everybody, long jumps were better for older people. Cricket had some benefits, but also had some negative effects on health due to the sudden bursts of running it required. The worst, however, in Dr Sen's view, was football and players apparently ran a higher risk of heart problems (*hrid-rog*).[40] The editors of *Swasthya*, on the other hand, claimed that '*vyam* differed according to nations and their physical health'. They lamented that traditional 'Bengali forms of *vyam*' such as *kusthi* (South Asian-style wrestling), horseriding, etc., were declining in popularity. They, too, felt that cricket was not very conducive to health due to its speed and scope for injury, while tennis was much better. Above all, however, the editors recommended billiards as a form of exercise 'admirably suited to the *bhadralok*'.[41] Dr Kalachandra Guha, on the other hand, denounced nearly all 'foreign' sports altogether, drawing attention to the negative economic and physical consequences of games such as 'bat-ball', football, etc. Instead, he recommended the cultivation of national Bengali sports as the appropriate form of *vyam*.[42] Similarly, in the case of *manasik vyam*, an attempt was made to codify different patterns of intellectual activity. It was claimed, for example, that studying late into the night was detrimental to health, but reading very early in the morning immediately after sunrise was healthy. Further intellectual activities for more than six hours a day were said to depress the body's vital powers.[43] In these six hours, a five-minute rest was necessary after every full hour.[44] The nationalization of the body therefore entailed not merely the encouragement for certain types of activities, but its inscription within highly structured patterns of behaviour as well as leisure. All of this was structured in the name and cause of the nation's future.

The nationalist project for building new and healthy bodies more capable of combating deadly contagions did not encompass everybody who lived in Bengal. Its particular focus was on the bodies of the middle-class youth and women (mostly in their capacity as mothers). It almost wholly ignored subaltern bodies of peasants and workers, often using them as counterpoints with which to berate the *bhadralok* and thereby stir the latter to participate in the active nationalization of the body. Some authors, like Mookerjee, went further to argue that certain types of occupations also led to 'predisposition' to contagion, thereby clearly demarcating subaltern lifestyles from *bhadralok* ones. He stated that potters, for instance, having to sit for long hours with their heads bent over, developed a predisposition to 'diseases of the head' (*shira-pirha*); cobblers and weavers, due to their having to lean over for long hours, developed a predisposition to intestinal complaints, etc. Dr Sen's discussion of *manasik vyam* aptly demonstrates the selective nature of the discourse by focussing the discussion almost solely on university students, arguing that they ruin their health by not studying regularly and then trying to revise everything shortly before the examinations. It must be noted, however, that the *daktari* writers also discouraged profligate lifestyles of the extremely rich. Mookerjee mentioned the debilitating effects of laziness and lack of any physical or mental activity, while Pulinchandra Sanyal, writing in 1916, mentioned how too much rich food and too little activity made one particularly prone to diseases like gout.[45] Another interesting apocryphal story that sought to shame the rich out of their lazy lifestyles was carried in the second volume of the *Swasthya*. According to the story, a *daktar* once came across an extremely lazy patient. When no amount of instruction from the *daktar* succeeded in making him change his lifestyle, he urged the patient to sit on his favourite chair for 15 minutes every day and beat himself with his fists. The lazy patient, however, got his servant to beat him everyday. The story concludes with the sarcastic quip that, 'some rich *babus* are so lazy that they will put up with the ignominy of being beaten by their own servants, but still not work'.[46] One of the most explicit as well as eloquent statements of this selective conception of the 'national body' can be read in Dr Sundarimohan Das' account of a brief visit to his native village in later life. Das was a professor at the Calcutta Medical School and a popular *daktari* author. On a brief visit to his native village, after a long time he wistfully wrote of his shock at the sight that greeted him. He remembered as a child that there were two groups of people in the village—the *bhodro,* or genteel, and the *ithor,* or plebeian. At the time of his departure, the two households of the genteels had grown to five and they had seemed to be flourishing; but on his return, he found that their numbers had dwindled drastically, while the *ithor* had flourished. 'The sole cause of the improvement of the so-called *ithor* class is due to their physical exercise', he wrote. However, instead of celebrating the good fortune of the latter class, Dr Das wrote of this as a sign of national decline and urged urgent action on the part of the District Board to improve the health of the village.[47]

The *daktari* prescriptions about *vyam* came, however, to be progressively overshadowed by the end of the nineteenth century by an attempt to locate a substantive basis for the weakness of the *bhadrolok.* Whereas discourse on *vyam* had recommended the development of more active bodies—the actualization of which depended upon the active participation of the patients—this new effort sought to reduce the patient's subjectivity to that of passive, objectified consumers whose weakness could be overcome by the *daktar* administering certain specific substances which the former's body was deficient in.

This substantive understanding of weakness had in certain senses coexisted with the prescriptions of *vyam* since at least the 1870s. Mookerjee had mentioned the necessity of *naitrojen* (nitrogen) in the Bengali diet in order to strengthen the body's defences and resist contagion.[48] It was however the researches of Professor David McCay at CMC in first decade of the twentieth century that instigated the efflorescence of *daktari* interest in bodily *naitrojen*. McCay had purported to prove by his study, which analysed the urine samples of 200 students and staff of CMC, that the Bengali *bhodrolok* were particularly weak due to the deficiency of nitrogen in their diets. *Daktari* authors responded to this damning racial criticism by challenging McCay's conclusions, but simultaneously accepting the need for urgent national dietary changes. Dr Devendranath Ray, for example, differed from Prof McCay in asserting that the nitrogen in the Bengali diet did not adversely affect basic metabolism; but he went on to clearly state that '…the blood of Bengalis is completely different from the blood of Europeans. This difference is solely the result of diet….The nitrogenous substances in the blood of the Bengalis is almost chronically under-nourished'.[49] Showing an awareness of the heterogeneous nature of the biomedical discourse on 'diets', authors like Ray made extensive use of the works of Russell Henry Chittenden to challenge McCay's conclusions.[50] Those authors who followed Ray's approach increasingly took up researches in protein digestion and the physiology of nitrogen absorption, going on to particularly investigate little-known diseases like acetonuria and indicanuria arising from imperfect protein digestion.[51] Others like Dr Mahendranath Ghosh sought to develop a more complex identity for the substance *naitrojen* itself. Challenging its substantial unity, Ghosh proposed that there were many different kinds of *naitrojen*. Of the total eleven *naitrojens* that Ghosh identified, eight were *jantob naitrojens* (animal nitrogen) and three were *udbhid naitrojen* (plant nitrogen). Each of them had different bodily functions.[52]

Naitrojen remained an important substance in *daktari* practice and writing till the 1920s. In the period between 1900 and 1920, however, two important changes affected it. First, whereas earlier authors such as D. D. Gupta had held that 'the plant kingdom had no dearth of nitrogenous foods', later texts such as Charuchandra Bhattacharya's immensely popular little book entitled *Bangalir Khadya* (The Diet of the Bengali) mentioned that flesh and fish were the main source of *naitrojen*.[53] Second, the recommended daily intake was lowered over time. Instead of the earlier 22.2 grams advocated by Gupta, for instance, Bhattacharya only recommended 16 grams.[54] The identification of *natirojen* with the more expensive foods like flesh and fish may have necessitated this reduction in order to keep the prescriptions meaningful for the middle classes.

The *naitrojen* of the *daktars* was not identical to the *nitrogen* of McCay and Chittenden.[55] D. D. Gupta, for instance, wrote that 'Nitrogenous [*naitrojen-gunabisistho*] foods are responsible for the development of all bodily "tissues" or "*dhatu*", therefore those who perform hard physical or intellectual tasks need to have a diet rich in nitrogenous foods. It is essential to daily consume at least 32 grams of nitrogen. Having any more than this, however, can cause other health problems'.[56] *Naitrojen* was thus recast as a *guna*—a kind of sublime, bio-moral fluid-substance used in some ayurvedic literature to designate a kind of fundamental bodily constituent.[57] Ayurvedic literature mentioned three *gunas*—*sattwa, rajah* and *tamah*. Many of the discussions on proteins and *naitrojens* prominently deployed these categories.[58] Moreover, the physiological role of *naitrojen* was understood in terms of the *dhatus*—once again, an ayurvedic concept designating the seven fundamental 'supports' (blood, bones, marrow, fat, muscle, chyle, semen) of the body.[59]

There is now a growing body of academic literature on the history of substance which seeks to de-centre the older essentialised understandings of substances.[60] While this literature promises to dislodge the anachronistic frame of reference whereby contemporary biochemical identities of substances are imposed on historical references—thereby eliding their historical specificities—most of this emergent literature focuses on pre- or early-modern substances and, hence, refers back to an epoch before the identities of substances became stabilised through technologies of identification based upon complex biochemical tests and powerful microscopes. It therefore leaves unchallenged the contention that these later technologies—at least since modernity—may have produced more stable and universally applicable substance identities. Substances are actualized as 'real' things only within networks of human and nonhuman actors. Within specific chains of human and nonhuman actors, they are capable of performing particular types of actions that they may not be able to transact within other networks. There is, hence, no reason to assume a single unified identity of substances, part of whose social lives are transacted within networks of biomedical identification. Nitrogen, when extracted from the networks connected to McCay's laboratories and inserted into Ray's research networks, begins to come undone and take on new characteristics and is capable of affecting the human body differently. In Gupta's writings it goes on to acquire the characteristics of a *guna*. These alternatives are each equally real within their specific networks of action.

The advantages of this substantive understanding of weakness for the *daktari* practice was that it allowed a quicker, more attractive (for patient's unwilling to undertake long term *vyam*) and commercially better-suited ways of addressing the problem. By 1920 the *Chikitsa Prakash* announced the availability of 'Nucleo-porotied [sic] Compound' tablets which helped to artificially raise protein levels in the body and make it stronger.[61] Nuctarlin was another such tablet with very similar capabilities.[62]

Towards the end of the 1920s and through the 1930s *naitrojen* and its related substances (proteins, urea, etc.) began to lose their preeminence to *bhaitameens* ('vitamins').[63] *Bhaitameens* were presented largely in the same vein as *naitrojen* had been—as a panacea for a range of ills, which worked through the revitalization of the body's defences, thereby making the latter more capable of fighting off contagions. Where *bhaitameens* proved more useful than *naitrojen* was that, since there were many types of *bhaitameens*, it allowed a complex economy to be mapped out that related different types of foods to different types of physical weaknesses.[64] In some ways this is the end that Ghosh's elevenfold classification of *naitrojen* itself had unsuccessfully sought to achieve. In fact, the failure of Ghosh's approach has important historiographic lessons. It shows the pitfalls of any radical postmodern approach to the history of medicine that might seek to treat all reality as a matter of representation. The simple reason Ghosh's classification did not work and vitamins did, was that reality is not simply a textual construct. Humans and nonhuman substances are both actors that allow each other—under certain specific conditions—to validly say ('articulate') certain things and not others. Though Ghosh's classification fulfilled the social and commercial roles that were required of a 'substance of weakness' in the given historical juncture, the reality of the substances concerned did not verify his classificatory schema. Vitamins, on the other hand, fulfilled the emerging need for a more complex, flexible system that would relate foods to bodily well-being as well as being capable of easy, passive, commercially driven consumption, while all along being verifiable by experimental techniques.[65] Put simply, therefore, *bhaitameens* were *real*, while Ghosh's *naitrojens* were a mere figment of his intellect. Reality and representation are not the same, but at the same time, reality too must be historicized.

Generally speaking, the substantiation of the discourse on weakness and the search for a techno-scientific solution to it since the beginning of the twentieth century encouraged the development of a patient subjectivity that was more passive and consumption oriented than the earlier prescriptions of *vyam*.

National Diet

One of the most prolific sites on which the strength/weakness dialectic was operationalized as part of a programme to nationalize the body, was that of 'national diets'. Numerous essays, tracts and books appeared on the role of diets in making bodies susceptible to certain kinds of contagions. This discourse, too, was highly selective. Prasad, in her illuminating recent article, has argued that, faced with a persistent lack of political power and an ever-growing social marginalization through extensive influx of non-Bengalis, the Bengali *bhodrolok* came to articulate a highly charged sense of embodied crisis around issues of diet and nutrition. This embodied crisis in turn allowed the *bhodrolok* to distinguish themselves clearly from the other groups with whom they increasingly had to compete as well as to aspire for social and political supremacy.[66] It focussed on the diet of certain groups in preference to that of others and articulated the project for changing their diets as a 'national' venture.

The relationship posited between the Bengali diet and their susceptibility to contagious diseases was neither new nor unique to the *daktari* discourse. Pratik Chakrabarti has shown that the necessity to improve the Bengali diet was a shared concern of many Bengali and British authors, even in the 1930s.[67] The roots of the discourse lie much further back in time. Early nineteenth-century authors such as James Johnson had advocated that Europeans adopt 'native diets' in India, as it was then thought to be better suited to the climate.[68] However, by the middle of the nineteenth century, the 'native' diet, and particularly the Bengali diet was being faulted for numerous real and imagined 'national' problems of the Bengali people. The blossoming discourse on Bengali effeminacy that depicted Bengalis as weak, lazy and sickly often overlapped and energized the discourse on the negative impact of the Bengali diet. It cropped up in numerous colonial discourses ranging from that on epidemic fevers to jail diets.[69] This need for 'dietary improvement' became one of the consensual grounds around which colonial discourses and fledgling nationalist and protonationalist ones started coming together, though within this consensus there remained significant scope for marking difference.[70]

The *daktari* discourse on diet drew upon both British authors and older ayurvedic traditions. In this latter respect, the corpus of texts known as *dravya-gunas* were particularly influential.[71] The plural roots of the discourse make it a rich and complex area of historical analysis. In the present section, however, we will restrict ourselves to only two aspects of this emergent *daktari* thinking on national diets. First, we shall look at a progressive numeralization of diets and second, we shall interrogate an almost paranoiac preoccupation with the adulteration/contamination of foodstuffs.

Numeralization of diets was basically the presentation of the daily dietary requirements of an individual in terms of the numerical weights of the respective 'necessary' foods, e.g., 139.7 grams of protein is a daily necessity for a healthy individual, or 30 grams of butter daily is required to maintain health, etc. One author went on to publish charts of how much mother's milk a newborn infant should to be allowed to consume.[72] Since the *daktari* writings were never targeted solely at scholarly readers, from the very beginning of the trend towards numeralization, there was also an attempt to present the data in easy visual formats. In the earliest instances, these took the form of simple tables of numerical values, but by the 1920s more innovative graphic methods had begun to emerge. These easily understandable modes of presentation of the dietary prescriptions were both a function as well as consequence of the populist nature of the *daktari* discourse on dietics. The graphic presentation also served to cement a dietary logic centred on an economistic notion of 'balance' of *aye* and *byaye* (lit: income and expenditure). Some of the charts gave details about how much of which foodstuff was expended during various times right next to the charts for prescribed consumption.[73] Chunilal Basu's *Manual of Hygiene* developed some of the most innovative and interesting graphic formats for the presentation of numeralized diets.[74] (Fig. V.)

The numeralization as well as the tabular form of the earliest *daktari* dietary texts clearly marked the continuities with the professional experience of the *daktars* in colonial institutions of confinement (jails, hospitals). Yet, whereas within the colonial institutions these dietary tables had been integrally linked to an objectifying regime of discipline, redeployed by the *daktars* into a register where to follow or not follow them was a matter of choice for the patients, these tables became technologies of self-formation.[75]

The economistic logic of *aye-byaye* (income-expenditure) also led to an obsessive concern with excretion. Inadequate excretion became one of the most written-about—by *daktari* authors—causes for contagious diseases. Several wrote to describe the physiology of digestion and the need and way of avoiding constipation. (Fig. VI.) Various numerical expressions of excrement were publicized through numerous *daktari* texts, e.g., 34 grams of carbolic acid needs to be excreted every 24 hours or 16 grams of protein waste needs to be excreted every day.[76] Though strictly speaking, excretion could take a variety of forms ranging from sweating to defecation, the *daktari* writings came to dwell disproportionately on constipation (*kosthokatthinyo*).[77] Dr Kulachandra Guha identified constipation as one of the most important factors that depressed the body's defences and made it prone to disease.[78] One author mentioned that if the bowels are cleared out every morning, 'diseases cannot accumulate in the body' and those whose bowels are regularly emptied are often found to be almost completely free from any affliction (*praye nirog*).[79] One Dr Annadamchan Gupta went so far as to state that constipation was the root of 'all diseases .[80] A related and widely held belief—which perhaps drew upon older ayurvedic traditions—was that suppressing an urge to excrete gave

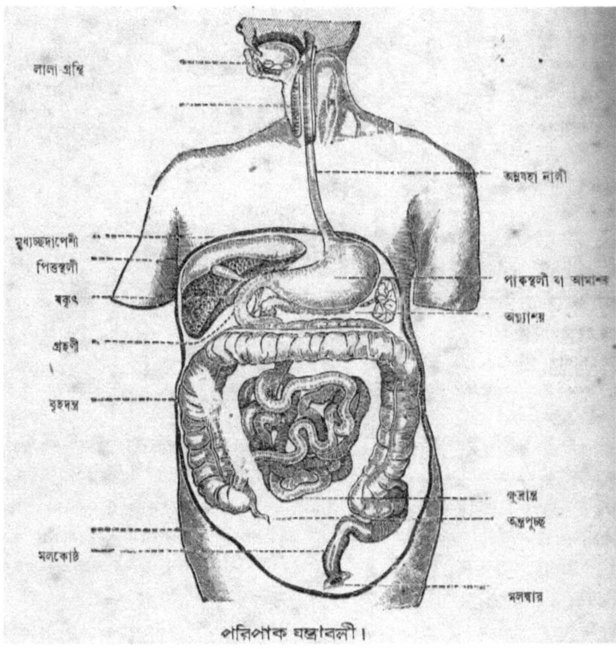

Fig. IV. "Paripak Jantrabali" (The Instruments of Digestion) in Dr Rameshchandra Roy, "Koshtoshuddhi" (Cleaning the Bowels), *Swasthya Samachar* 17, no. 4 (1928): 98.

rise to 'mechanical' faults within the body, which once again led to an increase in the predisposition to disease.[81]

This obsession with constipation also mediated a robust market for specifics for constipation. The innumerable advertisements in turn fanned the paranoia further and cemented the connection of contagious diseases to constipation in the popular mind. One remedy known as *Karpurashab*, sold by the *Nandan Ayurvediya Aushadhalay*, listed several serious ailments including cholera as being caused due to the improper clearing of the bowels.[82] Some remedies also linked it to other digestive complaints such as *ajirna*, which had been mentioned by *daktars* like Mookerjee in relation to contagions.[83] The *Ichhabhedi Batika* (The Pill That Knows Your Wish) claimed that 'emptying of the bowels makes the body full of energy and the mind full of joy…constipation makes one's breath smell bad, makes one feel tired and gives rise to feelings of embarrassment and guilt'. Constipation—reworked by the medical market—came to virtually acquire mythic proportions. The scatological obsession with balancing 'income' and 'expenditure' reached such proportions that it even inspired the humorist Sambuddha to write a comic, symbolic short story in

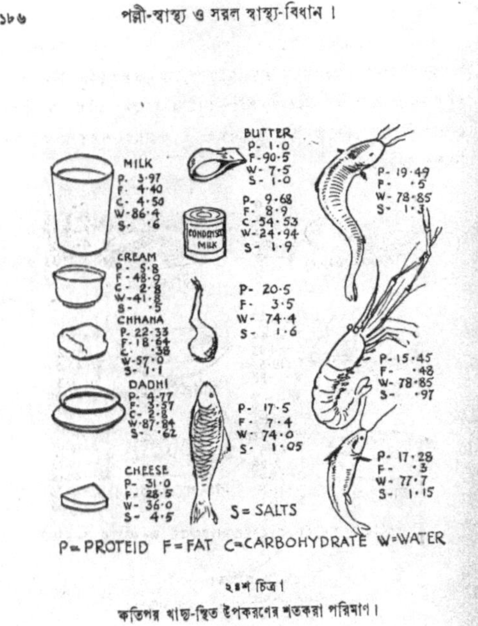

Fig. V. "Katipay Khadya-sthita Upakaraner Satakara Pariman" (The ingredients of a few foodstuff expressed in percentages) in Chunilal Basu, Village Sanitation and a Manual of Hygiene (Calcutta: np, 1931): 186.

the 1930s about a religious leader who was so obsessed with the fear of constipation after a particularly lavish feast that he ended up taking a massive overdose of extremely strong digestives despite the physicians' repeated efforts to dissuade him. The result: shocked devotees next morning discover that their leader had turned into a huge pile of excrement![84]

Once again, however, the general belief that people in Bengal suffered from particularly severe constipation seems to have been popular amongst some Anglo-Indian writers like W. H. Smoult and the much-better-known Edward J. Waring as well.[85] For these writers, constipation was usually related to environmental factors rather than to civilization, as it was by the 1920s in Britain.[86] Warwick Anderson's fascinating study of American 'excremental colonialism' has, in fact, brought to light a colonial 'poetics of pollution': a symbolic economy within which 'American colonial health officers [in the Philippines had come to use] the body's orifices and its products to mark racial boundaries….'[87] Though Anderson's study focuses on American colonialism in the Philippines, he does mention that the relationship of excrement and disease was present throughout the nineteenth century in 'western' medical tradition.[88] How then—if at all—is the *daktari* poetics of pollution distinct from the 'western' tradition? To answer this, we must see exactly how the *daktars* themselves said they differed from 'western' practices. Two particularly important points of distinction marked their excremental symbolism. In the first place, it was said that it was extremely harmful to resist an urge to defecate. Whereas the 'western' tradition accented being able to control one's bodily orifices and their rhythms, the *daktars* actively proposed—in line with certain ayurvedic traditions—giving in to these desires.[89] A second, more powerful point of distinction comprised the culturally specific post-excremental practices. Many *daktari* authors wrote on the harmful effects of using 'toilet paper' as 'westerners' did; instead, they advocated the use of water.[90]

The specificity of the *daktari* understanding of the link between constipation and contagion did not derive solely from either 'western' or 'eastern' sources. On the one hand, it repositioned the 'western' discourse by shifting the focus away from the objectifying environmental determinism to a more subject-forming focus on individual desire, action and practice. On the other hand, it aligned itself with certain 'eastern' discourses on post-excremental cleansing with water (*jalsaucha*) rather than the more subversive traditions that treated excrement as a sacral substance.[91] The specificity of the *daktari* thinking on the topic lay in selectively appropriating, aligning and contextualising these diverse discourses and praxes. Over the period of our study, there was a gradual shift—though nowhere as pronounced as that of the 'substances of weakness'—towards techno-scientific solutions to the problem, i.e. laxatives, specifics, etc.[92]

The paranoia about maintaining the dietary balance was matched—if not outdone—in intensity by the fears over the contamination/adulterations of foods. The limited political power that the *bhodrolok* enjoyed proved woefully inadequate in assuaging their concerns over food adulteration. The Bengal Municipal Act of 1894 and the later, more powerful Bengal Food Adulteration Act of 1919 both proved inadequate.[93] The journal *Gharer Katha,* ten years later in 1929, was still writing about the inadequacy of the municipal efforts. One author asserted that 'all citizens of Calcutta (*shaharbashi*) know that whatever foodstuff they buy—no matter how much money they spend—they are never sure that it is not adulterated'.[94] The fear arose, in part, as a consequence of the pervasive impact of colonial modernity and its attendant lifestyle changes. This specific concern about contamination/adulteration was directly related to a widespread consumption of commercially prepared food in the city. Whereas strict rules and customs had guided the eating habits of most people in their village homes, the rapid urbanization as well as the specific pattern of migration, whereby most men lived singly in city messes, meant that such rules soon started collapsing in the urban environment. In its place grew up a number of small commercial enterprises selling food. The most common form of such commercial food shops were the shops of the *moiras* (indigenous confectioners). Their staple ware comprised sweetmeats, but they usually also sold some hot snacks. Predictably, it was these sweetshops (*moira-r dokan*) that became the butt of the strongest *daktari* criticism. One author thus asserted that 'Of all the rules that need to be followed in order for a person to stay healthy, the *moira*'s shop follows not a single one of them'.[95] The author went on to demand immediate and strict action on behalf of the municipality to force the *moiras* to follow 'principles of hygiene'. The health journal *Gharer Katha* severely criticised municipal food inspectors in 1929 for having found only a third of all collected samples from *moira's* shops to be adulterated. The journal railed that all could see how the *moiras* had quickly replaced their thatch huts in the village with palatial residences in Calcutta due to their corruption.[96] In fact, even the faraway villages, it was said, were no longer safe from the *moira*'s shop, for ambulatory peddlers, or *pheriwalas,* bought up the *moira*'s unsold wares and peddled them in faraway villages, by which time they were stale and dangerous. It was not only the alien and unreliable context of *bajar-er khabar* (food from the bazaar/commercially prepared food) that made it a health hazard, often it was also the food itself. Thus Dr Sundarimohan Das lamented that the simple diets of his childhood, where people ate simple homemade snacks like coconut shavings and puffed rice, had been replaced by 'foreign biscuits' and ostentatious snacks bought at the *moira*'s shop. In the past, he claimed, even on festive occasions celebratory food was not ostentatious, consisting simply of village-produced rice and fish from the local pond. All this had been healthy and free from contamination. But the times had changed and, with it, people had taken to eating more complex foods that were not easily digestible.[97] Both Drs Sen and Guha attacked *bajar-er khabar* as being both contaminated and harder to digest (*guru-pak*) and claimed it was one of the most important causes of contagious diseases. Their attacks on *bajar-er khabar* also showed how 'predisposing' and 'immediate' causes of contagious disease could often collapse into one another and become, in effect, indistinguishable. Remarking on the obsession with adulteration and the blaming of *moiras*, *goalas* and other subaltern urban groups, Prasad points out, '*bhodroloks'* discourses of crisis over food were, therefore, simultaneously, calls for regeneration of health, critiques against colonialism and nationalism, and investment in identity formation that sought to hierarchically differentiate various social actors.'[98]

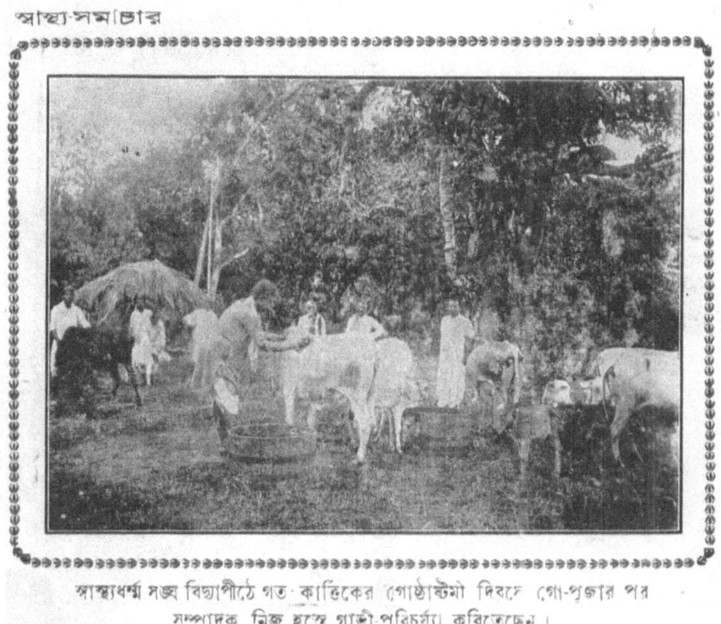

Fig. VI. "*Swasthyadharma Sangha Bidyapithe goto Kartiker Goshthashthami dibasey Go-Pujar par Sampadak nija hasthe gabhi-paricharja karitechhen*" (The Editor personally bathing cows at the recent cow-worship festival organized by the *Swasthyadharma Sangha* school on the occasion of Goshthashthami) *Swasthya Samachar* 16, no. 1 (1927): 18–19.

While most of the attacks on *bajar-er khabar* tended to also collapse the distinction between contamination and adulteration, in the case of milk this did not hold true. Diatribes against urban milkmen as being corrupt and deliberately adulterating milk were frequent and poignant. The Calcutta Corporation's food inspectors claimed in 1929 that of 1003 samples tested that year only 349 were adulterated. *Daktari* authors, though, contrasted the figures with what 'every Calcuttan knew', to conclude that the food inspectors were inept.[99] The importance attached to milk derived partly from the ritual associations with the cow and partly from being one of the major sources of protein for orthodox Hindus. (Fig. IV.) Its importance was also elevated due to its being the principal food for infants. Dr Guha remembered of his childhood that, 'milk was never sold back then. Nowhere as a child did I see milk being sold. It was thought to be a great sin [*mahapaap*] if one sold milk; but today, in that very place, I see adulterated milk being sold freely'.[100] As one poetically inclined author amply clarified, part of the importance attached to milk arose from the sheer range of milk-based foods that the average middle-class Bengali usually consumed:

> 'Milk is mixed with polluted water
> *Ghee* [clarified butter] is adulterated
> Butter and sweets are being daily corrupted'[101]

So important, indeed, was this concern, that even Dr Das' drama on urban hygiene, the publication of which was subsidized by the Calcutta Municipal Corporation, included a reference on the adulteration of milk.[102]

The passionate discourse against the adulteration of milk and the parallel longing for the 'milk of one's own cow' cannot be seen simply as dealing with a sanitary or economic problem.[103] It had an extremely important symbolic dimension as well.[104] As can be seen in Das' other essay published in the *Grihasthya Mangal* and cited above, the adulteration of milk derived its emotional appeal not merely from its actual importance in the Bengali Hindu diet but also through the rural nostalgia it articulated. [105] This nostalgia which Das felt on returning to his village after many years was not just for a rural idyll. It was a nostalgia for the comforts of a middle-class life in a slow-paced Bengali village. It encompassed both the material comforts which the rural middle class could afford and the symbolic prestige they enjoyed in rural society. All this, of course, appeared significantly more comforting after the experience of middle-class life in the colonial metropolis. Usually employed in lower ranks of the bureaucracy and being forced to live in an expensive city on a low income, they lacked in the city both the comfort and the status they had in their village homes. Moreover, a good many of these lower middle classes lived alone in the city, leaving their families back in the villages. The family cow was therefore also a symbol of the hearth where one's near-and-dear ones were. For the first-generation immigrants to the city, having the 'milk of one's own cow' connoted both longing to be 'home' where most of the family was and the middle-class status that owning a cow connoted. The nostalgia for the 'milk of one's own cow' came to symbolically represent the dual quests for both physical comfort and social status.[106] The commercialization and the adulteration of milk was not merely a simple health hazard; indeed, it came to stand—as is clear from the passionate prose of the *daktars* attacking it—for the sum total of the middle-class angst against urban modernity. It is perhaps no accident that Tagore's memorable prose-poem that immortalized the life and plight of the lower middle-class immigrant in Calcutta was, after all, named after a street (on which the main protagonist lives) which in itself was named after a milkman—*Kinu Goala-r Goli*.[107]

National Space

Like human bodies, the surface of the planet inhabited by those bodies has itself been a fruitful site for the theoretical elaboration of notions of contagion. Hamlin has pointed out that though contagion and miasma (which was usually more directly related to the surface/ground) are usually held to be distinct, many nineteenth-century authors did not demarcate them as clearly. In the process, notions such as 'contagious miasmas' were often found deployed by medical authors. Such usage can also be seen frequently in the case of *daktari* authors. Notions of contagion, miasma and even malaria would often be used in overlapping and overdetermining formulations. In recent years, some authors have pointed out that the changeover to bacteriological paradigms of disease transmission was an 'adaptive and additive process' rather than a series of irreconcilable conflicts.[108] The precise role of one's spatial environment was at the heart of these subtle reorientations. Doyalkrishna Ghosh's 1878 pamphlet titled *Malaria*, for instance, argued that 'malaria [was] a ground-loving poison' [*bhumi-priya vish*]. [109] Ghosh went on to clarify that the poison arose due to 'the chemical and structural composition of the earth' and to 'dissimilarity in the Geological constitution'.[110] Mookerjee, too, accepted a relationship between the surface, malaria, miasma and contagion.[111] In fact, in Mookerjee's influential early writings, each of the four categories—endemics, epidemics, pandemics and contagion—was described as a 'force' or 'power' (*shakti*) that could become associated with the earth's surface.[112] Even after the alleged watershed of the Germ Theory, numerous *doktars* continued to hold on to a vague idea relating contagions to the surface proper. Mookerjee himself had been aware of the early work on germs and had quoted the researches of Salisbury and Pasteur before eventually hesitantly asserting the relationship of contagions to the surface. Ray, writing much later and much more consistent in his conformity to the Germ Theory, still wrote that 'Some German doctors have proposed a separate category of Contagious Diseases entitled "Miasmatic Contagium". The English doctors do not approve of this. However, we see that whenever a patient is afflicted by Cholera or Enteric Fever, careful enquiry reveals that somebody or the other had been affected there at some earlier date. Though these diseases do not spread by touch from an afflicted person like Small Pox or Measles, yet it clings to the ground, water or air of an affected place and later affect others.'[113] He then went on to show by examples—mostly German—that such 'miasmatic contagiums' could cling on to the ground for decades. These writings, therefore, amply bear out Michael Worboys' argument that there was not one, but several germ theories and that these developed through adaptation and additions onto earlier epidemiological paradigms.

Some of the specificities of the *daktari* practice of germ theories, however, emerge through the discussions on endemics. Not only were some of the most serious diseases affecting Bengal thought of as endemics, but endemics, by their very characteristics, seemed to reinforce the posited relationship between landscape, contagion and, often, miasma. Deadly scourges such as cholera and malaria were believed to be endemically present in Bengal at all times, even when there was no epidemic outbreak. Their transmission, therefore, was both horizontally from one patient to another and vertically across generations. This overlap of horizontal and vertical modes of transmission and the characteristic problems raised by it were reflected in the Bengali translation of the word 'endemic' itself. 'Endemic' was translated by Mookerjee as *Daishik*, or 'Diseases of the Country'.[114] He even went on to state that there was some localized force or power (*sthanik shakti*) that lay at the root of endemic diseases. Later authors tended to use a slightly altered conjoint word *Desh-Dharmak* (characteristic of a country) instead of Mookerjee's early translation. The highly evocative word *desh,* however, was common in both translations. Usually the word *desh* designates a 'place of belonging'. Unlike the English 'place' or even 'country', it does not have possible connotations of emptiness. A *desh* is always already someone's *desh.* It belongs to someone and someone belongs to it.[115] Moreover, from the late nineteenth century, the word *desh* also came to designate national space. But this national territory had, once, again a very specific meaning within the usage of the Bengali literati. As Swarupa Gupta has recently shown, by creating a triangular grid of ideas composed of *desh, samaj* (community) and *jati* (a multivalent term designating various collectivities of birth—from caste groups to linguistic and national groups), the Bengali literati of the late nineteenth century 'discover[ed] and redefine[ed a] living link between the land [*desh*] and people [*jati*]'.[116] This organic link between the land and its people was both reflected in and renegotiated in the designation—*desh dharmak rog* (endemic disease).

Gupta also comments on the use of the concept of *dharma* as a fourth term that stabilized the transactions between the triad of *samaj, jati* and *desh.*[117] *Dharma* as a 'righteous way of life' was the key to the unity of the *samaj* (community). It was the inner logic that held the nation together and bequeathed it its unique character and genius. Endemics were not simply chronic ailments found to be ever-present in an anonymous geographic area; they were also afflictions that destabilized the very 'living link' between a land and its people and consequently hampered the unity and articulation of the national community. For the full blossoming of the national genius, therefore, the rectification of *desh-dharmak* contagions was unavoidable. Dr Kulachandra Guha, LMS, in a lengthy essay on the innate disease-preventive powers of the body against contagious diseases, wrote that the survival of the *jati* depended in equal measure upon the survival of its *dharma* (unique character/genius) and its *lok* (the actual people).[118] Drawing upon a variety of contemporary discourses, including that of Indian Aryanism, Dr Harimohan Sen, MB, lamented that 'We are the descendants of the mighty Aryans. Once we were 6 feet tall, today we are only 5 feet 5 inches…Our chests were 40 – 45 inches wide, today it has come down to a mere 30 inches. We used to live a 100 years, today we barely live to be 40. Once we had roamed happily on the plains of Central Asia in the shadow of the Caucasus and what sorry fate has befallen us in this diseased land!'[119] The unique character of the people—their bodily, intellectual and cultural genius—were all connected organically to the land they lived on. Inhabiting a diseased land was weakening the nation and leading it to its destruction. Dr Guha, in fact, commenced his essay by referring to a pamphlet by Dr U. N. Brahmachari—famous for his researches into the deadly Kala Azar—on the dwindling numbers of the Bengali Hindus, which was to later become a crucial text for Hindu revivalists.[120] To reverse this trend of decline and degeneration and to return the nation to its former glory, a combination of bodily and spatial rectification (*samskar*) was needed. Local spatial 'rectification' (*samskar*), designed to remove causes of endemic contagion, thus emerged as an important site of patriotic activity. But such projects of *gram-samskar* are hardly distinguishable from *samaj-samskar* and *shahar-samskar* (urban rectification).

This ethos of *samaj-samskar* was not in every case directly linked to political nationalism as such, but it formed part of a larger culture of 'national' activity. As clearly expressed in the term *samaj-samskar*, it was more keenly interested in the national community rather than the nation state as such. It was only in the course of the Swadeshi Movement of 1905 that these activities linked up more overtly with clearly 'political' agendas. After 1905 many of these activities once again disengaged with directly political activities, concentrating instead on what Sumit Sarkar has called 'constructive Swadeshi'.[121] All this is relatively well known in the historiography of Indian nationalism. But the links between this web of loosely organized patriotic activity and the thinking on contagious diseases has not been adequately explored. The relationship between the two, though, is extremely strong. Numerous local clusters of *samskar* actively drew upon what were by then popular notions about contagions like malaria (often thought of as a poison causing various diseases and not just a specific fever),[122] the Bengali predisposition to disease due to debility, consequent 'national' decline, etc. Just as the Bengali *daktari* writings were shaped by a commitment to 'improve' the nation's bodies and spaces, these 'bodies and spaces', the *nation* to which they were thought to belong and the ways in which to achieve 'improvement', were all in turn actualized through the *daktari* writings. This mutual influence is one of the most important axes of late nineteenth- and early twentieth-century Bengali *daktari* thinking about contagions and diseases. The examples of such mutual influence of *samaj-samskar* and thinking about contagious diseases are too numerous to list here, but let us cite one typical and quite well-known example, which itself inspired many others. In 1870 the charismatic Brahmo preacher and arguably the most influential man in Bengali middle- and upper-class life in the 1860s and 1870s, Keshabchandra Sen, returned after a lecture tour to Britain. His first action upon return was to establish a new association known as the *Bharat-Samskar Sabha*. Of the five fundamental aims of the association, one was to work for the improvement of the health of the local population. One of the first tasks performed by the *Sabha* in fulfilment of this aim was to designate Bijoykrishna Goswami to work in the suburb of Behala. According to one of the most important associates of Sen and Goswami, Shibnath Shastri, the historian, educator and reformer, 'Behala and the neighbouring areas were then reeling under Malarial fevers'. Goswami, moreover, was a direct descendant of Adwaitya Acharya of Santipur—arguably the most important figure of medieval orthodox Brahminism in Bengal—and the family was considered one of the highest Brahmin families in terms of ritual status in Bengal. It was therefore remarkable, and possibly intended as a symbolic gesture as well, that Goswami, of all people, should go and work amongst the low-caste, poor people in the malarious regions. Furthermore, Goswami had studied at the Calcutta Medical College. Every morning, according to Shastri, Goswami would rise very early. Having washed and meditated, he would soon leave for his *samskar* work with a bag of necessary medicines and dietary supplements. Till eleven in the morning he would work amongst the sick people of Behala. Returning at twelve noon, he would quickly lunch before rushing to teach at an adult education centre that, too, had been opened under the aegis of Sen. This example is particularly insightful in bringing out not only the personal commitment of the people involved in such patriotic *samskar* work, but also the close associations that were developing between medicine, religion and nation-building.[123]

Cities and Villages

The Bengali word *desh* has, however, yet another level of complexity. It can slip with ease between the 'local' and the 'national', depending upon the context of its utterance. A Bengali might refer to her native village where she has not returned for decades as her *desh*. She might also refer to the city she lives in, such as Calcutta, in certain contexts as her *desh*. Finally, she might refer to Bengal or even India (or in postcolonial times, Bangladesh) as her *desh*. This ambivalence meant that *desh-samskar* work could easily be translated into projects of different sizes inscribed on different spatial contexts. *Gram-samskar* (village rectification) and *shahar-samskar* (city rectification) both formed part of the larger project of *samaj/desh-samskar*.

This level of spatial inscription was also one of the most productive levels at which the *daktari* discourse functioned. It produced numerous specific sites, spaces and places of varying sizes. Villages, cities, village ponds, urban drains, streets, shops, toilets and even the very surface of the human body were just some of the numerous spaces the *daktars* spoke of. None of these spaces, however, had a fixed value. They came to acquire their value through juxtapositions and contrasts with other spaces. Villages, for instance, acquired their specific meanings through juxtapositions with cities and vice versa. Mookerjee, while discussing the *sthanik shakti* or 'endemic influence', mentioned that 'this poison is ever present in the huge cities (*vrihat vrihat shahare*). Tiny villages (*khudra khudra palli-gram*) and other relatively clean places are relatively free of this poison.'

Initially, in the late nineteenth century when *daktari* writing—properly labelled 'so-called'—came into its own, it painted a largely positive picture of the Bengali villages, in contrast to the malignant Bengali cities that were said to be seething with contagion. Mookerjee himself contributed substantially to this image. Apart from his comments about the *sthanik shakti* of disease causation in cities, he also added that there was another type of poison known as *daihik malaria* (bodily poison) which was secreted from human bodies through their exhaled breath, sweat, etc., and since cities were more crowded than villages, once again this 'poison', too, was much greater in the urban environment. Later authors like the eloquent Dr Harimohan Sen and the prolific Dr Kulachandra Guha built upon this foundation. Sen identified, for instance, eight main factors that, by either disseminating contagions or depressing the *jeevanishakti* (life force), promoted contagious diseases. Of these eight—air (*bayu*), water (*jol*), diet (*khadyo ebong potthyo*), dress (*porichhod*), bathing (*snan-adi*), exercise (*vyam*), enjoyment and sleep (*amod, alhad o nidra*), and finally intoxication (*madok dravya sevan*)—most were significantly worse in cities than in villages. The *bayu* (air) in the cities, for instance, was polluted by the 'exhaust of numerous factories, human excrement and rubbish, and much more'.[124] Other causes such as the lack of sleep, which was said to depress the *jeevanishakti* by depleting blood (since blood was said to be formed during sleep), were the result of peculiarities of the urban lifestyle.[125] Dr Guha similarly combined criticisms of urban lifestyles with other incidental factors such as overcrowding to argue that cities were particularly prone to contagions. The imperial capital city, Calcutta, came to be represented as a 'mighty crematorium' (*mohasmoshan*).[126]

The *daktari* writings in this regard undoubtedly drew upon older popular notions about the unhealthiness of the urban environment that had been developing since the beginnings of the rapid urbanization of Calcutta. Particularly potent among these popular notions was the notion of *lona-laga* or 'becoming salted' in a city. The belief seemed to be that there were some corrosive salts in the urban environment itself, or in the city water, that made people unhealthy. In his memoirs, Kartikeyachandra Ray, Dewan to the Raja of Nadia, gave a vivid description of the affliction he suffered as a youth during a brief stay in Calcutta in the early nineteenth century. Ray wrote that 'When people from the smaller towns [*mofoshwol*] travelled to Calcutta, they would often be afflicted by *ajirna* [an ayurvedic pathological category involving indigestion]. This affliction was known as "*lona laga*"...[Whilst I resided in Calcutta] even the slightest meals would make me sick and I therefore took to being very careful about my food. Despite this, within two months I lost my appetite and slowly my strength sapped away. Just as salt left in an open dish goes bland after a few days, so too did I lose all my strength. Even slight scratches made my skin peel off. When even medicines did not help, I took a boat home. From the very next day my health began to improve.'[127] By the 1860s, however, this concept as such was already in decline. The satirist, Kaliprasanna Singha, writing in the early 1860s, wrote that 'previously when people from the small towns travelled to Calcutta they used to be afflicted with *lona-laga*...'.[128] While the precise belief in *lona-laga* may have declined, the city persisted in being thought of as an especially malignant space. Plagued by overcrowding and poor water supplies, there was enough in the Calcutta of the late nineteenth century to justify such beliefs.

The *daktari* denunciation of the city reached its apogee in the plague years of the late 1890s and the opening years of the twentieth century. The critique of the city, however, was no longer a matter of simple objective presence of 'poisons' and 'salts'. It was now a much more comprehensive critique which touched upon urban lifestyles and mentalities. It found city dwellers greedy and selfish and thereby contributing to the unhealthiness of the city in general. One author, for instance, singled out the rising house rents in Calcutta as the cause of the urban contagions. The author argued that skyrocketing rents in the city forced people to live in cramped, damp and overcrowded conditions, thereby making them chronically ill. The rents in turn were said to be pushed by the ever-growing army of people seeking lowly paid clerical jobs in the city. This quest for clerical employment in turn was related to people's seduction by an ever-growing demand for luxury goods—good food, clothes, etc.—unlike previous generations who had been content to live on coarse rice and wear rough cloth.[129] Another essay in the same periodical criticized the 'selfishness of the city-dwellers' and argued that because Calcuttans invariably threw out their rubbish onto the streets in front of their neighbour's homes, this made cities 'hold out an open invitation to contagions'.[130] The city was ruining not only the national present, but also its future. It was claimed that the lack of sunlight in overcrowded lower-middle-class quarters affected the health of women particularly badly, making them susceptible to various contagions. This in turn affected their capacity to produce healthy children. The future generations of the nation being born of city-dwelling, unhealthy mothers were becoming ever weaker and more susceptible to contagions.[131]

By the end of the nineteenth century, however, there also began to emerge a more critical image of the village. Whereas early authors such as Mookerjee had spoken of the villages as relatively clean and contagion-free spaces, by the end of the 1890s, this beatific image was beginning to be fractured. The second issue of the *Swasthya*, for instance, had the editors warning readers about the corruption of drinking water in villages. Though it looked clean and often tasted better, 'the ease with which drinking water in the villages could be contaminated is much greater than that in the cities'.[132] Later in the same issue, the editors mentioned that 'With every passing day the condition of our cities is improving, it is a tragedy that at the same time the condition of our villages is declining…most educated *bhadralok* no longer want to live in the village…whatever other reasons there might be, the influence of malaria is the principal reason the better classes are deserting the villages'.[133] This discourse, however, did not become dominant until the second decade of the twentieth century. Until then, for every one article speaking of the unhealthiness of the villages, many more denounced the unhealthy cities. From the second decade of the twentieth century, the position became reversed. While the idea of the 'unhealthy city' was not wholly displaced, the 'unhealthy village' now became much more important.

Clearly articulating the changed emphasis, influential *daktari* author and the First Chemical Examiner to the government, Rai Chunilal Basu Bahadur wrote that '60/70 years ago many places in Bengal were healthy and prosperous…At that time people used to fear the very names of cities; leave alone live in cities, no one would venture into a city unless on an unavoidable business…Nowadays the reverse is true'.[134] Basu therefore appealed to Bengali villagers themselves to take up the project of restoring the health of their villages.[135] Other authors like Mukunda Das and Kaliprasanna Dasgupta also echoed Basu's exhortations.[136] It was undoubtedly in response to calls such as these that numerous patriotically minded young men now took up *gram-samskar* as a regular activity. The ethos for such patriotically inspired sanitary action was already there in the days of the plague—but it had then had urban spaces as its primary focus.[137] Increasingly, from the second decade of the twentieth century, this sort of ethos came to refocus on rural spaces. Partly, this inward turn was inspired by what Sumit Sarkar has called the ideology of 'constructive Swadeshi'. After the agitation against the Partition of Bengal along religious lines in 1905, some leaders and influential ideologues such as Rabindranath Tagore moved away from overt agitational politics and focussed anew on the villages of Bengal to 'build a new nation'. Many such leaders had already been influenced by British Romantic literature, and in translating the romantic sensibility into Bengali, came to acquire a new appreciation and understanding of the village. This engagement with the village, however, was not merely aesthetic.[138] A new generation, under the influence of Bengali Romanticism and following the conspicuous examples of men like Tagore, came to position the village as a site for specific patriotic activity.[139]

Though such activity was often organized by local charismatic youth organizers and associations and lacked, at most times, any centralized extra-local coordination, these activities came to acquire a very specific structure. There developed within the village, smaller, more specific sites and modes of action. An anonymous memoir from one who spent his youth in the village of Kherupara near Dhaka, brings out the way such patriotism actualized itself: 'Once every year we tried to recover the health of the village. We used to pull out water hyacinths from the rivers and ponds of the village. Dry them and then set fire to the lot. In the face of our concerted attack, numerous unwanted weeds and scrub too would disappear. We used to take up spades in a bid to improve the difficult muddy roads. Sometimes our heads would ache from carrying the heavy loads on them.'[140] The clearing of village ponds of water hyacinths (*pana*), levelling of village roads by filling ditches and removing of scrub around the villages were the acts which were repeatedly undertaken by numerous patriotic youth. These three acts formed the basic structure of *gram-samskar* activity.

As the 1920s progressed, *pana* clearance increasingly became the most dominant component of *gram-samskar*. Its real importance as a pernicious and fast-growing weed came to overlap with a range of symbolic investments in it that raised the threat posed by *pana* to almost mythic proportions. *Pana* now came to stand progressively for the 'decline' of rural Bengal. In 1923 the influential nationalist periodical *Modern Review* criticized the report of governmental committee to investigate the problem of *pana*.[141] By 1933 the Bengal legislature elected under the Montague-Chelmsford reforms of 1919 had introduced a bill for considerable state investment in water hyacinth removal.[142] In 1939, even while the province was being plunged into increasing religio-political turmoil in the run-up to its division and decolonization, one of the things the embattled Bengal ministry did was to declare a 'Water Hyacinth Removal Week' seeking to galvanize all into removing *pana*.[143] By the end of the mid-1940s, so great was the identification of *pana* with Bengal's decline that one author ascribed the loss of Bengal's 'old glory' chiefly to this one weed.[144]

British writers, too, recognized the overwhelming importance of the weed in rural Bengal. Significantly, however, British and Bengali authors differed on the nature of the problem. While British authors like C. A. Bentley insisted that it was principally an economic problem, which was lowering rural productivity, the Bengali authors—even when official subordinates in government service—continued to assert that there was a medical dimension to the problem as well. S. N. Sur, for example, refuted Bentley's contentions to reaffirm a connection between malaria and *pana*.[145] Once again, this is an example of how late-colonial discourse on *improvement* and nationalist *development* marked out their specificities within a consensual space.[146]

Hygiene as Culture

These individual and separate projects of village improvement or urban sanitation, physical and mental culture, etc., did not stand alone. Instead, they formed a single assemblage of activities often performed by the same group of people. One patriotic youth, for instance, from the village of Bojrojogini, near Dhaka, wrote wistfully in his old age, 'With what unflagging youthful exuberance did we take to improving our village! Exuberantly we built up a volunteer force [*Seva Dal*], built up gymnasiums for physical culture [*don-kusthi-r akhada*] and at the centre of all that we built up the Shantisudha Library!'[147] The *daktari* authors, too, often mentioned the whole range of projects in the same text. Bodily improvements, intellectual development and spatial rectification all came together in essays such as *Bangalir Shareer Poshon* by Dr Kulachandra Guha. Dr Guha advocated three important activities—promoting neighbourhood sanitation, regular physical exercise and 'mental exercise' [*manasik vyam*].[148] This entire assemblage of patriotic 'sanitary' and 'hygienic' activity, in time came to be framed as 'national culture'. Sanitation itself was equated to an ancient 'national' cultural practice that was only too often equated with 'Hindu national culture'. Every aspect of sanitation and hygiene was therefore found to be identical to 'ancient Hindu lifestyles'. Meera Nanda, in her study of the robust use of the idea of science by the postcolonial Hindu right wing has called this curious amalgam a 'reactionary modernity'. She points out that these arguments, which seek to align aspects of modern science with 'Hindu' antiquity, are not premised upon a rejection of modernity. Instead, they seek to reinscribe science and modernity within a specifically 'Hindu civilization idiom'.[149] In fact, the very scientificity of 'Hindu national culture' becomes one of its marks of distinction from the unscientific cultures of others.

Dr D. D. Gupta's periodical *Swasthya* [Health], devoted to 'Health and Sanitary Science', was particularly influential in this sphere. It developed, along with other influential medical periodicals, a notion of *deshiya swasthya vigyan* or national health science. Contributing authors sought to prove that modern sanitary ideas and practices were not alien incorporations, but rather an integral element of Bengali Hindu heritage and lifestyles. Though it drew heavily upon ayurvedic texts, this discourse was not limited to ayurveda alone and did not seek to match hygiene/sanitation merely to elements found in ayurveda. Its arguments were more far-reaching, and it aligned aspects of Bengali Hindu lifestyle, such as early morning ritual baths in the river Ganges or strict ritual rules about not eating from a plate that had already been eaten from, with hygiene. The recoding, therefore, was not limited to asserting that 'indigenous medicine' knew of 'modern sanitary science'. It went even further and posited an equation of a certain orthodox Bengali Hindu lifestyle with sanitary science. Habit and ritual practice thus automatically prefigured scientific practice. The journal *Swasthya* thus asserted that 'In order to know how much the people of a country [*desh*] know about the rules of health, we must observe their bathing practices [*snan*], food [*ahar*], houses [*vihar*], the cleanliness of the seating arrangements and attire [*asan basaner parichhannata*], their hatred [*ghrina*] for excrement [*mal-mutradi*]…it will be found that on every one of these aspects cited above, the ancient Hindus had kept an ever watchful eye…'.[150]

Central to this formulation of a 'national culture of hygiene' was a notion of decline. The idea of decline from a glorious past was available in a wide variety of discourses in late-colonial South Asia, and even formal political nationalism drew heavily upon this stock of images of the 'Golden Age'. Its deployment within the discourse of a 'national culture of hygiene' resonated with the intellectual ambience of its time and drew legitimation from the rich variety of 'Golden Age' tropes and discourses. At its most fundamental form, it argued that, the nation had in the past been much healthier and stronger and that the health problems faced in contemporary times was a consequence of modern changes, rather than longer-term factors. One author asserted that 'In the ancient times, in India [*Bharat*] maintenance of health [*Swasthya-rakshya*] was an extremely important concern [*gurutoro byapar*]. At that time devout seers [*dharmaparayon rishis*] were the legislators of every aspect of human life. In all their legislations, their chief concern was the maintenance of the health of the people. Their rule was so firm that it ensured total compliance and the rules of health became entangled with people's religious duties. Consequently people of that time used to follow the rules of health out of religious obligation and fear. In the fullness of time, however, the descendants of the Hindus, through contact with other nations have strayed off the track of their ancestors'.[151] It was this idea of a glorious Hindu past, where everyone was healthy due to their strict adherence to religious rules formulated according to laws of health, that underwrote the nationalization of the science of hygiene itself. The decline in their health was a cause of modern acculturation, and redemption, in this view, lay in a return to the pristine ways of the past. An essayist in the *Chikitsha Shommiloni* thus began his espousal of a *deshiya swasthya vigyan* by asking 'what is the main cause of the almost daily decline of the Bengali's physique?'[152] He then went on to identify 'malaria, cholera and a slavish mentality' as the main causes of the decline. While malaria and cholera directly affected the health of the Bengali nation, it was their slavish mentality that made them ignore the traditional ways of staying healthy and fighting these diseases. He sarcastically commented upon the numerous 'volunteer armies' (*shokh-er shoinyo*) that had grown up in villages and cities to spread the knowledge of hygiene and undertake 'rectification' projects. All this the author found mere slavish mimicry of British ways and almost totally futile. Instead, he explained that if the Bengali nation (*Bangali jati*) was indeed to reverse the trend of physical decline and fight off the deadly contagions like malaria and cholera which had laid them low, they had to 'return' to the long-established rules in ten distinct spheres of life. These were: religious commitment (*dharmey mansthapan*), air (*bayu*), diet (*ahar*), drink (*pan*), injustice (*avichar*), etiquette (*vyavahar*), dress (*paricchod*), exercise (*vyam*), occupation (*vyavsaya*) and sexuality (*abhigaman*).[153] Numerous authors identified a variety of Bengali Hindu customs with hygienic practice since the late 1890s.[154] This coincided with the decline of Brahmoism and the reabsorption of its critical rationality by an emergent neo-Hinduism most conspicuously identified with Swami Vivekananda.[155] In the 1920s alignment of Hindu custom with sanitary science was reinforced through the work of Bengali Gandhians like Dr Kartikchandra Basu.[156] Even those elements of Hindu custom that defied any direct 'scientific' explanation were said to have a deeper functionalist role in promoting *jeevanishakti* through faith, thereby fortifying the body against contagions. Dr Gyanendranarayan Bagchi's 'medical novel' (*daktari uponyash*) includes such an explanation of the hook-swinging during the *Chodok* festival.

It was this tendency to find functionalist scientific explanations for cultural traits peculiar to the Bengali (usually specifically Hindu) lifestyles that structured much of the discussion on *deshiyo swasthya vigyan*. The *daktari* use of the notion of *uchhishto*, or *ento*, is illustrative of this. This peculiar cultural institution, often referred to elsewhere in South Asia as *jhootha*, entails ritual and cultural taboos about not eating or offering cooked food or water that has been eaten or drunk by another to certain people. Usually there is an attendant ritual hierarchy which determines who can eat who's *ento* food or drink who's water. Not only did the editors of the periodical *Swasthya* use this notion in their writings about how to prevent contagion, they also proposed its conceptual expansion to include stale breath in crowded places.[157] Getting up early in the morning, which originally had ritual functions for some orthodox Hindus who performed *suryapranam* (making oblations to the sun) at sunrise, were equated to hygienic practice. The *Swasthya* wrote, 'That early rising is the key to good health and long life is indisputable. The ancient Aryan seers used to wake up just before dawn (*brahmamuhurtya*)'.[158] In yet another article in the same periodical, it was argued that ancient Hindu seers had laid down the rules for the building of homes and that they had done so 'strictly in accordance with the rules of health'.[159]

As already stated, this Hindu nationalization of sanitary science was cemented in the 1920s and 1930s through the work of Bengali Gandhians. Dr Kartikchandra Basu launched at the time a new, annually published almanac entitled *Swasthya-dharma Panjika* that sought to clearly align Hindu religiosity with sanitary beliefs within a popular idiom. The *Panjika* commenced with the lengthy dialogue in verse between Shiva and his wife Parvati in which Shiva explained the concepts of hygiene and sanitation, and their link to Hindu customs, and extolled the hapless readers to return to their ancient ways in order to fight the deadly contagions that preyed upon them. Shiva thus told Parvati:

> Let me tell you now of the life of germs (*Jeebanu-Jeebon*)
> Of various diseases who are the primary cause
> Ayurveda had called these sublime-worms (*sukshma krimi*)
> It is to kill these that the Yaju and Sama [Vedas] have given you spells
> All those Contagious, Life-Destroying Diseases,
> These creatures are their main cause.[160]

Shiva then went further to state that not only was Germ Theory of disease known to the ancient Aryans, but Hindu customs were directly tailored to avoid such contagion.

> The things that the West (*pratichya*) are saying today
> Long ago have they been said by the Aryans
> To avoid germs the Hindu was always cautious
> The rules of touch (*sparsha-bidhi*), customs of [post-excremental] washing (*sauchachar*) were followed with great care[161]

A range of customary practices came to be identified as both essentially Hindu as well as being effective ways of fighting contagions. One author, Dr Dheerendranath Haldar, gave a detailed exposition of this complex project involving nation-building, Hindu upper-caste hegemonization and contagion, in a mock dialogue between an eponymous king and a doctor. The king asked, 'Tell me, what types of *adharma* on the part of humans leads to the country's environment (*jal-bayu*) to becoming corrupt?' The doctor replied, 'Earning one's living dishonestly, dishonest actions, oppression, telling and acting out lies, lack of self-control, multiplicity of dietary choices, selfishness, jealousy, anger and other similar dishonest behaviour, needless and illegitimate cohabitation with women, ignoring the rules of the *Shastras*, disrespect to the elders etc all those forms of oppression which we see to be widespread in today's society, all these corrupt the air and water of a country.'[162]

Hinduism, however, is notorious for its plurality of practices. Different groups and traditions, all calling themselves Hindus, held beliefs that were often directly opposed to those customs which *daktari* authors like Basu or Haldar were seeking to promote.[163] A further categorisation was therefore needed in order to identify the specific set of Hindu practices that were to be aligned to the sanitary and nationalist projects. It was thus there emerged the overlapping notions of *suddhachar* and *sadachar*. Notions of culture, etiquette and *dharma* (righteous action) came together in these categories. Shiva said:

> When one decides to forsake *sadachar*
> Numerous Contagions prey upon him[164]

The politics of the category became clear in a serialized essay by Dr Kunjabihari Jyotirbhushan on *suddhachar*. He argued that 'we see many more people of the lower orders [*odhosrenir lok*] suffering from Contagious Diseases [*sankramak rog*] than the *bhadralok*'.[165] Since the *bhadralok* could not avoid coming into contact with these 'lower orders', every attempt had to be made to reform their behaviour and make everybody practice *suddhachar*. Sanitary education therefore entangled explicitly with projects of Hindu upper-caste hegemonization and the nationalization of the body. The consistent *daktari* insistence on individuals' capacity to resist contagion, had led to a focus on both individuals' subjective capacity to change, as well as on their lifestyles. By the 1920s and 1930s, the Bengali *daktari* discourse actualized nation bodies weakened by the ravages of contagious disease, but capable of redemption through 'reforming' their cultural lives and realigning themselves with upper-caste Hindu lifestyles.

Conclusion

Till this day, numerous modern Hindu homes follow rules that are doubly inscribed on registers of sanitation and ritual in parallel. The leaving of footwear on the threshold of the house, not entering the kitchen with shoes, daily morning baths are all part of average modern Hindu lifestyles that are believed by many to be grounded in sanitary science. This recoding of sanitation as (orthodox Hindu) lifestyle a defence against contagion was something that was first achieved amongst the *daktari* authors of the early twentieth century. The idea and practice of 'contagion' in all its numerous forms has been an immensely productive site for the elaboration and actualization of the nationalist project.

Contagion and anticontagion were not two mutually incommensurate poles between which medical rhetoric and practice remained trapped. The questions of susceptibility, immunity, heredity, etc., allowed disease transmission to become one of the most productive occasions for the intellectual and practical elaboration of a nationalist project. This project actualized bodies, beings, practices, customs, spaces, substances and sites. In short, it would not be unfair to call contagion the crucible for the nationalization of the body in *daktari* thought and practice.

Chapter IV

POLITICAL PLAGUE: DIAGNOSING A NEO-HINDU MODERNITY

David Arnold has described the plague epidemic of the 1890s as an occasion for an unprecedented 'attack on the body'. Plague, clarified Arnold, 'was specifically identified with the human body and thus occasioned an unprecedented assault upon the body of the colonized'.[1] Informed by the arrogance of what it believed to be 'scientific' practice, the British Indian state sought to intrude upon the colonized body as it had never done before. The forcible search and quarantine measures instituted by the government eventually led to widespread protests and violence and even the assassination of W. C. Rand, the Sanitary Commissioner of Pune. This account, however, has been largely based upon the experiences of the Bombay Presidency. Though mention is made of other regions across the subcontinent, the scope of Arnold's pioneering work did not include the interrogation of regional specificities. Ira Klein's demographic study of plague mortality and antiplague measures also focussed primarily on the western and northern regions of the subcontinent,[2] while Ian Catanach's studies highlighted the 'tensions of empire' that the politics around the plague brought to the fore. Apart from the conflict between the Pune politicians, Catanach highlighted the differences within the European medical community.[3] Rajnarayan Chandravarkar's study, based once again on Bombay, highlights the ways in which the 'epidemic' came to be constituted and the diverse and varied responses it evoked. He highlighted the absence of a generalized 'Indian reaction' even within the context of Bombay. He argued that 'epidemics do not represent a single, integrated phenomenon but signify different things to different people'.[4] Recently, Prashant Kidambi has revisited the Bombay plague to highlight the persistence of 'localist' theories of its causation, thereby pointing out the divergences within the Indian medical bureaucracy.[5] The only two studies of the disease that focus on the eastern flank of the subcontinent are Alok Sheel's study of the plague in south Bihar and Amal Das' account of the epidemic in Calcutta. Sheel's largely descriptive account, underpinned by a firmly biomedical understanding of the disease, highlights the role of local geographic, social and economic factors in shaping the incidence of the disease.[6] Das' account, on the other hand, while generally acknowledging the plurality of responses to the antiplague measures, concludes that the measures and the ensuing 'subaltern' rioting was a 'a symbol of protest by the Indian population against colonial domination and subordination, its exploitation, arrogance and policy of strong racism'.[7] Despite a growing importance of the 'local' in the studies of Chandravarkar, Kidambi, Sheel and Das, all the accounts accept without question that the disease in question was indeed the plague. There is consequently little engagement with the process of diagnosis and the history of the plague in India becomes, in varying ways, a part of a disease which, at various times has preyed upon nearly the whole of the Old World. What seems to mark out the Indian plague as being worthy of independent study, therefore, is not so much the disease itself, but people's reactions to it. Often the plague sparked a range of overt political actions—variously against state power, elite domination, etc.

Global histories of the disease thus continue to be written within a framework that accents the spread of a common disease. Even the dissonances highlighted within the colonial medical establishment by authors like Kidambi fail to register in these global histories. Myron Echenberg's recent study of the Bombay plague, for instance, presents a homogenous picture of the IMS as enthusiastically rushing to adopt the 'rat flea theory'.[8] This refusal to notice the conceptual plurality within the IMS is partly the result of choosing a small and elitist archive, and partly the complete faith in an abstract and value-neutral act of diagnosis. Echenberg and the highly influential William McNeill before him base their works on the assumption that the historian can know with relative certainty what was and what was not 'plague'.[9] It is this conception that allows Echenberg to assert that the plague in Calcutta till May 1898 was a 'threat [rather] than a reality'.[10] Sources, however, are not mere repositories of value-neutral facts. They are socially constructed objects that need to be read with reference to the context of their production. As we shall see later in this chapter, the act of determining plague (at least in Bengal) was not, however, such an uncontentious act.

Guy Attewell's study based on Delhi and the Punjab presents a very different picture of the plague. Attewell highlights how unani tabibs, faced with the enormous crisis of both human health and tibb's authority, urgently sought to adapt their practice and theory to develop a viable alternative to allopathic measures to tackle the epidemic.[11] Attewell's account, though functioning within the intellectual contours of unani tibb, is the only one to present a pathological category that cannot be wholly collapsed into the global category.[12]

In some ways, our study will follow Attewell's lead in challenging the implicit division between the variable 'local' perceptions of the disease and the seemingly stable 'global' identities. We will try to show how 'locally' specific responses could also shape the identity of the disease itself. This overlap between 'local' perception and diagnosis, however, could only operate when those making the diagnosis were themselves influenced by 'locally' specific responses to the epidemic, i.e., through the *daktars*.[13]

In many ways, Bengal presented an interesting contrast to both Pune and Bombay on the one hand and Delhi and the Punjab on the other. Bombay Presidency was amongst the last areas to be colonized and therefore retained a substantial presence of the precolonial elite, and their firmer social presence often gave the politics of Bombay Presidency an 'indigenist', antiwestern flavour. This was particularly true of Pune, the old capital of the Peshwas. Delhi, on the other hand, had a much larger—though severely disempowered and in most cases impoverished—Mughal aristocracy. Many of the sharif hakims who were at the forefront of the reconfiguration of unani tibb, were directly descended from the old Mughal courtly families. Bengal's old aristocracy based in Murshidabad, however, had been virtually completely marginalized in provincial politics by the 1890s. The imperial capital of Calcutta was itself a British creation. Its elite mostly owed their wealth to early cooperation with the British. In the imperial capital, the depth of British influence was also much more pronounced. 'Western'-style education had been introduced in Bengal for the longest period and as the middle-class Bengalis came to realize the importance of an 'English education' as a source of employment, an ever-increasing number of them took to it. As a result, by the 1890s the Calcutta elite were, relative to the other presidency towns, perhaps the most deeply indoctrinated in the 'western' sciences. The process was aided by the early establishment of 'western' educational institutions. The establishment of the Calcutta Medical College in 1835 was a part of this project. Over the years, as its ambit of courses was broadened, an ever-increasing number of Bengali medical personnel trained in allopathic medicine were produced. The colonial medical establishment thus soon came to have a disproportionate number of Bengalis in it.

The situation in Calcutta, though not unique, clearly presented some specific dilemmas. The strident Bengali professional classes that had celebrated the much vaunted 'Bengal Renaissance' and was at this time laying the foundation of a modern nationalism premised upon rationality, would not have been comfortable with the obscurantist rhetoric of some of the Pune protestors, while still needing to develop an idiom to oppose the violations of the colonial state. It is precisely this idiomatic difference that is glossed over in the Pan-Indian histories of protest against the antiplague measures, since they tend to ignore the actual idioms of protest. Partly, this is the consequence of an almost exclusive reliance on the government archive, an archive constituted principally to quell the protests which, in turn, erupted in the first place, at least partly due to the lack of understanding between the state and its subjects. By relying, instead, upon a variety of nongovernmental archives—literature, Bengali medical periodicals, pamphlets, etc.—we seek to retrieve the actual idiom in which the protests in Bengal were articulated.

Once the faceless 'protestors' are disaggregated, multiple fault lines emerge. The Bengali *bhodrolok*'s plague project was not merely a straightforward question of opposing government incursions; halting government violations were only part of the project. The challenge lay in doing so in such a way as to not having to completely repudiate the authority of 'rationality' and 'modernity'—and even more importantly, 'science' as a metaphor for both—for it was around these that the professional *bhodrolok*'s own identity had come to be based. In short, the dilemma for the *bhodrolok* was how to oppose the antiplague measures without having to say that the science it was based on was itself wrong or inapplicable. A second dilemma arose from allopathic medicine's proximity to state power—a proximity made more explicit in the antiplague campaigns. Arnold has demonstrated how allopathic medicine often became 'state medicine'. The profound challenge that faced the Bengali *bhodrolok* doctors during the crisis years of 1896–1898 was thus twofold. First, they had to find a way to oppose the plague measures without demolishing the authority of 'medical science' itself. Second, they had to reimagine the relationship of modernity (which was metonymically represented by allopathic medicine) and state. It was within these two challenges that the pressure to vernacularize allopathic medicine was further strengthened.

Resisting the State: The Politics of Diagnosis

In October 1896, W. J. Simpson, the controversial Sanitary Officer who had developed a highly antagonistic relationship with the city's elected Bengali municipal commissioners after the cholera epidemic of the 1880s, was once again at the centre of controversy when he insisted on forcibly examining the corpse of a woman who had died at home, allegedly of mumps. The *Hitavadi* called it 'oppression in the name of sanitation'.[14] The thought of the *Antahpur* (Zenana) being forcibly searched by complete strangers and the possibility of respectable Bengali women being physically examined by white doctors outraged the *bhodrolok*. N. Mukherjee, the chairman of the municipal commissioners, asserted that 'people would prefer to die of Plague rather than consent or submit to the removal of their mothers, wives, daughters or sisters to hospitals'. Moreover, the ignominy did not stop in this life. It continued after death. A Bengal plague committee memorandum in 1897 argued that even after death, since a plague corpse was the 'focus of infection', funerary rites had to be curtailed. The dreaded disease thus evoked not only the possibility of extreme humiliation in life, but also possible violations in the afterlife.[15]

The Bengali doctors of the time were caught in this crossfire. On the one hand, their affective ties with the cultural world of the *bhodrolok* inspired them to oppose the government's antiplague measures, while on the other hand, their professional commitments also urged them to oppose the orthodoxy and narrow political considerations of the *bhodrolok* politicians. It was within these dual commitments that they were forced to vernacularize their medical knowledge.[16]

The easiest way available to these doctors to protect their fellow men and women from forcible removal to a hospital, followed by a lonely and ignominious death, was to simply not diagnose the affliction as plague. It is not surprising that little evidence is to be found for such deliberate 'alternate diagnosis', since no form of documentation would have reported the 'original' diagnosis. Following Carlo Ginzburg, it is worth reiterating that the absence or minimal presence in the historical archive does not always designate that something either did not happen at all or happened very little.[17] The best way to shed light on the actual act of diagnosis is to move away from the theoretical and statistical accounts of the plague, and concentrate on individual case histories.

One of the best case histories in this regard is that of Ramlal Das of Darjipara. Das had been suffering from what was initially thought to be *baghi*—an ayurvedic disease category causing swellings. The *kaviraj* who was treating him, however, soon recognized the telltale signs of the plague: swellings at the roots of the limbs (armpits, groin, etc.), high fever, a heavy chest with slight phlegm, etc. The *kaviraj* advised the family of the situation and asked them to call in a doctor. Dr Satyacharan Ray, who was called in, however, continued to call it *baghi* and did not officially declare it a plague. Yet, while settling for an ayurvedic pathological category, he continued to treat the patient. Surprisingly, when Ray had to leave Calcutta for a few days, another doctor, an MB, Dr Nandalal Dey, was called in instead of reverting to the *kaviraj*. Even more strikingly, Dr Dey carried on, like Dr Ray before him, treating Das while calling his affliction *baghi*. The reasons they gave for nominally distinguishing *baghi* from plague seem tautological and lacking in conviction. Dr Ray argued that since no one had yet found 'plague bacilli' in the fluids from the true *baghi* (as distinct from plague) glands, the two diseases could not be equated. Ironically, if such bacilli were indeed found, it would no longer be true *baghi*. By means of a circular reasoning, Ray thus argued that every similar case was potentially *baghi* until proven otherwise and implicitly, since it could not be proved without testing and testing would not be undertaken for *baghi*, it could never become plague. However, at the same time, Ray also disputed the efforts by some *kavirajes* to claim that the disease was the same as the ayurvedic *bradhna*. In fact, he went to great lengths to establish that *bradhna, plague* and *baghi* were indeed distinct pathological categories.

Significantly, Ray's article goes to great lengths to oppose any obscurantist attempt to deny the 'advances' of allopathic medicine. He sarcastically reminded the *kavirajes*, who claim to find all answers in the ancient texts, that it was quinine that controlled the dreaded scourge of malaria in Bengal. He caustically asked them how they could even claim to speak of the plague, when it was a disease that they had never before seen, since it had never before occurred in Bengal. Like so many others amongst his readers, Ray was clearly fighting a battle on two fronts. On the one, he challenged the obscurantist who sought to reject modernity per se, while on the other, he attempted to resist what he viewed as an 'oppressive' and illegitimate, state-sponsored modernity. It is from this liminal space that Ray can confidently say that 'there is absolutely no mention of plague in their [the *kaviraj's*] ayurvedic texts', while at the same time asserting that though 'many today say that plague is caused by a specific bacillus, this is completely wrong'. In fact, he continues, it is caused by the imbalance of *bayu*, *pitta* and *kaaph*, but 'unfortunately' very few contemporary *kavirajes* any longer know the true nature of these *doshes*, while the doctors are misled by their bacilli.

Subsequently, Dr Ray also mentions another unnamed case where a lady had developed the dreaded signs of the plague. Here, Dr Ray prescribed for her under the perplexing and nonexistent medical category of *Kokhyastha Granthisphithi Rog* (lit: swelling of hidden glands disease).[18] Unlike *baghi*, which was an affliction known to ayurvedists, this latter designation was a complete novelty and given its lack of elegance, one suspects was made up at short notice—as a mere shorthand of the primary symptoms. Another medical author, Dr Girishchandra Bagchi, wrote to establish the plague cases in Calcutta as *ashangomik brodhno* or 'non-venereal bubo'—another modification of an ayurvedic category. However, for its treatment, instead of any ayurvedic method, he proposed a treatment regimen using arsenic and drawing upon the researches of one Dr W. C. Spencer of Westminster Hospital.[19] A third doctor, one Dr Gaganchandra Nandi, the Medical Officer-in-Charge of the Harisabha Charitable Dispensary in Chandernagore, diagnosed a patient suffering from similar symptoms as suffering from 'menstrual irregularities'.[20]

Leaving us in little doubt about the reasons for his diagnosis, Dr Ray went on to write immediately after his case histories that

> Recently the Health Officer of Calcutta. Dr Simpson. and Dr Cobb had together detected some cases of Bubonic Plague. Subsequently some doctors of the Medical Commission examined these cases and decided they were not suffering from plague. Had this not been so, Dr Simpson would have raised hell in the name of the 'plague'. I am not sure how good Dr Simpson is in his work, maybe his intentions are good. It is the part of the wise not to create a commotion or oppress but work silently towards the fulfilment of his ends.[21]

Clearly, he was not challenging the authority of the 'science' that informed Simpson's practice in the name of custom What Ray was saying was that he was suspicious of Simpson's professional competence in view of the latter's proven misdiagnosis, and that his approach to the situation was not 'wise' or appropriate.[22] Thus, from where Ray was standing, it was not his own, but, indeed, Simpson's diagnosis that was inaccurate. In terms of approach, too, Ray is clearly advocating a nonconfrontational approach rather than Simpson's controversial methods, which 'oppress' and cause 'commotion', in his view. In this he is clearly drawing upon his own cultural acumen to define how a 'wise man' ought to proceed in a given situation. Dr Amritakrishna Basu's compendious text *Plague Tattwa* makes a similar case. Dr Basu, while wholeheartedly supporting the allopathic treatment of plague as well as the need for segregation, gives a detailed account of how physical examination of plague is almost always totally misleading. He goes on to cite a case where, apparently, in his student years, all his classmates had 'misdiagnosed' two cases. According to him, given the 'extreme variability of the symptoms in plague', though some help in diagnosis could be found by judging the mental and the physical signs exhibited by the patient as well as talking to their relatives, no amount of physical evidence could be conclusive.[23]

Even Dr D. D. Gupta, editor of the *Swasthya* journal and one of the otherwise staunchest supporters of sanitary and public health measures, mentioned that of the 125 reported cases of Plague (in 1897), he reckoned that several were erroneously diagnosed and were actually some other disease. Dr Gupta was also quick to point out that the *Sannipathic Jwar* (tri-humoural fever) of some ayurvedic author's was very similar to the plague. The usually circumspect Dr Gupta therefore argued that, though some cases amongst the 125 may well be 'true plague', it would be wrong to call it an epidemic.[24]

It is cogent to guard against any belief that, somehow, the actions of Gupta, Ray or Nandi alone were politically informed and 'incorrect', whereas the actions of British doctors like Simpson and Cobb were 'objective' and apolitical. Indeed, another case history amply demonstrated how far Simpson and Cobb were willing to go to diagnose cases as 'plague'. In this case, the patient was one Bepin Behari Dutt, a labourer at a small enterprise at Raja Rajballabh Lane in the Bara Bazaar area of Calcutta. Dutt had initially been treated by a Bengali *daktar* called Dr Kishori Mohun Mukherjee, who had not diagnosed the case as plague. Mukherjee held on to to his diagnosis even after the patient's death, and was instrumental in bringing the actions of Simpson and Cobb to light by helping a reporter of the nationalist daily, the *Amrita Bazar Patrika*, to find and interview witnesses who had been present during the forced inspection of the patient by the British doctors. A number of local witnesses testified that Drs Simpson and Cobb had, without any prior permission, inspected the patient and drawn blood from several incisions made on his person in order to carry out the tests. The details of their gruesome and heartless investigation of the sick man were published in the newspaper in the form of lengthy first person interviews with the witnesses. Subsequently, when responding to the public outcry occasioned by the publication, the government decided to investigate the matter, it transpired that Simpson had further, almost certainly, conspired to suppress his role in the events. He had not filed an official report on the matter, as he was duty bound to do by virtue of the same regulations he so zealously sought to implement, until the morning after an official letter of enquiry from the Government of India to the provincial government following the report in the *Amrita Bazar Partika*—nearly a month and a half after the events. He had moreover obviously misstated the extent of his physical examination when directly questioned by Municipal Commissioner Nalin Behary Sircar. Subsequently, despite the Medical Board not finding any evidence of the case actually having been plague and Brigadier Surgeon Lt Col D. D. Cunningham informing the Medical Board that the blood analysis carried out by Lt Col Cobb and Simpson were utterly unreliable due to extreme contamination of the samples, Simpson still went ahead and published articles in the local daily, *The Englishman*, claiming that 'true plague' had been detected in Calcutta. The government eventually severely reprimanded Simpson for his actions and forbade him to publicly write on the matter.[25]

If Ramlal Das' case brought out the politicization of diagnosis on the part of the Bengali *daktars*, Bepin Behari Dutt's case brings out the difficulty of trusting the diagnosis of British doctors. Even without imputing overt malfeasance, it is clear that plague diagnosis in contemporary Calcutta was a contentious issue, where the physician's subjectivity was crucial. The fact that Kishori Mohun Mukherjee was at the forefront of the fight to bring Simpson to book shows that he did not consider his own diagnosis in any way incorrect and was willing to stand up for it, just as Simpson, despite all his official sidestepping, was willing to risk departmental censure and still write about it. It is not the motive behind the diagnosis that we seek to highlight here, but the mere fact that diagnosing plague itself was a contentious and political (in the broadest sense of the word) act and, hence, without engaging with this crucial aspect of the history of plague, any decision on how many people in Calcutta had been afflicted with the plague would remain a misguided question.[26]

Subjectivity of Diagnosis and the Importance of Place

Though there is now a grudging awareness amongst many scholars about the subjectivity of diagnosis of mental illnesses, there still seems to be a fair amount of scepticism about accepting the subjectivity of diagnosis in the case of somatic illnesses. It is often taken to be a more or less subject-neutral operation of medical logic upon an equally neutral object of perception. However, as Byron Good has pointed out through his fieldwork amongst students of the Harvard Medical School, there is a culturally specific process through which physicians are actually tutored to construct the 'persons, patients, bodies, diseases and human physiologies' in certain culturally specific ways.[27] Using Ernest Cassirer's theory of 'symbolic forms', Good argues that 'medicine is a 'symbolic form' that 'mediate[s] and organize[s] distinctive forms of reality'.[28] These 'symbolic forms', Cassirer argues, are an amalgamation of 'imagination, perception and activity', which together constitute a thoroughly historicized 'image world', by engaging with which, observers actively constituted the reality they witnessed. This is not to argue for some kind of extreme idealist position where the reality and materiality of the world have been replaced by pure idealized forms. It is merely to underline that the basic units through which perceptual data is comprehended and categorically understood, varies. As Good himself points out, 'molecular medicine' and 'epidemic medicine', for instance, approach the same set of realities from very different angles and constitute the subjects of their actions differently. Since the historically fashioned image-worlds through which medicine constructs particular objects were culturally specific, even the basic perceptual first stage to diagnosis cannot be purely objective and culture- neutral. Thus, the difference in the ways Kishori Mohun Mukherjee and Simpson saw Bepin Behari Dutt arose not necessarily because one was lying about what he saw; it may well have been due to the fact that the two physicians were approaching the case in front of them through two distinct image-worlds. How they saw the patient in turn depended upon what sort of information about the patient they had access to.

One conspicuous difference in the way they approached the question of diagnosis was that while doctors like Simpson tended to concentrate on the body of the patient alone, the *daktars* tended to look at the case within a particular spatial context, especially the patient's house and the houses he visited.

In 1901 the influential journal *Swasthya* published an editorial in which, while commenting on the renewed reports of plague from the other Indian cities, it asserted that, basically, the disease had reappeared everywhere in the same localities and even in the same houses which had been afflicted previously. It therefore proposed that the government take immediate steps to 'send its usual messengers of death' to these particular houses and get these cleaned.[29] This accent on the place of affliction rather than the afflicted body was visible in the earlier texts on the subject. In November 1896, for instance, one Dr Devendranath Ray, writing in the *Bhisak Darpan*, organized his essay around a discussion of the places where one would be most likely to contract the dreaded diseases. Rejecting in broad cartographic determination, Dr Ray clarified that this disease was to be encountered anywhere from the beaches of the Levant to the mountaintops of Kedarnath. It had, he added emphatically, absolutely no connection with low-lying, humid lands. Instead, he mentioned that two types of places were the most dangerous with regards to plague: first, small crowded houses where there was little circulation of fresh air; second, houses where cattle, pigs or goats were kept close to the windows.[30] Ray also mentioned that the people of Kumaon and Garhwal—amongst whom the disease was already known—abandoned their houses once they realized the epidemic had started. Though the disease was not carried to the new place, Ray added that those already infected might actually manifest the symptoms up to fifteen or twenty days later. Yet, he believed that taking the old clothes and bedding along from the old house did not carry the disease. D. D. Gupta argued that 'Plague germs (*bijanu*) cling to the floor, walls or other objects in the house where Plague cases have been reported'.[31] The greater susceptibility of Bombay to the disease than Calcutta was ascribed to the habit of poor Bombayites of living in overcrowded *chauls*.[32]

The importance of the spatial context of diagnosis was not wholly absent from the writings of European doctors either, though, relatively speaking, they continued to attach more weight to the plagued body as such. Thomas Corrie Rutherford, who served on plague duty in Punjab, Lucknow and Burma and wrote a dissertation on the plague in South Asia, stated, for instance, that a 'history of exposure' was often crucial in determining whether a case was plague or not.[33] In many cases which Rutherford discussed, even though the most prominent signs of the disease had been absent upon the initial examination of the patient, what had made him diagnose the case as one of plague was a previous 'history of exposure', i.e., presence in spaces—especially houses—where plague had been known to have raged. Rutherford also admitted that bacteriological blood analysis could only detect plague in 50 to 70 per cent of instances, and not in all cases. Diagnosis, for Rutherford, depended eventually upon a 'history of exposure to infection, the severity of general symptoms and on microscopical examination'.[34]

'History of exposure', understood to be the houses which the patient had lived in or visited in recent times, thus formed a crucial component of the final diagnosis. Obviously, the degree to which such histories of exposure could be determined with any certainty depended upon the degree of trust that existed between the physician and the patient. If the patient did not give the physician accurate details about where he had been, or if the physician mistrusted the patient's testimony, there was scope for misdiagnosis. In Rutherford's case, for instance, he mentions one case of a Sowar (cavalry trooper) in the native regiment with which he was serving at the time, who had picked up the infection while 'visiting a house in which plague had occurred for purpose of illicit intercourse with a woman'.[35] Such information about their patients would almost certainly not be given up freely to Simpson or Cobb, but might very easily have been available to men like Kishori Mukherjee.

The importance of the 'history of exposure' brings to light not only the subjectivity of the physician in the act of diagnosis but also the extent of trust which the patient might have had in the physician. The reports about the case of Bepin Behari Dutt repeatedly asserted that Simpson and Cobb did not speak to any of the other witnesses present. Gopalchandra Basu, the manager of the factory Dutt worked in, Gurupada Bhattacharya, a writer in the factory, Ram Sevak, a fellow employee, Beharilal Das, another employee who had nursed Dutt in his illness and Dr Mukherjee, all of whom had been present during Dutt's examination, testified that the British doctors had spoken to none of them.[36] The latter may well have felt that speaking to these witnesses was immaterial, as they would not be giving the truth of the matter in any case. The signs legible on the body were, therefore, the only reliable witnesses that Simpson and Cobb could speak to, and they had absolutely no way of determining the 'history of exposure' which Mukherjee could easily have had access to. The divergent diagnosis—in part, at least—was the result of the very different relationships *daktars* and European doctors came to occupy in colonial society and the differential access they had to information.[37]

Swadeshi Atmashakti and Bengali Plague Medicine

In Sumit Sarkar's classic study of the Partition of Bengal in 1905, he has suggested the need to disentangle the varied idioms of participation in the Swadeshi resistance to the partition. Sarkar broadly identified three trends within the movement: one which increasingly fell back upon 'moderate' methods and sought the state's support to develop the nation exemplified by Surendranath Banerjee's newspaper the *Bengalee*; another, represented by Rabindranath Tagore among others, sought to almost totally ignore the state and pursue nation-building on a voluntarist basis; and finally, that strand which would by 1908 become the ideological bulwark of the 'revolutionary terrorists'—for a time nominally represented by the meteoric Aurobindo Ghosh, the future spiritual guru Sri Aurobindo. The last two of the three strands, in Sarkar's brilliant reading, came to share a bivalent, or perhaps even polyvalent, concept of soul force or *atmashakti*. Its interpretations varied from a personal heroic pursuit by the militants to an individualist spiritual quest in the later Aurobindo. Tagore's notion of state-independent national development also resonated with the notion of *atmashakti*.[38] The logic of *atmashakti*, we will argue, was already visible in its rudiments a decade before the momentous Partition of 1905 in the Bengali *bhodrolok*'s response to plague.

A discourse was developed on *Pratirodh Shakti*, or the power of resistance, that would keep on resonating in Bengali *bhodrolok* consciousness throughout the early decades of the twentieth century. Its basic premise was based upon the idea of prevention rather than cure, but it was continuously elaborated upon and given a variety of dimensions. In its most basic form, it was stated by one author who asserted that, 'even though plague is an infectious disease, it cannot attack if the body is healthy. A healthy body can resist not only plague, but a number of other contagions.'[39] However, defining and describing the 'healthy Bengali body' was no easy task, and over the next two decades it became one of the most powerful and polyvalent intellectual tools to be articulated by the Bengali *bhodrolok* physicians.

We have already seen in Chapter III that the *daktari* discourse had long been engaged with a multicausal model of disease causation and continued to give significant importance to the predisposing causes in the patient that made them susceptible to contagious diseases. The discourse on *Pratirodh Shakti* was an overlapping but slightly different notion. Instead of susceptibility, it looked at the patient from the point of view of his or her innate power to fight or resist external contagions. The belief in the body's innate power to—if not always resist—cure itself once afflicted had been popular amongst an earlier generation of 'western' authors as well. William Cullen himself had often drawn upon the idea of a *vix medicatrix naturae*, and its use by the *daktari* authors did not, therefore, stem from any essential cultural peculiarity, but rather from their situation in history where such ideas 'articulated' with their historical context.[40] One of the earliest essays on the subject was written by Dr Hemchandra Sen, MD. Dr Sen argued that since the same bacillus could produce different diseases in different people, the disease causation actually depended on the strength of the individual's *Swabhabik Rog-Badhok Shokti*, or the patient's normal disease-preventive power. 'The same Plague Bacilli causes different types of Plague in different people,' he continued. 'People who have a strong Normal Disease-Preventive Power are never afflicted by the dangerous Tubercule or Plague Bacilli'.[41]

Dr Sen's essay also resonated with older anxieties about the physical weakness of Bengalis/Indians. Malaria, which had emerged as an important and polyvalent image and metaphor for this 'racial weakness', especially amongst Bengali *bhodrolok* writers, was directly invoked, thereby lending further cultural connotations to the discussions on plague.[42] Sen's essay slipped easily between Bengal and India on the one hand and malaria and plague on the other. He wrote that 'Due to the destruction of the Disease-Preventive Power, the weakly population of India is being ravaged by such dangerous diseases as Malaria, Dyspepsia and Plague. To try to reverse this ought to be the doctor's foremost duty.'[43] His solution for the problem was even more redolent with wider cultural anxieties of the Bengali *bhodrolok*. He advocated the injection of 'testicular emulsions' to promote disease-preventive powers. Drawing upon the writings of one Dr Brown Shepherd and a French doctor named Dr Arsenevalle, he argued that an emulsion made from crushed testicles contained a certain active principle called 'spermatin' or 'testiculin' and that these, when injected into people, could promote both physical (*sharirik*) as well as mental (*manoshik*) strength. It was this strength that prevented disease.[44] By slipping easily between physical and mental strength and then positioning this 'power' as the prime factor in preventing plague, Dr Sen's essay was clearly being framed by the cultural anxieties around the notorious 'Bengali effeminacy'.[45] As we have seen repeatedly in Chapter III and shall see again in subsequent chapters, and as historians of gender have well documented, the Bengali *bhodrolok*'s anxieties about racial and national effeminacy remained a redolent theme in the latter's cultural mindscape. Popularized in the first half of the nineteenth century by British authors such as T. B. Macaulay, it became internalized by the end of the century and rearticulated in a variety of ways. It was also to be observed in some of the redefinitions of the Swadeshi search for *atmashakti*. Indira Chowdhury, for instance, has shown how the rhetoric of revolutionary terrorist youth in Bengal was replete with references to Bengali effeminacy and the need to cultivate 'strength', or *shakti*, to overcome this debilitating powerlessness.[46]

The discourse on *Pratirodh Shakti* clearly deemphasized the effectiveness of the state in preventing or controlling the plague epidemic. By accenting the agency of the individual in maintaining health, it also proposed a very different relationship with the state than the one that seemed to inform the antiplague measures of Dr Simpson and others. A lengthy editorial in the *Swasthya* clarified that plague could not be prevented by the government, despite their 'unquestionable good intentions', as long as the people remained ignorant about the disease. It pointed out how little the government had done to make available information about plague, specifically on issues like 'What is Plague? How can it be cured? And what can be done to prevent it from affecting one?' The only information available was either in the form of difficult-to-access 'Parliamentary Blue Books and Reports' or, at best, in ephemeral daily newspapers that were never preserved. Instead, the editors recommended that the government ought to implement its plague measures through disseminating free pamphlets that would educate the public. In the absence of such government initiative, they themselves undertook to do what they could in this regard.[47] The discourse thus came to acquire a conspicuously didactic approach. In most cases it started being organized in the form of bullet-point injunctions like:

- Do not remain on an empty stomach when you are hungry.
- Do not fast on any grounds.
- As far as possible, try to avoid work that is likely to tire you.
- Do not allow any blood in your body to be wasted.
- Do not consume food which you know to be bad for you.[48]

The format of this discourse, which is explicitly directed at Bengali householders themselves, is very different from the Plague Regulations promulgated by the municipal authorities. Instead of a 'Dos' and 'Don'ts' format that placed the initiative for disease prevention squarely with the individual subjects themselves, the Regulations gave explicit powers to the Health Officer and his officers to directly intervene—with due safeguards of intimation and forewarning—upon any Bengali home. Unlike the didactic instructions of the *daktars*, the Regulations addressed the individual subjects only to let them know the limits of their rights and to inform them of how and where their rights might be superseded by the Health Officer. For example, where D. D. Gupta urged his readers, 'Do not live in crowded dwellings', the Plague Regulations informed them that 'When a dwelling is so overcrowded…as in the opinion of the Health Officer, to make the inmates especially liable to an attack of the Bubonic Plague, the Chairman may…require the owner or the occupier…to abate the overcrowding'.[49] Arguably, the goal of both directions were identical, but where one relied upon the self-reflection and judgement of the householder, the other was premised on the municipal authority's right to suspend the householder's rights through the judgement of the Health Officer.

The *daktari* injunctions were often also thematically redolent with older ayurvedic notions of *Din-charya*, or daily routine. These notions—as we saw in Chapter III—had, moreover, been partly adopted and identified with normative Hindu middle-class lifestyle and therefore resonated on multiple cultural registers for the overwhelmingly (though never solely) Hindu Bengali *bhodrolok* medical authors. The editors of the *Swasthya*, for instance, while advocating daily baths, added 'every Hindu bathes daily in any case, but merely the habit of daily bathing is not sufficient, you must always keep your body and your clothes clean'.[50] The most overt statement of this Hinduization of *Pratirodh Shakti*, however, appeared in an essay on the effect of *sankirtan* (singing of religious hymns) on plague. While admitting that there was no direct link between plague and *sankirtan*, the essay argued that it was 'undeniable by any one conversant with medical literature that faith (*bishwash*) can cure disease' and that the stronger the faith, the better the effect. It argued that this strong faith promoted the individual's ability to resist, and thereby prevent, the disease or even recover from it.[51] In the very year (1896) that the plague scare reached Calcutta, another author writing in the *Chikitsa Sammilani* went even further and quoted a variety of press reports from Europe on séances, hypnosis, theosophy, Christian faith healing, etc., to argue that 'divine power' (*daivya shakti*) could act to cure diseases in human beings in a mode akin to mesmerism and hypnotism. The author, Surendranath Bandopadhyay, rhetorically asked: Was there no Force of Gravity before Newton? Why then can there not be such powers which we do not yet understand but whose operation we witness?[52] Both *sankirtan* and *daibya shakti* worked, therefore, through the mediation of a power within the body—a power to defend itself against disease and to cure itself once afflicted.

The religious affiliations of these interdictions become even more obvious upon a brief comparison of these writings of the *daktars* and the Plague Manifesto of Swami Vivekananda. Written in May 1898, the Manifesto included bullet-point injunctions such as:

- Always keep the house and its premises, the rooms, clothes, bed, drain, etc., clean.
- Do not eat stale, spoiled food; take fresh and nutritious food instead. A weak body is more susceptible to disease.

- Always keep the mind cheerful. Everyone will die once. Cowards suffer the pangs of death again and again, solely due to the fear in their own minds.
- Fear never leaves those who earn their livelihoods by unethical means or who cause harm to others. Therefore, at this time when we face the great fear of death, desist from all such behaviour.

It also asserted that the mind should be freed from fear and faith placed in God. It ended with the final injunction: 'In order to remove the fear of the epidemic, you should sing Nâma Sankirtan every evening and in every locality'.[53]

The hero of the novel *Bagher Baccha* also advocated a similar approach to matters of custom and faith. He commented that instead of fighting 'superstition', doctors should try to utilize the patient's faith in cure. A strong faith, according to him, dispelled fear in the patient and therefore strengthened his/her powers to fight off disease and ill health. This framing of disease in terms of a binary of weakness and strength and the cultivation of an 'inner power' for recovery or immunity from disease is a redolent theme in Hindu Bengali culture of the early twentieth century. It also coincides with the birth of a Neo-Hinduism, most notably through Vivekananda, wherein science and religion are sought to be reconciled. This Hindu insistence of faith and inner strength was not narrowly communal on the face of it, for it asserted, for instance, that both Hindus and Muslims should freely take part in the numerous communal *sankirtans* organized in Calcutta during the plague years. It also stressed that people's faith was reinforced by participating in such communitarian activities. However, that it remains Hindu in its idiom is clear. In this alliance of religion and science, there is also an attempt to add the legitimacy of either term to the other term. Science thus benefits from being seen to be unopposed to religion, and religion also gains a new legitimacy in view of its own 'scientificity'. Along with this legitimacy, there is also an implicit espousal of superiority. To assert that Hindu practice is 'scientific' is to also implicitly argue that Muslim practice is not scientific. To say that Hindus, as a rule, bathe every day and are clean is to implicitly say Muslims are unclean and do not bathe regularly. Customary practices in general, but cleanliness—or claims to it—became markers. Therefore, not only of community identity, but also of the scientific functionality of religious customs. Dr Basu, for instance, who was a staunch allopath in his professional loyalties, went on to argue that the Europeans in reality knew nothing of the reality of plague and everything that was salutary in allopathic treatment of plague, including segregation, had already been incorporated into Hindu medicine and custom by the '*Arya rshis*' (Aryan seers). Moreover, he claimed that this was recognized by all honest and compassionate Englishmen. To prove his case he quoted

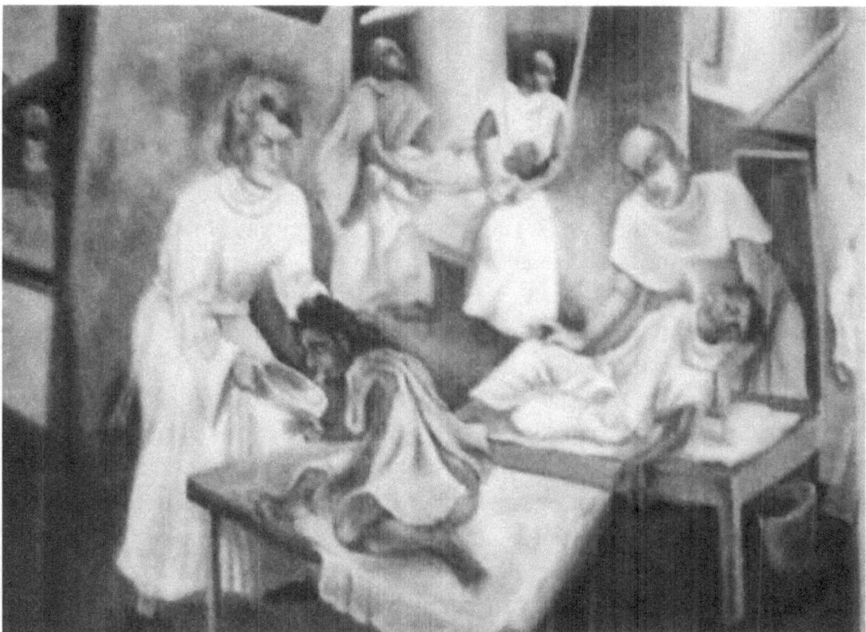

Fig. VII. A contemporary popular representation of the work of Sister Nivedita and the Neo-Hindu monks during the Calcutta Plague, available at www.uttishthata.org, accessed on 24th October 2008.

a letter from one Sir Bradford Leslie, who mentioned that the Bengali Hindus were 'perhaps, personally the cleanest race of people in the world. They all bathe once daily at least…'.[54]

Plague and the Community

However, it was also through this communitarian impulse within the discourse that the individual pursuit of *atmashakti* could take on a more social aspect. As in Vivekananda's own case, the individual pursuit of strength eventually spilt over into a voluntarist vision to make the community itself strong. Thus, organized under Vivekananda's closest disciple, Sister Nivedita (previously known as Margaret Noble), a group of young Bengali men volunteered to serve the victims of the plague by going into plague-ridden ghettoes and 'manfully' cleaning the houses and provide succour to the dead and dying. (Fig. VII.) The Hindu Satkar Samiti was born from amongst these volunteers to ensure the proper cremation of the Hindu dead. These acts clearly and emphatically rejected the role of the state in controlling the plague. Instead, they sought to take the onus upon themselves. They cremated the dead as quickly as possible and thus fulfilled the demands of sanitation, but did so according to Hindu ritual injunctions and, therefore, also assuaged anxieties of plague-corpses being cremated without proper ritual. Religion and science were once again brought together, not as individual pursuits, but as voluntarist social action. This voluntary social service became a quasi-religious activity in itself. In Saratchandra Chattopadhyay's novel *Grihadaha*, published in 1920 but serialized in the *Bharatborsho* since 1916, the morally ambiguous *daktar* Satish, on finally seeing the folly of his ways and being ashamed of his previous attempts to elope with Achala, the wife of his boyhood friend Mahim, leaves to pay for his sins by voluntarily working amongst rural plague victims where he eventually dies of the dreaded disease himself, nursed by Achala. The moral value of working amongst the plague victims, as well as Satish's choosing to do so, knowing the risks, as an act of penance (*prayashchitta*), clearly depicted the emerging overlaps between religion and medico-social work. Significantly, a subplot in the novel revolves around the contrast between Achala, a Brahmo woman, and Mrinal, a Hindu girl married to a much older man, but perhaps actually in love with Mahim. By contrasting Mrinal's selfless sense of duty for a husband she cannot truly love with Achala's impetuous and somewhat selfish 'independent spiritedness', Saratchandra also subtly described the superiority of a specifically *Hindu* 'sense of duty'—the same sense of duty which eventually surfaces in Satish's *prayaschitta* and thus, he hopes, redeems his amoral life. It is this whole cluster of ideas about duty, Hindu identity, selflessness, finding religious merit in social work, etc., that started to coagulate on the site of the Bengali response to plague.[55]

One of the key digits of this voluntarist movement was the articulation of space. We have already mentioned that when diagnosing, whereas the British doctors sought to concentrate upon the body of the afflicted, the Bengali *daktars* accented the spatial context of exposure to disease. This emphasis on particular places was further developed into a powerful idea of local and domestic cleanliness. Once again, the anxiety over cleanliness was shared by both British authorities and the *daktars*, yet their modus operandi differed radically from each other. Further, this difference found resonance in both their practical injunctions and their theoretical writings.

Ironically, while the British sought to use the plague to breach the privacy of the Bengali home through enforced searches and removals, the Bengali doctors sought to turn the Bengali homes and localities into fortresses against contagion.[56] They spoke energetically of the need to protect the home against *Galij*. The etymology of the term is obscure and it is not usually used in Bengali.

Though translated by authors as *filth*, it was in effect a broader concept that included, apart from what we recognize as 'filth', such other entities as 'bad odours', 'darkness', 'crowds', etc. One author clarified, 'For plague to occur there must be two causes present in tandem. First, the plague germs must be present, and second, both our bodies and our homes must be receptive to such contagion; that is, our homes must be unclean, disorganized, malodorous and without sunlight or fresh air'.[57] Authors, therefore, sought to inspire people to undertake voluntary cleanliness drives.

The drives were, of course, expected to start at home, and everybody was expected to keep their own homes in a sanitary state. Strikingly, where the government's Plague Regulations completely disregarded the sanctity of the threshold of a Bengali home, advocating supervision and, if necessary, forcible action by the Health Officer, the Bengali doctors elevated the sanctity of the home and reposed full faith in the householder and the community-at-large to keep homes clean. They advocated taking off one's shoes and clothes every time one returned home and immediately bathing and washing the clothes taken off. The boundary wall was also to be regularly slaked with lime and painted. Thus, the home was to be a veritable fortress of cleanliness. All household garbage was to be expelled from the house and deposited somewhere far away for collection by municipal garbage collectors. Proper flow of fresh air in every part of the house was to be ensured and, most importantly, it was to be ensured that every inch of the house received daily sunlight. Sunlight, it was believed, could dispel germs most effectively. The number of members in families was also to be reduced wherever possible to reduce overcrowding.[58] Some even suggested that the house should—much like a moat—be surrounded on every side by a nice garden with fragrant flowers.[59]

Despite these precautions, should a family member still fall prey to the plague, the *daktars*, instead of removal and hospitalization, advocated segregation in a special room within the house. Only the indigent, it was said, would benefit from hospitalization.[60] It was clarified that, first, the existence of caste restrictions (*jatibhed*) and purdah (*aborodh*)—amongst both Hindus and Muslims of distinction—made hospitalization impractical for Bengalis. Second, Bengalis, it was claimed, did not have the same sense of public good that inspired an Englishman to leave his home and remove to the hospital. Finally, it was asserted that even if a Bengali were to go to the hospital, he would never receive the good care that an Englishman receives there.[61] All this made it impracticable for them to go to the hospital; it was therefore much better for the Bengali to be cared for within her/his home.

Yet, what, asked one author, can be done to safeguard against the plague if your neighbours continue to lack sanitary sense? What if some orthodox neighbour ignored sanitary science and continued to keep his yard full of foul rubbish? What if down the road the milkmen continued to have a filthy cattle shed? It was here that the cleanliness drive needed to be taken beyond the home and needed to become a community project.

It was within this context that in 1899 Vivekananda instituted his 'sanitary mission', where volunteers of the Ramakrishna Mission formed voluntary squads and undertook to clean the city.[62] He had responded urgently to the plague and had seen in it the workings of God. It was an opportunity for him to give his particular vision of Neo-Hinduism, based upon a vision of voluntary community work as worship, a concrete shape. Nivedita recalled that upon hearing of the panic struck by the plague, Vivekananda had said, 'There are some who scoff at the existence of Kali. Yet today She is out there amongst the people. They are frantic with fear, and the soldiery have been called to deal out death. Who can say that God does not manifest Himself as evil as well as good? But only the Hindu dares to worship Him in the evil'.[63] However, not only was this vision conspicuously Hindu in its idiom, it was also framed within a slightly different politics of masculinity.[64] While the talk of inner strength accented an individual quest for manliness, here the 'daring' lay in worshipping God's work amidst danger, i.e., going into the midst of the plague voluntarily to effect sanitation and care for the ill. It also had a pronounced class aspect to it. Nivedita glowingly mentioned how Vivekananda sought volunteers who would 'devote themselves to Indian pariahs'. She also wrote of how he exulted in 1897 on seeing his Brahmin devotees nursing low-caste patients.[65] The upper-caste, middle-class volunteers thus became the saviours of their lower-caste, lower-class neighbours. Yet their actions, crucially, were said to be animated by a 'love' and 'religious piety' and not power.

The intellectual resources that frame Vivekananda's project are all present in Bengali medical writers on the plague. The class dimension, for instance, is most prominently present in several writers. One writer mentioned that plague affected the 'unclean'. It started with rats and thereafter affected the lower classes because of their unclean habits, and only seldom affected the rich. The author, therefore, sought to inform the *bhodrolok* of the dangers posed by such 'dirty people' (*nongra lok*) and possibly inspire them to either shun the latter's company or seek to reform them.[66] Another author mentioned that the reason the government's cleanliness drives failed was because they were executed by unthinking, low-class 'coolies'. Moreover, he wrote that the expensive foreign disinfectants could easily be replaced by homemade quicklime if only it were properly supervised. The crucial element is that there must be enlightened supervision, as a consequence—from the perspective of the author—making the *bhodrolok* indispensable in the fight against plague.

They would have to be educated in the proper sanitary sensibilities and thereafter be expected to supervise the cleanliness of their homes and localities. They must be expected to not only keep themselves free of *galij*, but also to supervise the actions of their servants and inferiors and be vigilant towards the actions of unsanitary neighbours.[67] Even the ethics of love and care within which Vivekananda sought to code his project can be observed in Bengali medical writings. It was often asserted that plague victims needed tender and loving nursing during their convalescence. Gupta, for instance, writing in 1898, mentioned that there is no real medicine for plague other than tender nursing (*sushrusha*).[68] Even Vivekananda's reference to the goddess Kali occasionally cropped up in medical writings, such as when Gupta equated plague germs with *Raktabij*, the demon whose severed head Kali's idol is seen to hold in her hands.[69]

Interestingly, many of the same ideas about religious identity and worship through medico-social caring may have been developing within the oral traditions of popular Bengali Islam at the same time. Plague, of course, was known to the world of classical Islamic scholarship through their Abrahamic intellectual roots in west Asia. A popular faith-based Islamic healing tradition known as the *Tibb-e-Nabi* (Medicine of the Prophet), based upon the sayings and actions attributed to the Prophet, which had developed through both oral and textual lineages in the Islamic world, had thus developed a fragmentary discourse on the plague and Islam. Such texts were definitely known in certain circles in Bengal, and there is also reference to one incomplete effort to translate these texts into Bengali by a Muslim Bengali doctor—Dr S. G. M. Choudhury. However, no definite documentary evidence of *Tibb-e-Nobi* texts in Bengali had not been found until very recently. Overtly, Islamic medical literature in Bengali, though, is one of the most neglected areas of archival preservation in the region, and the existence of such texts cannot be wholly ruled out. Recent texts, which clearly draw on earlier oral traditions, hint strongly at such a possibility. Two recent texts mention the plague *hadiths*. One eponymous text called *Tibb-e-Nobi* recommended that all Muslims immediately leave an area afflicted by plague.[70] The other, however, which is probably closer to popular Bengali Islamic culture and purports to be a history of the nation of demonic beings known as *djinns*, showed remarkable similarity with the views espoused by Vivekananda. This latter text mentioned that the plague is the work of *djinns* and, hence, all true Mussalmans ought to see it as a *jihad*. Serving and caring for those afflicted by the plague, therefore, is a religious duty and even death in its pursuance will be regarded as martyrdom. On the other hand, he who leaves the area blighted by the plague will be considered to be in breach of his religious duty and having fled from a *jihad*.[71] In the absence of clear documentary evidence however, such tantalizing parallels within the popular Islamic tradition would have to remain merely a strong possibility.

It is not our intention here to argue for a causal relation between Vivekananda's work and writings and those of Bengali medical authors. In the absence of detailed biographic information on many of these early doctors, such a claim can hardly be made. However, what we have been trying to describe is the way in which the Bengali response to the plague cannot be understood in terms of a simple Power-versus-Resistance paradigm. It involves a much more complex process of cultural translation of medical modernity. This process of vernacularization is, moreover, not limited to physicians alone; influential cultural and religious leaders also actively participated in this project. This widening of the social and professional groups engaged in the process of translation also leads to a much more complicated location of medical authority. It does not derive solely from the state. This is a crucial and important point. Because of the close relationship that has hitherto been documented between public health and the state in colonial medicine, the latter's authority has been seen to derive principally from the state. Even studies of 'Indianization', therefore, stress the process of taking over of the state apparatus by allopathically trained doctors in the twentieth century. However, this cannot totally explain the huge cultural legitimacy and authority that allopathic medicine has since come to acquire amongst certain sections of the postcolonial population.

Cleanliness Drives and *Bhodrolok* Authority

Sudipta Kaviraj and Dipesh Chakrabarty have both attempted to relate issues of garbage and filth disposal to the changing forms of state power.[72] Chakrabarty has argued that the flow of garbage was a process of performatively enacting the boundaries between the inside and the outside. The outside was always seen as a threatening space where transactions had to be controlled within familiar social ties established through patterned linguistic incorporations into fictive kinship relationships or through appeals to supernatural forces. The obligations that the colonial and, later, the national state, sought to impose upon this threatening open space, thereby seeking to tame it have, in Chakrabarty's reckoning, largely been rejected. The acceptance of mutual obligations that could make this 'open space' safer, without the necessary social mediation, would effectively transform them into 'public spaces' and validate the state as the sole arbiter of these norms. But that, Chakrabarty points out, has not happened. However, in the time of the Calcutta plague, the modern state was not the only candidate for wielding modernist authority on 'public spaces'. The voluntarist movement sought to create a different location as well as idiom of modernity. This modernity was aligned to the older language of appeal to supernatural forces (worship of Kali, the destruction of *Raktabij*, etc.) and sought to work within an affective domain of love and caring. Its logic did not derive, ostensibly, from the pursuit of power for power's sake, but flowed out of love and concern for one's own. Ralph Nicholas and Ronald Inden have argued that the Bengali kinship network operates along a notion of 'love'—not surprisingly, the precise word repeatedly used by Vivekananda to define the relationship of his volunteers and their patients. This Bengali notion of 'love', Nicholas and Inden add, 'causes them [those within the kinship group] to desire one another's well-being *(mangal, kalyan)* and to obtain it by selflessly "caring for" (*palan*), nourishing (*poshan*) and supporting (*bharan*) one another. Following this code of conduct, kinsmen are thought to retain their solidarity with one another and therefore attain pleasure, delight and gratification *(ananda, tripti, santosh)*'.[73] Much of the plague rhetoric was couched explicitly in this idiom of familial love and kinship solidarity.

The difficulty in seeking to apply too strict a binarism between state and Civil Society is that is often obscures from view other locations of power, particularly in societies that traditionally have operated upon multiple rationalities organized in multiple idioms around multiple forms of solidarities. The family is one such important form of solidarity with its own affective logic. The common image-world of both our *daktars* and Vivekananda's volunteers often drew, extended and operationalized this affective domain of the family.

Inscribing the community within an affective domain does not imply equality in any respect. As any one conversant with the Bengali family would know, they are notoriously hierarchic, and seldom is there any question of equality. While the solidarity is governed by a logic of love and mutual obligations, these obligations themselves are structured along stringent hierarchies of gender, age, etc. Thus, when the affective logic of the family was sought to be extended, its hierarchic dimensions were as crucial as its idiom of mutual support, caring, nourishing, etc. The hierarchies are clearly brought out in a little-known but important text in the medical history of Calcutta from the early 1890s. The *Munisipal Darpan*, written by the Medical Inspector and Professor of Sanitary Science at the Calcutta Medical School, Dr Sundarimohan Das, MB, on the request of his superior, Dr W. J. Simpson, was an attempt to translate the vexatious aspects of municipal sanitation into an idiom recognizable by the townspeople.[74] The *Darpan*, which borrowed a popular generic form and was organized around a series of twelve scenes, provides interesting reading for anyone seeking to understand the process of vernacularization of 'western' medicine in Bengal. Every scene is structurally almost identical. It begins with somebody lamenting or cursing the municipality/government (which, by the way, is still referred to as the 'Company'). Thereupon enters the enlightened Rameshbabu who works in the municipality and takes it upon himself to point out the wisdom of the municipal regulations to all who would listen. He then gives a detailed account of the exact regulations on the matter at hand and the scene concludes with everyone acknowledging the magnanimity and wisdom of the 'Company'. What is interesting here is that in every case, Rameshbabu is either a friend or a relative or an acquaintance of the people concerned; at the very least, he establishes a fictive kinship tie by addressing a stranger as his 'elder sister'. Following Chakrabarty, we can see how this is very similar to the way in which transactions in the *bazaar* are made less threatening through fictive or real kinship ties. Even the white doctor is shown to be thwarted by the obdurate Bengali householder until Ramesh intervenes. Clearly, medicine can only be 'translated' by Dr Das by creating a fictive Ramesh who can vernacularize Simpson's good intentions within an acceptable affective domain. However, equally visible is the stark inequality of Ramesh's enterprise. Not only is it to be witnessed in the modes of address he uses towards subaltern interlocutors such as Dukhi, the washerman, or the eponymous Jeleni (woman who sells fish), but also in the content of his message itself. When the fishmonger tells him that she has had to borrow money at a high rate of interest to buy the fish and if it is taken away by health inspectors it would ruin her, he simply tells her that while that may be so, stale fish can endanger several lives and hence needs to be confiscated. He does not even spare a kind word for her plight. Similarly, while speaking to Dukhi, he mentions how Baburam, the washerman's son, had turned up for work despite suffering from cholera. This apparently had led to Nilubabu's ten-month-old son contracting the disease and dying. 'Even hanging such washermen like Baburam's son would not be enough punishment!' ends an irate Ramesh. There is not a word for the plight of the young boy who had to still work for a living while suffering from cholera. Clearly, people like Dukhi are within the affective domain and are seen as family dependants, but there is no question of equality.

This personal affective dimension, which is seen to be the crucial ingredient that is lacking in the measures undertaken by the public health authorities, is most clearly spelt out in Dr Basu's voluminous and often seemingly contradictory work as well. Time and again, Dr Basu highlighted the importance of the actual people who implemented the policies of the government, their personal ties and compassion. He even identified a few isolated British officials whom he found particularly compassionate and held them up as the ideals through whom the allopathic treatment of plague could succeed. In effect, these few compassionate officials turn out to be those who had closely identified with the *bhodrolok* opinion or, indeed, had been personally close to the author himself. While almost the entirety of the colonial establishment is passionately denounced for its lack of emotional attachment to its citizens, a few isolated Europeans, such as Dr Evans, Sir John Woodbarron, Lt Col Dr Sweeney, etc., are praised profusely.[75] The linchpin of their compassion, however, is always proximity to either the *bhodrolok* opinion or, indeed, to individual representatives of the *bhodrolok*. Their claims of medical prowess and praise are based, therefore, not upon their medical skill per se, but rather upon their emotional attachment and support of the *bhodrolok*.

The translation of plague medicine—in order to be successful—must be relocated within an affective domain structured according to the affective logic of a Bengali family, with the *bhodrolok* occupying the position of head of the family. Power, underwritten by sanitary modernity itself, is therefore not rejected. What is rejected is the anonymized, bureaucratic location where this power is inscribed. From the closing decades of the nineteenth century, the *bhodrolok* had increasingly come to be socially marginalized in its very bastion—Calcutta—through the influx of numerous non-Bengali communities and the increasing commercialization of the agriculture.[76] In the absence of any political power and their persistent inability to articulate a politically significant regional/Bengali nationalism (as opposed to a nationalism which constantly slipped between larger Indian, Hindu and, lastly, Bengali nationalism) meant that the only way to seek to resist their social superiority was to recast it as something other than power: to cast it as 'loving care' of an extended family which included everybody.

In marking out his disagreement with Partha Chatterjee's earlier formulation, Vinayak Chaturvedi has argued that the nationalist elite had 'accepted the coming of the modern state, not as a form of surrender, but as an opportunity to continue dominating…within the postcolonial nation'.[77] This is as true for the *bhodrolok* as it is for Chaturvedi's *Patidars*. However, the exact idiom in which this relationship of domination is phrased also needs specific investigation, for in it lies locked the particulars of the distinct regional modernities that mark the nationalist consciousness. The specific idioms also constitute the forms of citizen subjectivities that inhabit the modern state. In this case, those who are seen to be the citizens of the modern state understand and articulate their own relationship with it in terms of an affective domain of familial sociality. Their relationship to their subalterns cannot be understood solely through a logic of power, though power and authority are, of course, elements in the familial domain as well. Like Gandhi's *Patidar* compatriots, the *bhodrolok* disciples of Vivekananda would perhaps never have accepted that they even secretly wished to wield power over their subalterns. The difference is that the latter might actually have been telling the truth. Yet, the irony was that their 'loving care' was no less 'domination' than, say, that of a dominating father's concern for his prodigal daughter! Sincere altruism, unfortunately, is often much more ruthless and brutal than Machiavellian power-seeking.[78]

Plague and Folk-Healing

The enormity of the plague paranoia meant that it was not limited to the *bhodrolok* alone. Our *bhodrolok* authors and their projects of reform and sanitation projected the subaltern classes in various ways as insanitary, dirty wretches in need of control or sanitary salvation. Occasionally, they were also seen to be gullible dupes peddling rumours like that of a 'plague car' with poisonous walls that the government used to kill hapless victims.[79] Hardly any records are available of how they sought to tackle the affliction as a health problem.

One way of recovering the subaltern medical responses from the *bhodrolok* sources is to look at those cures which are coded as 'folk' remedies (*totka*, *tuno*, etc.). With the development of the Bengali medical public sphere from the late nineteenth century, there was an ever-increasing attempt to appropriate the medical knowledge base of the subaltern orders (this included medical knowledge traditionally possessed by women of the family, i.e., grandmother's remedies).[80] Regular columns or essays appeared on the subject in most of the medical periodicals. Occasionally, pamphlets and tracts on the subject also appeared. Thus, while textually derived elite 'indigenous' medicine became coded as 'classical' ayurveda, there also emerged the category of 'folk medicine' within the Bengali medical public sphere.

The *Chikitsak* published from Rajshahi mentioned a few such folk remedies from the region. These remedies, even in the truncated anecdotal forms in which they appeared in print, provided interesting insights into the logic of popular or subaltern medical ideas. They also dispelled any notions of the 'folk' as a realm of 'pure' premodern wisdom. Surveying the cures clearly shows how 'folk medicine' appropriated new objects and things within its own logic in an attempt to find an accessible cure for a perceived medical crisis. Lakshminarayan Mallick, for instance, contributed a set of remedies based upon the central ingredient of bovine urine. He mentioned that drinking half a cup of cow's urine daily prevented plague. An afflicted patient could be similarly cured through the application on the buboes of a mixture of soil and cow's urine taken from the cowshed. A serious patient was also to be made to drink the urine at regular intervals. If the patient was too ill to drink, the urine was to be massaged all over the body. Significantly, the urine of the cow is sometimes used in traditional Hindu rituals (particularly in purificatory rituals)—as are most other parts of the cow—and the belief may have been connected to such practice. But another cure recommended by one Pandit Sankarnath used ingredients that were clearly of a recent vintage. He said drinking lemonade daily, or at least a sherbet made from lime juice, would prevent plague. Moreover, in a passage reminiscent of numerologically coded texts on pulse diagnosis known to be popular in the area, he said that various mixtures of carbolic and sulphuric acids and water were affective against the plague. A 1 per cent solution of carbolic acid and water, he claimed, killed the plague germs in ten minutes. A 1/2000th solution of sulphuric acid killed them in five minutes. Finally, a 1/100th solution of sulphuric acid killed the germs immediately. Significantly, he used the English terms for 'lemonade', 'carbolic acid' and 'sulphuric acid'.[81]

Another undated, cheap low-brow text published from Calcutta dealing with magical spells and herbal remedies mentioned that the application of a paste made of crushed spinach leaves (*pnui shaak-er pata*) and the leaves of a variety of pond algae (*jol keuteh sheola-r pata*) on the armpits and the groin prevents plague. It was also said to be effective against the 'fear of plague' and could allegedly also cure those who are already afflicted.[82]

Stanley Tambiah has argued against seeing ritualized or 'magical' healing practices as arising out of the 'ignorance' of 'simple' or 'primitive' people. He suggests, instead, that these practices be judged in terms of their own logic. This logic, argues Tambiah, operates on two axes. First, metaphorically it makes abstract comparisons equating one thing to another, and second, it metonymically reduces an object to what is believed to be its constituent parts. A combination of these two holds the clue to unravelling the logic that determines what looks like senseless practice to us. However, in order to understand this operative logic it needs to be understood within the totality of the experiential context of the community which uses it. Moreover, Tambiah further suggests, the failure to see how two things that might be seen to be equivalent within the logic expressed by the healing ritual might actually be an artefact of the observer's own cultural blind spot.[83] The societies that we inhabit today have—under the impulse of capitalism—undergone a significant segmentation of social labour and the attendant production processes. This parcellization of our experiential world makes it impossible for us to comprehend the associations that might be made by societies whose experiential domains were significantly less fragmented.

In the absence of more detailed information about the contexts in which these remedies were developed and used, it would be impossible to seek to reconstruct the logic which informed them. However, some provisional conclusions might yet be drawn from them. The *pnui shak*, or spinach and algae, both formed precious sources of nutrition for the Bengali rural poor. Tarashankar Bandopadhyay's famous novel *Hnashuli Bnaker Upakatha*, based on a marginal Bengali rural community called the Kahars in the early twentieth century, mentions that their staple food was spinach growing in the corners of their houses and snails they caught at the local ponds.[84] The Rev. Lal Behari Dey's English novel *Bengal Peasant Life* also mentions the centrality of spinach in the diet of the Bengal peasantry. Though algae are not explicitly mentioned, *The Cambridge World History of Food* mentions that algae is one of the most easily available sources of nutrition worldwide, and was extensively used by the poor across the globe with textual references from neighbouring China, Southeast Asia and further afield in Japan, dating from over a thousand years ago.[85] Bengal's long-standing connections with Southeast Asia through the Bay of Bengal, and Tibet and China through the northern passes of Sikkim and Bhutan, are often ignored while studying Bengal as an extension of South Asia alone. There is no reason therefore to believe that the region was not influenced by its East and Southeast Asian neighbours as well. In any case, whatever the sources of the practice, the use of cheap and easily available foods like spinach and algae must have been heightened during the famine and food scarcities of 1897. The role of these two food sources as agents for the preservation of the lives of the rural poor in times of hardship and crisis clearly lent them to being seen in the same light at the time of the plague crisis.

In this, then—despite the *bhodrolok*'s own disinclination to see the symmetries—the basic logic of the healing remedies of the poor were not very different from that of the *bhodrolok*'s. It sought to promote the body's powers to combat the contagion by promoting what it knew to be life-preserving foods.

The two other sets of remedies recommended by Pandit Sankarnath and Lakshminarayan Mullick also have their own internal logic. However, that they were reported in the polite press and not published in the world of lowbrow print also hints at further refractions of these remedies through polite conventions Mullick's advocacy of cow's urine is an interesting aspect through which to explore both the logic that informed the creation of such a remedy as well as its polite narrative refractions through which it has become available to the historian. Cow's urine had traditionally been used in orthodox Bengali Hindu rituals as a purifier of sins. Its associations with purifying the body in a more literal sense were therefore not surprising. Moreover, it was also used in ayurvedic medicine and must therefore have been known or believed to have some medicinal properties. Traditionally, ayurvedic literature prescribes its usage in conjunction with several other ingredients in cases of

Slipada—an affliction caused by the dampness of the air in the vicinity of ponds and lakes and causing, amongst other symptoms, the swelling of the groin. Both the ritual and ayurvedic uses of bovine urine may have encouraged its associations with, the plague.[86] Though the learned *kavirajes* tended to relate plague to *Baghi* or *Bradhna*, in the popular mind, any disease with similar symptoms or alleged causes may have become associated with it, and by a classic demonstration of the dual process of abstract equation and metonymic truncation, the most easily accessible ingredient of the medicines used for *Slipada* may have come to be associated with the cure for the plague.[87] However, while multiple sources of cultural aura of bovine urine as a healing substance cannot be ruled out, its precise form of usage bears striking resemblance to shamanic magico-religious healing practices of heterodox peasant religions in Bengal. Anwarul Karim's vastly informed anthropological study of Bengali shamanism points out that the use of urine in general is quite common in Bengali shamanic magico-religious healing. Some of the uses observed by Karim are strikingly reminiscent of the plague cures we have met with. In the case of a patient suffering from severe headaches, Karim observed the shaman first uttering a chant:

> In the name of Allah-Hari!
> Oh Mother Earth!
> You are my mother; I am your son.
> Whatever you may do, Mother, do as you like. You are my mother, truly

Thereafter, writes Karim, 'the shaman…used sticky soil soaked by urine and rubbed the affected part of the body of the patient. After some time, the patient was cured of his headache'.[88] The whole process of applying a paste made of urine and soil upon the affected parts of the body is clearly reminiscent of Mullick's plague cure. Mullick's recommendations of the ingestion of cow's urine, too, had shamanic parallels. Once again, Karim observed fakirs drinking urine and intoning the following chant to cure stomach pains:

> Guru is True!
> Thakur is True!
> Hari is True!
> Your body is rid of the disease!

Once again, the practice, without the chants, which may not have been reported in the *bhodrolok* press, is strikingly similar. The only difference lay in the displacement of human urine by cow's urine. Karim mentions that the use of urine to cure was mainly practised by the heterodox peasant religions of the *Bauls* and *Fakirs*. These religions and their practitioners were usually frowned upon by orthodox Hindu and Islamic Bengali society. One of the reasons for the disgust they evoked in orthodox circles was their usage of human excreta and sexual fluids in their rituals. The use of these substances marked their symbolic inversion of elite/orthodox mores. Most of these religions denied the orthodox gods and sought to find God in the very corporeality of the body that the orthodoxy saw as an impediment to fulfilling spiritual life. To reappropriate their practice within a polite narrative and cultural economy therefore necessitated a critical renegotiation of these elements of conspicuous subaltern difference. Mullick's cures, therefore, succeeded in effecting this renegotiation by displacing the *Fakir*'s markers of difference from the human body to the body of the cow—an animal redolent in its associations with the orthodox Hindu sacral symbology.

The power of lemonade, carbolic and sulphuric acids, on the other hand, may have been seen to lie precisely in their novelty. The use of English names suggests their exoticness in the popular context, and it may have thus come to be related to the new disease that, too, was seen to be an exotic phenomenon. Carbolic acid may already have been encountered though the government's attempts to control the cattle plagues in the 1860s.[89] Its association with lemonade and sulphuric acid arises, perhaps, from the sour taste that each of these have. 'Indigenous' ideas about the nature and curative power of substances was organized according to the dominant taste of the substances. Regionally popular texts such as the *Rajballabhiya Drabyagun* written in the late medieval period had attempted to codify these ideas. The belief that sour or lemony things cured digestive complaints was also common and are occasionally also found amongst *bhodrolok* authors. By 1890s that such ideas were being used even by *daktars* can be seen in their writings on cholera. The popular mind may thus have made a similar association between lemonade, carbolic and sulphuric acids and taken it to be an effective cure. Their association may also have arisen from their being introduced into the region at the same time and perhaps by similar people. Whatever their individual histories, it is clear that the 'folk remedies' for plague were not the simple knee-jerk reaction of hapless, ignorant people at a time of crisis.

Conclusion

The binary framing of the history of the plague as a moment of colonial imposition and 'indigenous' resistance is clearly limited. The epidemic was also an impetus for the rapid vernacularization of 'western' medicine in colonial

Bengal. The work of this translation was not limited to *daktars* alone and involved a range of other actors as well. While cultural ideologues such as Vivekananda actively emerged at the forefront of such vernacularization, the *daktars*, too, utilized a range of intellectual, political and narrative resources which went beyond strictly medical registers.

The process of vernacularization, moreover, connected and renegotiated the relationships between many distinct chains of signification. Not only was the relationship between religion and medicine remapped in the wake of these renegotiations, but, indeed, new identities and visions were produced. A particular and peculiarly neo-Hindu blueprint of a society organized around a logic of one extended family became the template on which both religion and medicine could now be defined.

Other chains of signification such as the market, however, did not always become completely subsumed by this template. While certain aspects of the 'folk' practices that were part of neither the neo-Hindu self nor its clear Other were indeed disciplined into a closer conformity through the censorial mechanisms of the popular press, other undisciplined possibilities continued to poach on the opportunities of the market in low-medical print by publishing manuals of magic spells, prophetic healing and self-diagnostic domestic remedies.

Chapter V

ENDEMIC COMMERCE: CHOLERA AND THE MEDICAL MARKET

The existing rich historiography on cholera in India can be divided into three distinct, albeit occasionally overlapping, strands. David Arnold has looked at how cholera was seen as a disease connected to disorderly crowds. His work has analysed the role of cholera in the imperial British-Indian state's efforts to 'control' spaces where large numbers of Indians gathered.[1] Harrison's account of cholera, though also interested in issues of 'control', gives greater weight to the numerous internal tensions within the Anglo–Indian medical ureaucracy in speaking and writing about cholera. He gives particularly detailed descriptions of the varied positions maintained by different authorities on the question of the transmission of cholera. Harrison also points out how, being closely implicated in imperial politics, the eventual triumph of any one of these many views depended largely upon political considerations.[2] Dhrub Kumar Singh uses a very similar approach to accent the difference in the medical response to cholera in Britain and India.[3] Apart from these two major strands accenting, respectively, the politics of control and the politics of translating heterogeneous medical opinion to medical policy, a third strand investigates the demographic impact of cholera. Ira Klein's work is particularly significant in this regard.[4] The scope of each of these studies reflects the massive administrative importance that a deadly endemic such as cholera had. Each of these studies draws upon administrative archives of the colonial government and therefore critically reflects the major concerns of those who compiled that archive.

As a longstanding affliction and one causing massive destruction, the disease has left its traces in other archives as well. The experience of suffering, not as an administrative disorder, as a matter of public health policy or as statistical demography, but as a personal crisis can be found in numerous nongovernmental archives. Literary accounts, personal memories, healing treatises, etc., abound that frame the disease as an extremely personalized, human crisis shared by many in the region. The Bengali *daktars* who treated cholera patients had to work within this milieu. Their writings were shaped by their own position within this very different archival framework.

This chapter looks primarily at how the Bengali *daktars* fashioned their own distinctive discourse and practice around cholera. Since the *daktars* worked within an extremely competitive medical market for cholera cures, the chapter also looks at some of the other healing options that competed with *daktari* medicine.[5] Instead of drawing a clear line between the 'rational'/'medical' cures offered in this market and the 'irrational'/'magical' cures, this chapter seeks to understand the different logics and rationalities which shaped the varied understandings and cures of cholera.

Origins of the Bengali Discourse

The scale and rapidity of what was then believed to be the first outbreak of cholera in 1817 caught the British government totally off guard. In the ensuing panic, matters of disciplinary or racial boundaries—which in any case were yet to crystallize—seemed to temporarily count for less than trying to bring the disease under control. The government began to encourage any form of treatment and sought to build up an archive on the subject at the same time. Apart from seeking information from its own doctors, it also urged the district magistrates to encourage 'indigenous' healers to contribute to the effort. They were urged to not only treat cholera patients, but also to write down detailed descriptions of the disease along with what courses of treatment they had followed. These were to eventually be forwarded to the Medical Board through the district magistrates who in turn would reimburse and reward the physicians for their efforts.[6] Even the secretary of the Medical Board, James Johnson, included inputs from the local physicians into his authoritative views on the disease.[7] In many cases, 'indigenous' physicians were also taken directly into government employ. The terms of employment, however, varied widely and while in some cases they were given a fixed monthly salary for the period of their employment, usually at the rate of Rs 8/- per month, in other cases they were paid according to the number of cases cured, i.e., at a rate of two annas per cured case.[8] This gave the Kavirajes not only a widespread familiarity with the disease, but also a direct cause to write about it, since they had to submit reports to the district magistrates stating the numbers of cases treated and the course of treatment followed. Some of these physicians proved extremely successful. Nausher Kaviraj, for example, cured 85 of the 109 patients he treated. Bykuntha Kaviraj cured 97 of his 150 patients. And Ramjoy Kaviraj cured 98 of his 148 patients. Some of the more successful ones such as Tincowrie Kaviraj, Kamal Kaviraj and Gobinda Kaviraj were also temporarily deputed to other areas beyond their usual sphere of activity.[9] Their modes of treatment, however, did not derive solely from 'indigenous' sources. The School Book Society tract which gave a summary of the treatment methods compiled from the writings of these early Bengali cholera specialists showed that 'traditional' remedies such as mixtures of opium, camphor and black pepper were being used side-by-side with clearly nontraditional remedial measures, such as giving the patient peppermint or brandy, and even bleeding them in some cases.[10] Seema Alavi has rightly pointed out that '[m]anaging of the cholera epidemic and the inoculation drive created a shared but often contested public health space in which British doctors and Hindustani [and Bengali] healers came together to share their medical practice…'[11]. Though this experiment in using 'indigenous' physicians as a matter of policy proved short-lived, it did set a tradition for Bengali writing on the disease. Further, as we have mentioned in Chapter I, the practice of employing 'locally entertained native doctors' during cholera outbreaks as a popular ad hoc measure continued right up to the twentieth century. In fact, as late as 1913 we still find occasional references to local medical practitioners being temporarily appointed at times of cholera epidemics.[12] Even when such local practitioners were not given government employment, they were often given subsidies. Babu Panna Lal, a 'medical practitioner', was, in 1903, reimbursed his travelling costs for travelling to Champaran during a cholera epidemic even without being actually given an appointment.[13] Naturally, this promoted an expectation amongst local medical practitioners that, should they be able to prove their medical practice in an area, they might receive support from the government. This expectation can be seen in the petitions sent by the local practitioners asking for support.[14] Taraprasad Sarkar, for example, petitioned the government in 1913, asking for medicines to help him treat a local epidemic.[15] This tradition of employment, and even wider expectation of such, might have done much to encourage numerous Bengali physicians to write down their treatments of the disease. Alavi, in fact, mentions the continual institutional instigation to British doctors to produce texts. Especially in the case of cholera—a disease particularly identified with India—British doctors could often use their Indian experience and the texts written about them to establish themselves as cholera authorities in metropolitan Britain.[16] James Adair Lawrie or Charles Turner Thackrah, for example, by the successful articulation of their Indian experience, emerged as 'experts' during the cholera outbreaks in Newcastle, Gateshead and Tyneside.[17] Such practices may, in turn, have inspired a degree of 'mimicry' amongst those such as Panna Lal or Taraprasad Sarkar who, while not employees of the state, did attempt to share some of its authority. Sarah Pinto, working on a later period, has called such people 'ersatz doctors'.[18] Pinto argues that such people, placed on the fringes of the state's medical apparatus, seek to tap into the aura of state-backed medical authority by performing certain acts associated putatively with state medical functionaries. The Bengali cholera narratives—especially in this early period—were produced both by direct state instigation and an urge to tap into this aura.[19]

The Bengali cholera narratives were qualitatively very different from their English counterparts. Most conspicuously, whereas the English writings tended to look upon cholera as a 'disease of disorder' and passionately debated its mode of communication, the Bengali writings used individual cases as their main focus. Until the middle of the 1920s, the use of statistics—a signature feature of the English writings—was minimal in Bengali.[20] Instead, a single case was described in great detail and within an overtly familial and emotional context. Anirban Das has pointed out that the use of medical statistics allows for the articulation of a *universal body*—where differences can be coded as divergence from a common norm; the tardy use of statistics, therefore, points to a recalcitrance in *daktari* practice towards the framing of an *universal body*.[21] The structural difference was factor of the distinct positions the *daktars* occupied in the economy of health. Whereas the *daktars* functioned either privately or very low in the government hierarchy—thereby lacking the resources to collect or use statistical data—those who wrote in English usually worked sufficiently high up the medical bureaucracy to have access to statistical datum. Spelling out this difference, Surgeon Major Hamilton wrote in 1885 that 'each local observer necessarily receives different impressions in accordance with facts that have come within his observation… In opposition to the local observers we have the statistician surveying the facts from a central office, comparing manifold observations…numbers, dates of attack, and progression…'.[22]

The dread disease, as noted by the English commentators as well, was especially feared because of its rapidity, its unexpectedness and its singularly undignified symptoms.[23] Doctors repeatedly noted how a patient who was happy and healthy in the morning could fall ill in the evening and be dead before the night was out. They also noted how, just when everyone had given up all hope, a patient could miraculously recover. One doctor went so far as to advise colleagues never to hazard a comment to the family about the patient's chances of recovery, for chances were, no matter what the prognosis, they might eventually be made to look a fool. There was also something singularly undignified and inhuman about the way the disease made one's will to live almost leak away.[24] Violent and increasingly involuntary evacuations accompanied by a deathly pallor and an eerily nasal voice signalled the workings of the fearful disease. The Bengali cholera narratives, like their English counterparts, while noting these aspects of the disease, also commented frequently upon the human suffering and the experience of these sufferings. Where the English narratives concentrated their medical gaze upon the patient's body, the Bengali narratives could not avoid being drawn into the familial affective domain within which the patient lay. Signalling perhaps the very different affective ties that Bengali physicians came to have with their patients, the doctors commented on the anxious queries of the husband of a patient, the heart-wrenching cries of a bereaved father and the hopeful prayers of an afflicted mother's son. One particularly heart-rending episode is reported by Dr D. N. Chattopadhyay.[25] In writing an extended essay on the disease, he recalls a case in Rangpur. He had been visiting the local landlord during *Durga Puja*, the Bengali autumnal festival. Towards the end of the five-day festival, cholera cases started breaking out in the village. Arnold has pointed out that the disease was preeminently depicted by the commentators writing in English as a 'disease of disorder' that often arose where there were fairs or festivals and hence big crowds. Dr Chattopadhyay, however, does not comment on the crowds or the festival or, indeed, the disorder. Instead, he organizes his narrative around the recollections of one particularly tragic case. A young wife had fallen ill and was in quite serious condition when he was called in. Once the diagnosis, which had already been guessed by the unhappy family, was confirmed, the young husband eagerly asked if he should send a telegram to his father-in-law in Calcutta advising him of the situation. This practice of sending telegrams to all one's near and dear ones as soon as cholera was confirmed seems to have been the norm even in the 1930s.[26] The premise presumably was that the chances of survival were so uncertain that all who might want to be with the patient, should she die, were given the best chance of getting there in time. Dr Chattopadhyay told the husband that the situation was pretty grim. Later that evening, the patient's distraught father arrived from Calcutta. As everyone busied themselves in caring for the young woman now at death's door, the father refused to eat, and sat and wept next to his daughter's sickbed. Dr Chattopadhyay could not but be moved by the sight. He tried to reason with the father in an effort to get him to eat something. Yet even after agreeing to eat, distracted as he was with grief, he was utterly unable to eat anything. Next day the daughter, almost miraculously, began to recover. But the family's joy was short-lived as, by the evening, the patient's father had come down with the disease. While the daughter's recovery continued steadily now, the father rapidly deteriorated and was dead in less than a day. The human tragedy of the narrative is not unique to Chattopadhyay's essay and is often seen in many other Bengali cholera narratives.

Comparing these with the English case histories of cholera patients amply brings out the difference. The English cases give the bare minimum of details about the patient's background. Only the name (that, too, sometimes reduced to mere initials), age, caste/religion and occupation are given. There is absolutely no mention of the patient's extended family.[27] Thereafter, times, dates, mode of treatment and the patient's response to it are presented in disjointed staccato prose. This becomes even more striking once we remember that the case history as a genre was devoted to only dealing with a single case, whereas the Bengali texts are more like essays and introduce the individual cases anecdotally. It would seem more likely that the genre more exclusively devoted to dealing with particularities—in this case, the case histories—would be better placed to introduce biographic details. The case history as a genre was popularized amongst English physicians in the eighteenth century by authors such as Sir John Floyer.[28] The eighteenth century popularization was, moreover, selective. As Christina Alvarez Millan has pointed out, both Galen and Hippocrates had supplied earlier models for the genre, but the eighteenth-century writers preferred the Hippocratic model which was thought to be more 'objective' than the Galenic model.[29] There is enough evidence to suggest that the genre was used by British physicians in India. John Peter Wade, for instance, published many case histories that he had maintained during his practice in India.[30] Indians who came into contact with English medicine would have been exposed to the genre. The very first modern case histories written by an Indian appeared in late eighteenth century and were written by Athar Ali Khan in English.[31] Yet, there seems to be no clear parallel genre in Bengali medical writing. When discussions of individual cases exist—as they do most prominently in the cholera cases—they are immersed within larger treatises and describe the patient within an affective network rather than as a mere biological entity. Harriet Nowel-Smith argues that case histories actually contribute to the objectification of the patient, and it might well be possible to read this *daktari* recalcitrance to writing case histories as growing out of a context in which the doctor–patient relation itself was less objectifying than that which existed between a British doctor and his Bengali patient.[32] It is perfectly plausible to contend that, given the relations of power as well as linguistic difficulties, the relationship between a British doctor and his Bengali patient would be more distant than that between a *daktar* and his Bengali patient. Bengali *daktars* lived, practised and treated their patients within an affective milieu and their writing reflected their position both in its logic and its form.

Dr Jadunath Mukherji's[33] compendious manual on cholera treatment also commenced with a case history framed by the anxieties of the patient's relatives.[34] Mukherji, in fact, went further and gave these affective ties a therapeutic value that in his view made the difference between life and death. When the elder brother of Dr Mukherji's patient asked him anxiously, 'Is there any chance of his surviving?', Dr Mukherji's immediate response was, 'that depends on how many people you can find who will care for him'. The brother eagerly said, 'if it'll make him live, the whole *para* [locality] shall be at your disposal'. Dr Mukherji went on to explain that the only way a cholera patient can pull through is if they receive continuous careful nursing. 'Thus', he wrote, 'whenever a physician is called in to see a cholera patient, the first question to ask is how many people do they have at the patient's disposal [*lok-bol kemon ache?*]'.[35] Anonymous jostling crowds of the English writers are replaced here with large affective networks and instead of causing the disease, it is this large gathering which will save the patient.

The language of the Bengali cholera narrative was often highly emotionalized, using rhetorical questions, onomatopoeic representations of the patient's distress, a generous helping of sentences ending in exclamations or dashes, etc. There was an almost total absence of statistics, precise dates, ages, etc., which were an integral part of the English cholera discourse. Moreover, the cases narrated were not only within a familial domain, but also—though cholera was often said to be indiscriminate in its choice of victims—the narratives tended to be almost exclusively focus on the death of younger members of the family. The grief of the elderly at the suffering of the young was thus seen to be even more poignant.

This curious selection of always describing young victims hints at the influence of Bengali literary conventions of the day on Bengali medical prose.[36] The lamentations of the bereaved parent for a child lost to cholera had come to encapsulate one of the most commonly found tragic-romantic tropes of Bengali literature of the time. Bengal's national poet, Rabindranath Tagore, who had himself had to haplessly watch his favourite son die of cholera, used the image several times. In his critically acclaimed novel *Gora*, two cholera deaths are mentioned and both are young boys at the height of their youth.[37] His short stories in *Galpaguchha* also mention parents, such as Anondi Boshtomi, who lost young children to cholera.[38] Given the immense influence of Tagore in the cultural landscape of Bengal in the early twentieth century, it would be very probable that our doctors would have been well aware of his works. Furthermore, the trope might not have originated with Tagore. It might have been much older. Tagore's friend, the historian Dinesh Chandra Sen, had argued that the Bengalis as a nation were singularly emotional. Significantly, to elucidate his point about the 'national emotionalism' of Bengalis, Sen used as an example a medieval legend that an actor playing the part of a father whose son had just been forced to leave home for fifteen years apparently got so involved in his role as a bereaved father that he actually died of grief![39] The ultimate trope of Bengali pathos was therefore the picture of a parent mourning the loss of his child.

The point is not to argue that the *daktars* were deliberately choosing to frame their narratives along the lines of Tagore's and Sen's. What we are arguing here is that the writings of the *daktars* are primarily narratives and, therefore, need to borrow from the narrative conventions of the time. These conventions, in turn, draw upon shared symbols, tropes, metaphors, i.e., historically shared ways of seeing and making sense of the world. Faced with the immensity of the human suffering of the patients and their families that the doctors were forced to deal with close at hand, a certain pathos informed their experience of the disease. Their narratives of the disease sought to express that pathos and, in so doing, borrowed commonly shared images of pathos from their shared cultural repertoire. The image of the suffering parent came to embody the sum of the pathos of the impact of cholera upon the affective domain.

Even the *Munisipal Darpan*, a drama written by a Bengali physician in government employ at the request of his British superiors to popularize ideas about sanitation, used the image of a father grieving for his dead infant to convey the depth of the tragedy and the extent of the blame of the person from whom the infection had spread.[40] By the 1920s, when the structure of the Bengali cholera discourse had begun to change significantly, it remained an article of faith amongst *daktars* that, 'cholera mainly strikes the youth'.[41]

From the mid-1920s we begin to find Bengali *daktars* occupying important bureaucratic positions continuing to write in Bengali.[42] These new *daktari* authors had access to statistical data and made some limited use of it. At the same time, new practices of combating cholera through techno-scientific strategies, such as vaccination, injections, etc., also contributed towards a greater objectification of the patient. (Fig. VIII.) Yet, the story of the heroic or tragic individual still found its way into *daktari* cholera narratives. Brojendranath Ganguly, for instance, narrated a tragic story of how in a village called Narayanpur a single man had refused—despite much persuasion—to take the cholera vaccine and how he alone had succumbed to the disease soon after.[43] Heroically, Chunilal Basu mentioned how an unnamed lawyer in Basirhat had read his book and then personally gone around the village explaining to villagers how to protect themselves from cholera and how, as a consequence of one man's efforts, the villagers had been saved.[44] Albeit these stories are very different from the previous stories of individual suffering—they may even be apocryphal—but they retain the structure of the narrative as one centred on a single 'hero' and his/her troubles and efforts. In so much it is structurally akin to a novel.[45]

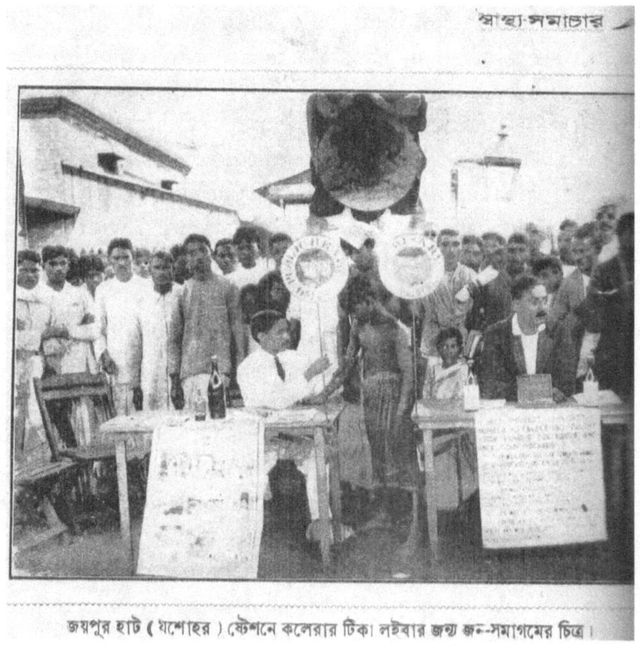

Fig. VIII. "Jaipur Hat (Jessore) Station-e Kolerar Tika Laibar Janya Janasamagamer Chitra" (A Picture of the crowd gathered to receive vaccination against Cholera at the Jaipur Hat Station in Jessore), *Swasthya Samachar* 17, no. 2 (1928): Unnumbered page.

Naming the Disease

Unlike diseases like the plague, which had come to be identified overwhelmingly with 'modern' western categories, cholera was often sought to be connected to older social memories of other afflictions and thereby older 'indigenous' names. The very first vernacular tract on the disease, printed by the School Book Society and written by Peter Breton, commenced, therefore, by establishing a long list of linguistic equivalences.[46] The opening lines of Breton's tract introduced the disease by saying that 'This is that disease which is known as *Cholera Morbus* in Latin, *Hayja* in Arabic, *Thchbala* in Persian, *Ukal—Pukhal* in Hindustani, *Bishuchika* in Sanskrit and *Olautha* in Bengali…'[47]. These various names, however, did not always refer to the same disease. Jagannarayan Mukhopadhyay's early Bengali dictionary, published in 1838, still referred to *Bishuchika* as either a name given to 'symptoms of diseases' (*upasarga*) or constipation, whereas *Olautha* was identified with another category, '*Naamutha*' and signalled by the symptom of acute diarrhoea.[48] The earlier Bengali–English dictionary of Rev. William Morton had also followed a similar format, identifying *Bishuchika* with 'symptoms' in general and *Olautha* with *Naamutha*. Additionally however, Rev. Morton had identified *Naamutha/Olautha* with 'cholera'. Yet, he did not relate this to *Bishuchika*.[49] The even earlier 'vocabulary' of HP Forster, published at the turn of the nineteenth century, described *Olautha* as 'Flux attended with vomiting', while *Bishuchika* was wholly absent.[50] Breton's equation therefore was clearly not universal.[51]

When writing about the disease thus, the first decision that confronted the physician-authors was which name to use. Though these reasons were not always clearly stated, they can easily be inferred by looking closely at the text as well as the professional identity of the physician-author. Since each of the names evoked particular social and professional memories and associations, when called upon to choose or relate these names to each other, the physician-authors had to reconcile these complex and distinct memories within a particular vision of society and medicine. The choice of names thus, in itself, becomes a window into the professional and social politics that framed the disease in a particular author's writings.[52]

Dr Kunjabihari Das, for instance, denied the existence of the disease in lower Bengal before the onset of colonial rule. He argued that the affliction had been introduced into Bengal by Lord Hastings' troops who had acquired it while fighting the Marathas in the 'valley of the Indus'.[53] Das, therefore, could not accept the name '*olautha*', as it would acknowledge a long popular memory of the disease. However, accepting the term 'cholera' would also place him at a disadvantage, as it would mean that the European representations of the disease, which he now sought to challenge, were more valid by virtue of their longer acquaintance with the disease. He therefore chose to use the Sanskritized term, '*bishuchika*'. This allowed him to argue at one and the same time that the disease was not prevalent in precolonial lower Bengal and that it was well-known to the ancient Sanskrit authors writing in other parts of India. This manoeuvre also positioned him ideally as far as treating it was concerned, since he had access to both Sanskrit wisdom and European medical theory. The significance of Das' text lies in his paradoxical urge to, on the one hand, deny the stigma that Bengal was the deadly cradle of cholera, while on the other hand, try to argue that his unique professional identity made him better equipped to deal with cholera than his European peers. Das' text is also significant, since Mukherji's before him had grappled with the same paradox. Mukherji, too, had proposed that his own identity as a Bengali *daktar* gave him unique opportunities for treating and understanding the disease. He chastised those who 'neither consulted the latest European works, nor the ancient Sanskrit classics'.[54] Making the centrality of professional politics in cholera narratives clear, Mukherji added that it was because of the lack of guaranteed success in cholera cases that 'real' doctors and quacks could not be told apart by the public. The only way doctors would achieve their due status in society, he felt, was through the successful treatment of cholera. Like Drs Das and Mukherji, another cholera author, Dr Mitra, also chose to use 'cholera' and '*bishuchika*' as his designations of choice. However, in Dr Mitra's writings, '*bishuchika*' appears only rarely and cholera is by far the term of preference. In terms of Mitra's professional identity, it is significant that he had what was still considered a rare privilege for a Bengali—a European medical education. He amply displayed his European credentials by littering his text with innumerable quotes from contemporary European doctors and scientists. Moreau, Koch, Kuhane, Sedgwick and many others were mentioned, even to the point of distracting from the piece itself. Yet, within this highly Europeanised framework, too, the sparse mention of '*bishuchika*' allowed Mitra to lay claim to the classical Sanskritic heritage which made him stand apart from the luminaries he quoted by giving him a special professional advantage.

By contrast, an anonymous essay, which sought to argue for the spontaneous generation of cholera germs in certain specific villages in the vicinity of Bahrampur, used the designations '*olautha*' and 'cholera', ignoring the term '*bishuchika*' completely. Once again, however, the choice makes perfect sense in terms of the professional politics of the text. The author sought to use his in-depth local knowledge—to display it, he gave detailed descriptions of individual cases, including the victims' habits, their lives and even the internal organizations of their houses—to demolish the established allopathic theories of cholera-transmission. Since the text claimed to base itself on the long local memory of the disease, *olautha*—the popular designation—was indispensable to the logic of the text.[55] Similarly, Chattopadhyay used both designations, 'cholera' and '*olautha*'. Predictably, the twin axes he based his professional claims on were, respectively, prolonged acquaintance with Santhali ideas of the disease through practice in the tribal areas and his acquaintance with the *daktari* tradition.[56]

Authors continued throughout the nineteenth and into the twentieth century to disagree on which names could and which could not be equated with cholera. In 1880 Radhagobinda Kar's *Bhisak Suhrid* described his chapter on the disease as '*bishuchika ba olautha*'.[57] In 1885 the first Bengali encyclopaedia published by Rangalal Mukhopadhyay and Trailakyanath Mukhopadhyay categorically stated that *bishuchika* was not the same as cholera.[58] Yet, when Professor Ramendrasundar Tribedi, an eminent scientist and essayist, sought to produce a Bengali scientific vocabulary as part of a project undertaken by the *Bangiya Sahitya Parishad* (an influential Bengali association of men of letters), he exclusively used the word '*bishuchika*' as the Bengali word for '*cholera morbus*'.[59] Leaving little doubt that the decision to exclude other names such as *olautha* was a deliberate choice, Tribedi mentioned that he had used a copy of Breton's vocabulary as his starting point.[60]

Kaviraj Prasannachandra Maitreya, on the other hand, used the term '*olautha*' almost exclusively and avoided the term 'cholera'. He commenced the first instalment of his serialized essay by attacking the 'modern trend' of being fascinated by the 'western sciences' and ignoring the great wisdom of India's past, before going on to attack those who claimed that nothing about *olautha* had been mentioned in the ancient ayurvedic lore. However, for him, 'tradition' itself was more of a lived inheritance than merely textual citations. He mixed popular superstition, veneration of ancient texts as well as local herbal lore in his vision of 'indigenous tradition'. He quoted from obscure, locally available, medieval Sanskrit texts such as the *Madhumati*, but not from the ayurvedic classics like Charak Samhita, Susruta Samhita, etc.[61] As a Kaviraj with a rural practice, Maitreya was following the age-old Bengali medical practice of using a motley collection of local healing practices organized within a Sanskritized framework. Significantly, later, in another piece, when Maitreya is trying to directly respond to the allegation that the ancient ayurvedic texts mention nothing of *olautha*, he chooses to use the term *bishuchika* and claims that the reason people have not found any references in the ancient texts to *olautha* is precisely because they were looking for the wrong name and ought to, indeed, look for *bishuchika*.[62] Maitreya's texts, therefore, clearly show how the same author could choose different names for the disease depending upon the nature of the argument of a particular text.

Though authors such as Maitreya often equated *olautha* and *bishuchika*, such easy correspondences were not without its problems. The most obvious divergence between *bishuchika* and *olautha* is, of course, the associations of the local Bengali goddess Olabibi or Olaichandi with the later category. Olabibi is a goddess conspicuous by her absence in the vedic pantheon, and by her widespread popularity in lower Bengal. Though Arnold mentions the beginnings of other cholera divinities in northern India in the nineteenth century, none match Olabibi in her ready recognizability and antiquity as a cholera goddess.[63] Moreover, though there are wide variations in descriptions of her identity by votaries of her cult, by most accounts she is a Muslim gentlewoman. Ralph Nicholas gives two stories of her alleged origins, related by two groups of village performers. One describes her as the avatar of Narayan born to a virgin Muslim princess in order to convert the princess' father to her cult, and the other portrays her as a composite of two demonesses who had been given permission by Krishna in the name of Allah to cause death and destruction wherever the praise of God was not sung.[64] The openly cross-cultural shades of her cult as well as the seemingly 'irrational' and faith-based nature of the explanations of disease would have made the disease and its memories quite difficult to reconcile with the *bishuchika* of the Sanskrit tradition. However, this is precisely what Kavirajes like Maitreya sought to achieve.

One of the reasons the term *olautha* became increasingly out of fashion with Bengal's scientific men was its overt associations with the nonclassical, non-Hindu and irrational legacies. All of these associations were anathema to the new image of science emerging in Bengal. *Olautha* was problematic because of its close proximity to popular Islam, and the increasingly Hindu tinge to *daktari* writings.[65] Amarkrishna Chakrabarty has pointed out that to this day, despite the overwhelming Hinduization of the cult in certain parts of western Bengal, the priest who performs the worship of Olabibi continues to be either a Muslim fakir or, even more radically, a young Muslim woman.[66] Its 'irrationality' and its proximity made *olautha* an increasingly unpopular choice amongst the majority of *daktars*.

The sheer plurality of the world of Bengali printing, however, ensured that this growing *bhodrolok* dislike did not totally suppress the use of the word in print. Abdur Rahim, who wrote a genealogy of the Nawabs of Dhaka, writing within an expressly popular Islamic idiom in 1906, however, devoted about a third of his text to describing the ravages of cholera in Bengal by consistently using the word *olautha*.[67] A radical peasant leader, mystic and pioneer journalist, almost ignored by his contemporary *bhodrolok* peers, Kangal Harinath Majumdar—better known as Fikirchand—also wrote songs on cholera using the name *olautha*. Fikirchand was a close associate of the radical Sufi mystic Lalan Fakir. Both Rahim and Fakir, though their politics were completely different from each other, came to use the word *olautha*, not only by virtue of their location outside the *bhodrolok* milieu, but also their shared framework of supernatural explanation of the affliction. While the conservative Rahim saw it as a divine punishment for the transgression of social laws, the radical Fikirchand saw it as a divine visitation sent to humble false human hubris. Fikirchand thus proclaimed:

Olautha is the principal among all diseases
Even British science [*bilati bigyan*] has been defeated by it
Hakimi [unani tibb] and *Daktari* [allopathy] both
The ayurvedist [*boidyo*] goes about searching in his books
But there is no mention of this in his books
. . .

Kangal says citing proof
Brother Scientist, leave it be, leave it be
Leave your scientific pride [*bigyan obhiman*]
He who creates, when He himself kills, there can be no medicine[68]

The attitudes of Kangal and Rahim are both reminiscent of Rudyard Kipling's Teshoo Lama's views on cholera. The Lama had believed 'that the dung of a black horse, mixed with sulphur, and carried in a snake skin, was a sound remedy for cholera; but [and here lies the crucial similarity with Kangal and Rahim] the symbolism interested him far more than the science.'[69] Cholera here becomes a damning sign, one that marks out the body as having been damned by a power which lies beyond human manipulation.[70] Dipesh Chakrabarty sees such coding of epidemics as signs and symbols of divine damnation as resisting the reconstruction of the premodern body as modern, individuated, anatomical body.[71] The 'modern' state with its distinct modes of power, argues Chakrabarty, needs to reimagine the body as isolated from other social ties and subordinated preeminently to the organized violence of state power alone.[72] Preserving the name *olautha* in such registers of meaning therefore becomes a mnemonic device that resists the operationalization of 'modern' state-power.

The name *olautha* also remained popular amongst the ruder forms of *daktari* texts and advertisements. At this level, enlightened self-image counted for less than the need to express oneself in words likely to be understood by the largest number of people. Clearly, far more people were likely to comprehend the vernacular *olautha* than the classical *bishuchika*. Fakirchandra Basu's 1878 book *Karyasadhok Aushadhgyan* (Knowledge of Medicines that Get the Job Done) predictably used the terms *olautha* and cholera without any mention of *bishuchika*.[73] Dr Syed Abul Hossein, MD similarly advertised his specific *Sinkuasa*, allegedly made from ingredients brought from Tasmania, using the popular term *olautha*. Advertisements of the *Cholera Cure* also used the term *olautha* throughout their texts except in the name of the medicine. However, since commerce was the primary motive for the choice in these texts, they could often shift. *Sil's Cholera Camphor*, for instance, only used the English designation though written in Bengali, while Nafarchandra Datta's eclectic manual published in 1905 used all three terms—cholera, *olautha* and *bishuchika* as synonyms.[74]

After the 1920s however, the use of either *bishuchika* or *olautha* became rarer amongst respectable Bengali *daktari* authors. 'Cholera' had by then taken on a sufficiently recognizable vernacular identity as *kolera*.[75] Though occasional use of the former names continued—especially in other non-*daktari* registers of use.

Cholera Ethics

As we have mentioned above, the cholera debate in Bengali *daktari* writing was usually not over the mode of transmission of the disease as was the case in English. The principal debates in Bengali were over the modes of treatment to be followed. The modes of transmission tended to be glossed over with reiterations of general precautions against all possible sources of contagion, i.e., food, water, air—everything. There was none of the bitter controversy between water-borne and air-borne theories. Dr Harinath Ghosh, MD, for instance, in his lengthy essay on the topic, satisfied himself with merely saying in the span of a single paragraph that 'three important causes' needed to be present together for the disease to occur, i.e., 'food corrupted by evacuations' (*mol-dushito khadyo*), 'drinks corrupted by evacuations' (*mol-dushito paniyo*) and 'air corrupted by evacuations' (*mol-dushito bayu*). He spent the next five-and-a-half pages, however, dilating upon the description of the disease and his preferred treatment of it.[76] Dr Kunjabihari Das went so far as to suggest that even sitting next to a cholera patient or touching her/him might cause the disease, but again did not dwell upon the transmission.[77] In Mukherji's hundred-fifty-odd pages, too, he hardly discussed anything about the modes of transmission.

There were two reasons for this lack of importance to modes of transmission in *daktari* writings. The first, a conceptual reason: the persistent *daktari* insistence on the body's powers of resistance rather than contagion as factors in causing disease. Second, a practical outcome of the position of the *daktars*: placed as they were, either in private practice or in the Subordinate Medical Services, they did not have the power to make public health policy. All that they could do was hope to persuade their patients. Hence, even when they did concern themselves with modes of transmission, its expression came close to the discourse on strengthening the body's resistance. Both axes—the writings on powers of resistance and those on avoiding the chance of contagion—combined to form a didactic discourse which can only be described as a 'cholera ethic'.

The *daktari* discourse, unlike the discourses at the upper end of the IMS was aimed directly at the patients and, lacking the necessary power to compel, was persuasive in its tone. It sought to persuade people to do or not do a range of different things. In effect, it reordered lifestyles and established a comprehensive ethics of how to live and behave in society in order to avoid dying from cholera. The *dos* and *don'ts* ranged from avoiding drunkenness to the need to stay happy. Chattopadhyay, for instance, mentioned that one should not get drunk during a cholera outbreak, should always stay happy and not be anxious about anything, should never leave for work without having eaten something, however little, etc.[78] Harimohan Sen went on to state that, 'for whatever reason, when the body goes limp, the life-force (*jeeboni shokti*) is depleted. That is when people become prone to fall ill. Drunkenness, extreme heat or cold, keeping late nights and mental ennui—these are what invite the disease'.[79] Das gave an even more elaborate list of things to avoid. He even advised against 'fresh fruits such as cucumbers, *knakur*, watermelons, guavas, coconuts, etc., which young children loved to eat', 'dry fish, salty fish or meat', stale sweetmeats, any stale food, 'British brandy', and also against being worried or depressed. The redoubtable Mahendralal Sircar mentioned a long list of foods that should be avoided. Sircar, echoing Das, mentioned in this list unripe or overripe fruit, things cooked in *ghee* (clarified butter), fried food, very salty or saltless fish, newly harvested paddy, etc. Apart from these, drinking alcohol or keeping late nights was also bad. Of all these though, alcohol was the worst and consuming it was said to 'almost invariably land the person at a stage just prior to the affliction'.[80] Not only foods, but even one's emotional states were medicalized and, as we have seen, most writers impressed on the reader the 'need to be happy'. Das went so far as to state that, 'should you find yourself feeling depressed upon waking in the morning, immediately give yourself five grains of the Sulphate of Quinine'.[81]

This ethico-moral dimension of the cholera discourse had even struck roots amongst practitioners in Britain.[82] T. M. Greenhow, who treated innumerable patients in the Tyne Valley during the first major epidemic in northern England in 1831 mentioned that 'predisposing causes' of the disease could be divided into 'natural' and 'acquired' causes. Of these, the latter comprised 'whatever has a tendency to debilitate moral or physical health'. He went on to add that 'it is not easy to draw a line of distinction between moral and physical agents.. it is evident that they act in concurrence or have a mutual reaction upon each other'.[83] Such symmetry is not surprising, considering the fact that India-returned doctors played an important part in British cholera medicine and, like Greenhow, confessedly borrowed from the practice of old India-hands such as Dr Johnson and Dr Bell.[84] In fact, many of the concerns such as those over fresh fruits, drunkenness, etc., are also identical to the Bengali prescriptions. Yet, the actual list of these 'moral' causes differed between Bengali and British doctors. Drunkenness, for example, which was uniformly condemned by all Bengali physicians, had a more ambiguous position in the practice of British physicians. Greenhow himself condemned it in the strongest terms. His friend T. K. Fife, another busy Newcastle doctor, however, asserted that he could not 'consider powerful predisposing cause, though for the sake of morality it is well to favour this opinion'.[85] For Fife, drunkenness was clearly a moral evil, but it was not a medical cause for cholera. James Adair Lawrie, who had practised both in India and the north of Britain, similarly wrote that he could not admit that drunkenness was the 'principal, much less the sole' cause of cholera.[86] The proscribed foods, too, were, of course, different. In place of *ghee* and paddy, we find cheese and bacon, raw apples and other autumnal fruits.[87]

Whereas most of the authors like Das, Sircar, Chattopadhyay or Bagchi developed their cholera ethics as part of the project to strengthen the body's powers of resistance, the writings of Harinath Ghosh, show clearly how this concern about powers of resistance did overlap obliquely with issues of transmission as well. Ghosh mentioned five essential things to avoid. Underlining the didactic nature of these texts, his injunctions were put down in numbered point form:

1. Avoid drinking water everywhere.
2. Be very sure of the purity of the food you eat.
3. Keep the patient in a clean place sufficiently separated from the rest of the family members.
4. Destroy all clothes which have been soiled by the patient's evacuations.
5. Report all cases of cholera to the local authorities at the earliest.[88]

Unlike the governmental concerns about preventing the transmission of cholera that tended to speak in terms of large, anonymous 'populations', which were to be monitored, controlled and isolated from sources of Contagion, the *daktari* discourse advocated an ethics of self-care. It sought to cultivate in the prospective patients themselves a sense of caring for the self that would determine their food, leisure and even their emotional states. Even after the 1920s when the *daktars* became more vocal about adopting techno-scientific solutions such as vaccination, their discourse was aimed at persuading patients to get themselves vaccinated.[89]

It would be unhelpful to see these two discourses in the Power/Resistance framework, for there can be little doubt that the *daktari* discourse itself was clearly didactic. Instead, it is better to see them as different forms of power operating through different modes of expression and on different subjects. The *daktari* discourse, owing to the institutional matrix within which it operated, however, objectified patients to a lesser degree than the more policy-focussed or erudite English writings on the subject.

Independently of how and on whom the power of the *daktari* discourse operated, the contents of its message also had other points of interest. Many points mentioned in it 'articulated' (in Latour's sense) with a range of similar positions in other spheres of contemporary Bengali society, ranging from social reform to 'indigenous' medical practice.[90] Drunkenness, for instance, was a common injunction in most *daktari* writings on cholera, but drunkenness had also become a major issue of social reform and 'national' uplift. Keshab Sen's *Bharat Samskar Sabha* had included fighting drunkenness as one of its foremost aims. Numerous tracts had been published on temperance, and many of the leading social reformers and ideologues of the day were involved in popularizing temperance. Popular tracts and propagandist plays preaching temperance were plentiful in late nineteenth century Bengal.[91] Though the original popularity of the cause undoubtedly had close links with Victorian temperance movements, the importance of the contemporary Bengali activists in fashioning the *daktari* concerns cannot be overlooked.

The concerns about drunkenness also formed part of a larger concern with *gurupak* foods. The seemingly strange lists of foods to be avoided that we come across in the *daktari* writings are actually assembled according to the category of their being '*gurupak*'.[92] Many traditions of 'indigenous' medicine had come to see digestion as the main arbiter of good health. All ill health, therefore, was related to forms of indigestion.[93] Pointing out the centrality of diet in lay perceptions of disease and treatment, Mark Nichter has pointed out that, '[f]oods are thought to enhance and facilitate the action of medicines, and provide a means of balancing the extreme qualities of medicines.'[94] Nichter further points out, that, the 'popularity' of the 'indigenous' physician is often a consequence of the latter's greater willingness to engage with 'popular' dietary categories. Numerous *kaviraji* authors in the nineteenth century wrote extensively on foods in general and the deleterious effects of *gurupak* foods in particular. *Gurupak* foods came to signify those foods that were considered difficult to digest. Cholera was always considered as disease of the stomach. Visible irregularities of evacuations strengthened its connections to faulty digestion, and many nineteenth century authors proceeded to link *gurupak* foods with the incidence of cholera.[95] Some of these *kaviraji* authors such as Prasannachandra Maitreya even contributed to *daktari* periodicals and wrote on the subject in them.[96]

Interestingly however, while there are thus clear points of correspondence between *daktars* and nineteenth century ayurvedists on the matter, the relationship between diets and *bishuchika* is not as clear in the older ayurvedic literature. Gobindo Das' *Bhesaja Ratnavali,* arguably the best-known medical text to be written in the eighteenth century in eastern India, did not, for instance, make any putative connection between diets, mental states and *bishuchika.* Neither did Kaviraj Binodlal Sen, writing nearly a century later. However, the lack of an explicit connection does not mean that the ideas were not present in these earlier texts. The two paragraphs in the *Bhesaja Ratnavali* preceding the discussion on *bishuchika* stated that those who are given to 'excessive physical exercise, excessive sexual activity, fond of travelling or riding horses as well as those who are tired…thirsty, disturbed by hiccups and wind…as well as those who have not slept at night or those whose stomachs are empty, for them it is advisable to sleep even during the day'.[97] Sleep and adequate rest are said to promote digestion and thereby cure digestive complaints. Since *bishuchika* in the late nineteenth century came to be seen as a stomach ailment, these earlier ideas may have easily been mapped on to the disease.[98] The use of lemony (*omlo*) drinks as a prophylactic are also similarly shared concerns in nineteenth-century *daktari* and *kaviraji* writings without having a direct precedent (in relation to the cure of cholera) in older ayurvedic literature as such.[99]

Scholars like Wujastyk, Pitman, Ecks and others have rightly highlighted the importance attached to digestion as the seat of major illnesses in 'indigenous' ideas about illness and healing.[100] In the case of cholera, however, this concern came to be shared by British practitioners as well. Most early British physicians who dealt with cholera patients underlined the role of faulty digestion in causing the disease. The prolific Thomas Michael Greenhow wrote in 1848, after nearly seventeen years of practice amongst cholera patients in England, that '[f]rom considerable experience…we are enabled to speak, with some confidence as to the indigestible character of some articles of diet…nothing more surely predisposes to cholera'.[101] British doctors were especially keen to discourage overeating and vehemently urged moderation in diet.[102] Greenhow even mentioned that Christmas feastings and the consequent overeating were instrumental in cholera breaking out at Gateshead.[103] Another contemporary of Greenhow, Charles Searle, who had practised in India for fourteen years before working with cholera patients in Warsaw and finally in Britain, asked his readers to '[r]emember the purpose [for which] you have a stomach is simply to supply the waste and excitement of the system…'.[104] This correspondence is highly likely to be a direct consequence of the import of Indian ideas about cholera into Britain, but it also drew upon popular older ideas about moderation in the six 'non-naturals' as a way of preserving health.[105] The British practice accented moderation but linked it to digestion. Its insistence on identifying specific foods that were difficult to digest (*gurupak*) also remained of minor importance compared to the Bengali discourse. Both British and Bengali ideas and practices were therefore realigned through their mutual entanglements.

It is therefore important to guard against any interpretation of *daktari* writings which presents it as being derived from a sphere of 'authentic indigenous' practice. It was more a matter of a complex realignment of multistranded traditions in ways that would reinforce similar ideas and practices within each other.[106] The prophylactic use of the 'cholera belt' provides an excellent illustration of such mutually reinforcing realignments that defy a search for origins.

Kunjabihari Das mentioned the utility of a 'cholera belt' made of flannel and worn around the waist as a protection from cholera.[107] Jadunath Mukherji too advocated the covering of the patient in flannel. Chattopadhyay, while not arguing for a covering as such, advocated flannel compresses to the waist for cholera patients. The origins of this curious practice go back to the eighteenth century. Early British doctors at the time had thought that the cummerbund worn by the elites in many Asian countries had a medical function. Since cholera came to be thought of principally as an Asian disease, many advocated the use of a belt similar to that seen in Asia as a prophylactic.[108] Authors like James Johnson, writing in the early decades of the nineteenth century in India, had advocated it.[109] Through the nineteenth century however, the practice had fallen into disuse, especially through the ascendance of the germ theories of disease. The persistent use of the belt in *daktari* writings, despite their acquaintance with various germ theories, is thus a telling example of how practices and ideas may evolve through misunderstandings and mistranslations as well as a search for legitimacy from neighbouring practices without being in anyway 'authentic' or 'indigenous' to the region.

The structure of reasoning that might have led to such mimetic legitimations and seeming symmetries was clarified in an essay on 'originality' in *daktari* writing by Jogendranath Mitra. Mitra, like many others, sought to inspire his fellow *daktars* to stop blindly following the teachings of their European teachers and books and develop their own originality. Mitra's quest for originality, however, did not stop at mere exhortations. He actually developed a method of 'independent thinking' as he called it. In it, he proposed that there were only two basic modes of original thinking—*sannikarsha* (contact) and *sadrisha* (similarity). According to Mitra therefore, in order to develop an original mode of thought, *daktars* needed to cultivate the faculty of finding similarities within their entire experiential world, i.e., everything they came into contact with.[110] It was this search for originality through similarity that provided the intellectual method for developing mimetic legitimations.

Treating Cholera

Once all the prophylactics had failed, the body's power of resistance been trounced and the patient afflicted with cholera, the *daktars* had to treat them. Correctly diagnosing and treating cholera, however, was another contentious issue. While most agreed on the basic symptomatology of the disease, they differed widely on the mode and timing of treatment.

Though most physicians agreed on the basic symptoms and the course of the disease, diagnosis remained a tricky affair. DN Chattopadhyay suggested that there might be more than one strain of cholera in the region.[111] There were also other complications whose variations complicated the act of diagnosis. These included 'remittent fever', '*aambath*' (allergic sores), '*baman*' (vomiting), '*hikka*' (hiccups), '*anidra*' (sleeplessness) and 'uraemia'.[112] Jogendranath Mitra also mentioned many of the complications that often made diagnosis unreliable.

Mostly, however, the doctors, irrespective of 'systemic' affiliations, tended to agree that there were at least three distinct stages of the disease. Some added an introductory stage of slight stomach problems. This 'introductory stage' was particularly viable commercially. It allowed enterprising patent-medicine sellers to depict even everyday stomach complaints as probable 'introductory stages' of cholera. Advertisements for *Chlorodyne* thus suggested that even stomach cramps and tiredness might be the 'introductory stage' of cholera and therefore advised would-be consumers to take a dose of the medicine immediately.[113] The three main stages were defined by the colour of the evacuations, the patient's state of consciousness, etc. The treatment was to depend upon in which of these three (or indeed four) stages the patient was found. One homoeopath named these four stages: stage of invasion, stage of development, stage of collapse and finally 'reaction'.[114] Mukherji, in an attempt that was not to be repeated in later authors, also sought to find ayurvedic correlates for some of the stages. Most of the authors also tended to agree on the basic description of the disease.

In terms of the characteristic symptoms of the disease, though these usually follow the English descriptions of the disease fairly closely, there is one significant additional symptom. Cholera patients were said to have their 'limbs locked' [*haathe paaye khil dhora*].[115] This symptom is described by nearly all *daktari* writers, and the phrase itself, though common in Bengali, has no accurate English translation. Its incorporation into the *daktari* symptomatology underlines the way in which the *daktari* authors—both idiomatically and in their mode of thinking about the disease—remained implicated within the very characteristic Bengali ways of experiencing the body.[116] Occasionally, some *daktars* described still other similarly untranslatable symptoms, such as when Pulinchandra Sanyal spoke of '*sharirer jhna jhna kora*' (very roughly, means 'feeling a buzz all over the body') as being a sign of the onset of cholera even before the first recognized symptoms appeared.[117]

Unlike in the case of the symptoms, however, there was very little agreement between different *daktars* over the precise mode of treatment. As Mukherji pointed out, 'If a cholera patient is seen by four or five different physicians, each of them advises a totally different mode of treatment—we are sure that our readers would agree with this statement from their own experience. The reason for the disagreement is that there is no consensus on how to treat cholera patients'.[118] Writing over thirty years later, Sanyal still said, 'Some say heavy doses of Calomel are the only medicine, others say making the patient ingest salts would help. Still others say, "give the patient cold water". Yet others hold that giving the patient medicines to make the stools stop will help. But, once again, others disagree and advocate giving laxatives.'[119] There was, indeed, little agreement between the different *daktars* on the precise mode of treatment to be followed.

There were two major points of disagreement. The first was whether it was better to stop the characteristic and involuntary evacuation seen in patients by *dharak* medicines or to wash the system out by giving more laxatives? Second, at which stage of the disease was it best to give the treatment? Thus, Jagadbandhu Basu, MD wrote, 'I believe, it's not just with allopathy, but with in fact any medical system, that there is no fixed medicine for this disease: no fixed medicine that can cure all types of *olautha* at all times in its career. Medicines have to be administered with reference to the particular stage that the disease happens to be in'.[120] Mahendralal Sircar, too, mentioned how important it was to get the timing of the medication right, just as it was, of course, to get the medicine itself right.[121] Even in the late 1920s when cholera treatment regimes were flush with techno-scientific prescriptions of injections, intravenous saline, vaccines, etc., debate still continued about what medicine to administer at which stage.[122]

Three medicinal substances, along with their derivates, were frequently at issue in these discussions of treatment. These were mercury, particularly mercury (I) chloride, or calomel, camphor and opium (principally as morphine). Some of these were also recommended by non-allopathic practitioners. Camphor, for instance, had been popularly held to have had some curative value with respect to cholera. Affirming this belief, Haridas Chakrabarty mentioned that keeping a piece of camphor on one's self and occasionally sniffing it might act as a prophylactic as well.[123] This view was supported in 1920 in an anonymously published letter to the editor of the *Chikitsa Prakash*.[124] Kaviraj Prasannachandra Maitreya also advocated its use in the first stage of the disease. An anonymous homoeopath, writing in the *Chikitsa Sammilani*, also mentioned that a few early drops of camphor could check the deterioration of the patient.[125] Sircar himself, who straddled both homoeopathic and allopathic traditions, advocated its use, but advised extreme caution in the timing, writing, 'about camphor, many experts have held many views, in our view, however, its indiscriminate use at anytime in cholera is neither advisable nor safe'. He thereafter went on to discuss the diametrically opposing views of Dr Hempel and his Venetian student, Dr Rocco Rubini, in the matter before finally even qualifying Hanneman's own prescriptions about camphor. Kunjabihari Das went to the extent of suggesting regular camphorated fumigation of the entire house where there were cholera patients.[126]

Similarly, the curative powers of opium or morphine were affirmed by *daktari* authors like Chattopadhyay, Basu and Sanyal.[127] When an anonymous *kaviraj* sent in a case history of a young man successfully treated of cholera with opium to the *Chikitsa Sammilani*, the editor, Avinashchandra Kabiratna, wrote that all good physicians knew and respected the worth of the drug in the treatment of cholera.[128] Significantly, Kabiratna clarified that his co-editor, Annadacharan Khastagir, concurred with him on the issue.

As in the case of the instructions on cholera ethics, so, too, in the case of the actual medicinal substances, there seemed to be, at least on the surface, a degree of agreement between various forms of treatment available in late-nineteenth and early-twentieth century Bengal. The shared prescription of the same medicinal substances, despite differences in the mode of application, no doubt further affirmed popular beliefs (already quoted by *daktars* like Chakrabarty) in the curative powers of these substances in cases of cholera. This led to the use of these substances in numerous remedies which claimed to operate outside of systemic boundaries. A *daktar*, Basudeb Ram, for instance, wrote to the *Medical Reporter* to inform its readers that he previously used a patent medicine by the name of *Chlorodyne* in treating cholera patients, but had found it to often have harmful effects, since patients, hoping to cure themselves sooner than expected, often took larger than the prescribed doses, with disastrous effects. Ram had then discovered that the main ingredient in the medicine was morphia. He had since stopped using *Chlorodyne* and had found a very effective curative in turpentine oil.[129]

The publication of such writings, as well as the numerous advertisements which drew upon popular beliefs by prominently displaying its ingredients, eventually led to the use of these substances by a range of 'quacks'. In fact, texts like those of Sanyal's were targeted specifically at 'untrained' *daktars*, who were said to be able to benefit from such 'trainers'. Instead, by popularizing the reputation of dangerous drugs like opium and mercury derivatives, these 'trainers' often had tragic consequences. One such tragic case that elicited a lot of debate was that of a seven-year-old boy called Sricharan. Sricharan's family were very poor leather workers in the Mechuabazar area of north-central Calcutta. Sricharan was taken to a local physician called Dr Habibar Rahman on 4 September 1899 after suffering from loose motions for a few days. Though Rahman did not hold any recognized medical degrees, he had long practised in the area and he prescribed opium for the boy, diagnosing it to be a case of cholera. After a slight improvement, however, Sricharan's condition rapidly deteriorated. Ultimately, another unqualified local practitioner called Dr Joibhushan Sarkar was called in. Sarkar suspected opium poisoning and advised immediate removal of the boy to the Calcutta Medical College. He was admitted to the Medical College on the morning of 5 September 1899. His condition, however, remained unstable throughout the day and he died the next morning. Dr Gibbons conducted an autopsy and an analysis of the remaining mixture that Rahman had given. Though he could not conclusively prove opiate poisoning in the autopsy, Dr Gibbons did establish from the remnants of the medicine bottle that a dangerously high proportion of opium had actually been administered to the boy. A case was filed against Dr Rahman and he was taken into police custody. The principal of the Medical College, Dr Bomford and Prof Bird both appeared as expert witnesses for the prosecution. Most tragically, perhaps, it transpired that Sricharan had not even been afflicted by cholera. He had actually suffered from tuberculosis, which, along with the diarrhoea, had misled Dr Rahman.[130] It was cases like that of Sricharan, which, in subsequent months, inspired *daktars* like Dr Abdul Ajed Khan Choudhury to start lobbying for stricter governmental controls on the sale of opiates.[131]

What Sricharan's tragic death proved was that, though the space of Bengali medical practice was heterogeneous, there were still numerous overlaps between different levels and spheres within it. Kaviraji, homoeopathy and allopathy overlapped and mimetically legitimized each other and bowdlerized versions of these commonly held ideas and beliefs percolated down to the level of the Rahmans and Sarkars. Though ill-understood and tragically executed at those ruder levels, it is unquestionable that the practice itself had similarities with the more polite practices of the college-educated *daktars*.

The Cholera Market

Cholera was, if one were to be cynical, one of the most *market worthy* of the major nineteenth-century afflictions. Cholera was known to be a great leveller of all physicians, since all were equally ineffective. As Pulinchandra Sanyal put it, 'When faced with cholera, the physician's wisdom (*gyan*), glory (*gaurab*), learning (*vidya*), intelligence (*buddhi*)—all is turned to dust. In the presence of cholera, allopaths, homoeopaths, hakims and kavirajes are all the same. Be it a qualified doctor or a quack—at the crematorium they all look the same. Cholera is that great crematorium.'[132] Reduced to such utter helplessness, Mukherji pointed out that patients thought any healer was as good as the next and often desisted from calling in a renowned doctor, viewing it as a pointless waste of money.[133] Viewed from the perspective of the medical market, this was an immense opportunity. Whereas in the case of other afflictions people might have had their preferred modes of treatment, and better-known healers and physicians could easily dominate the market; in the case of cholera people were willing to try whatever was available.

The medical market as such comprised a range of commodities from medical books and periodicals to medicines, charms, spells and even more specific and bizarre commodities such as the 'cholera belt'. The producers and the consumers who transacted their business in this market were diverse. The best way to understand the dynamics of this robust market is to concentrate on its two crucial aspects: innovation and plurality.

Anne Digby's work on early-modern England has shown how the medical market encouraged innovation.[134] Nichter has added that amongst the less expensive practitioners of the bazaar—especially in multitherapeutic contexts such as South Asia—medicine is eclectic. He calls it *masala medicine*: a mixture of allopathy, homeopathy, ayurveda, unani and just about anything else that might have some value in the eyes of the lay medical consumer.[135] But the pressure and opportunity of innovation in colonial Bengal cannot be understood without reference to the massive urbanization, especially of Calcutta, and the significant growth of the print industry. Between 1800 and 1851, the population of Calcutta went from a mere 57,041 to a whopping 165,301.[136] This massive increase in the size of the population brought with it, alongside its attendant new health problems, a crisis of older forms of medical authority. As new people crowded into an ever-growing city, it became impossible to know which healers or physicians were 'good'/'reliable' and which were not. It also became much easier, in the relative anonymity of a huge and constantly expanding city, for dubious healers and physicians to evade detection by constantly reinventing themselves and their medical reputations. Kaliprasanna Singha's numerous anecdotes about the confrontation of medical students and 'quacks' and 'magicians' claiming healing powers mentioned in Chapter I, might also be seen in terms of the vast market for healing.

In order to make an impact in this vast market, every physician sought to outdo his peers through innovation. Subrata Pahari has therefore mentioned that the early nineteenth century was a period when the 'discovery of numerous new *kaviraji* medicines and the aspiration to make a fortune by their sale, went hand in hand with the rampant adulteration of [A]yurvedic medicines in the hope of making even bigger fortunes'.[137]

In the case of cholera, this spirit of innovation continued right into the twentieth century. Moreover, this spirit of innovation was not limited merely to unscrupulous 'quacks'; many physicians in government employ also dreamed of discovering an effective cholera specific. Dr Bajle Rahman Miah, for instance, the doctor-in-charge of the Chandpur Dispensary in Khulna, had developed his own 'patent medicine' called *Choleradyne* which he was advertising in 1895.[138] A retired professor of chemistry at the Scottish Church College, Calcutta, Pandit Khirodeprosad Bidyabinod, also 'invented' his own cholera specific called *Lymodyne.*[139] Dr Shamsuddin J. Sulemani, the Chief Medical Officer of the native state of Boroda, developed his own treatment regime and urged other doctors to try it in 1900.[140] In fact, Dr Sulemani's method was adopted and advocated enthusiastically by Dr Kunjabihari Das.[141] Hemchandra Banerjee, who treated cholera patients with his own discovery in the winter of 1875, even petitioned the government of India to draw attention to his discovery and undertook to supply the medicine to the government gratis for distribution amongst the poor.[142] As pointed out in the Introduction, the market was neither opposed to the medical profession/bureaucracy nor excluded from it. It constituted a 'heteronomous' domain of activity but one that often intersected and overlapped with the state.[143] Contrary to the usually assumed oppositional orientation of the state and the medical market, in the nineteenth century, we often find the market utilizing the state—both practically as well as discursively—to its own ends. A well-known Calcutta drug seller, D. Gupta & Co., for example, successfully sued two men—Nandalal Ghosh and Bimalacharan Majumdar—for selling medicines which looked like Gupta's in the immediate vicinity of the former's shop.[144] Similarly, Lalmohan Saha of Babu Bajar, Dhaka, sued Kailashchandra Bandopadhyay for having sold medicines resembling the former's.[145] What was most interesting, however, was not simply these examples of the market using the state and its laws to protect its profits, but rather, repeated use of the decisions of the courts in the advertisements of the victorious party as a kind of tacit state approval of its drugs. The court cases therefore had two lives. One, as a practical instrument to enforce power in the medical market; and another, as a rhetorical device which sought to derive some of the state's legitimacy for operators on the medical market.

The second crucial aspect of the cholera market was its plurality. The nineteenth century had witnessed the progressive marginalization of popular (*lokayata*) traditions of 'indigenous' medicine in favour of more classicized and textualized versions of 'indigenous' medicine. In 1858, for instance, three members of the Calcutta elite, Prasannacoomar Tagore, Jan Mohammed and Jaumat Ali Khan, petitioned the government to prevent all indigenous physicians from practising who had not studied either the 'medicine of the Veds [sic]' or the 'pharmacopoeia of the Greeks'.[146] Textuality came to be seen as an indispensable aspect of the 'rationality' of 'indigenous' medicine.

The Bengali *bhodrolok*, which increasingly prided itself on their rational, classical heritage, came to increasingly reject the nontextual, nonclassical, 'irrational' aspects of their cultural heritage. Yet in the case of cholera, *daktars* were often found enthusiastically incorporating 'folk' remedies into their treatment. This, in turn, ensured the textualization and further dissemination of these fragmentary knowledges. Dr Bibhutibhushan Tarafdar, for example, mentioned having successfully used a paste made from two local herbs in a case involving a seven-year-old girl called Araitan Bibi.[147] Similarly, Dr Satyaranjan Das mentioned following local belief in using an emulsion of banana in the case of Jhagri Mandal of Dhaka.[148]

Spells, charms and magic cures proliferated alongside local herbal cures. But the access to printing and the demand for cholera remedies encouraged such fragmentary local knowledges to be put in print and disseminated. The *Prankrishana Aushadhavali*, based upon the eclectic recipe books of Prankrishna Biswas, published several cholera cures.[149] Biswas had worked as a diwan to the British Collector of Cooch Behar in Northern Bengal in the late eighteenth century and had confessedly picked up many of his recipes there.[150] Later, Biswas' book was read and referred to by Abdus Sobhan in his *Elaj-e-Lokmani*, published from the old quarter in Dhaka.[151] This practice of nonmedical officers compiling encyclopaedic collections of 'recipes', or *nushkhas*, was also to be observed among some early English officers such as Edward HC Monckton.[152] But whereas in the hands of the English officers they were either 'sanitized' through rigorous laboratory work or, instead, remained merely in personal collections, in the vernacular print sphere these often appeared in print and spread widely—as was the case with Biswas' remedies.[153] Thus, the market in cheap medical books ensured the survival of many *lokayata* cholera cures and their dissemination into new regions. Two small pamphlets by Gobindachandra Basak, published in the 1880s, are good examples of how the market in cheap medical books was drawing on localized, fast-disappearing modes of treatment and motoring further dissemination of them. One of Basak's pamphlets drew upon remedies ascribed to the siddha saint, Lolimbaraj, while the other was based upon local traditions of hydropathy.[154] It is cogent to note that the remedies in these texts often did not maintain the divide between the medical and the magical.[155]

A good example of how printing and the market were helping to sustain and disseminate cholera cures beyond their immediate contexts can be seen explicitly in a letter published in the *Grihastnya Mangal* of 1927. Satishchandra Bala sent in two cholera remedies in a letter to the editor, requesting their publication. Bala mentioned that he had found the remedies while clearing out his father's old papers. They had originally been collected and published by the *Education Gazette* in 1877. Bala's father, who was in the habit of keeping cuttings of medicinal recipes published in newspapers and periodicals, had cut them out and kept them amongst his papers. Though there is no hint of where the original publication had obtained their remedies from, their publication, preservation and republication in 1927 in a widely circulated periodical, clearly bring out the role played by commerce and publishing in disseminating 'local' cholera cures beyond their immediate precincts.[156]

Cholera charms and spells were another important commodity on the medical market. Numerous manuals, like the recipe books, collected and disseminated fragmentary localized knowledges. Dipesh Chakrabarty has noticed that the connection posited between a negative supernatural influence (*durdaibya*) and an epidemic, usually helps to articulate both a sense of social ownership of the individual body as well as a sense of 'locality'. Chakrabarty observes that epidemic deities such as Olabibi, Mariamma, etc., are usually invoked to protect small, well-defined areas. The rituals associated with their worship therefore helps to articulate a sense of 'locality'.[157] The insertion of these divine powers within a medical market, however, continuously served to de-centre this locality and make it indefinitely reproducible. Cheap books detailing the rituals and *mantras* of disease deities were popular fare in the book marts of the nineteenth century. These allowed for the reproduction of the sense of locality indefinitely and over widely dispersed spaces.

The most common form of 'supernatural' cholera cures, were charms and spells. Mostly such charms and spells are usually dismissed by scholars as simply 'irrational modes of thought through which people, in the grip of a crisis they did not really understand, sought to grapple with it. Even when rare attempts are made to understand these texts as 'rational' texts embodying a distinct rationality, these readings tend to ignore the historical context of their occurrence and rely instead on 'ancient' symbology.[158] The cholera spells and charms, however, cannot be seen merely in terms of the ancient symbology that is alleged to have fashioned them. They were produced for a specific medical market, and unravelling their rationality in terms of the market also reveals, in turn, some underlying structural truths about the market itself. One popular cholera spell for example was:

Om Hrang Hring Rang Ring Bishnu Shaktaye Nomoh
Om Nomoh Bhogoboti Bishnu Shoktimenong
Om Horo Horo Noy Noy Poch Poch Moth Moth
Uthshadoy Uthshadoy Duri Kuru Swahah
Himbonthong Gochho Jeeb Shoh Shoh Shoh
Chondromondologotohoshi Swahah[159]

At the very outset, there are structural characteristics which prove the redundancy of a classical Tantric framework in understanding this spell. According to classical Tantric beliefs, all ritual action is categorized into one of six categories—*Shatachakra*. Of these, curative spells fall under the category *Shantikarma*. In this category, all spells are supposed to end in the words *Namah* or *Swahah*. Two of the six lines of the above spell follow this rule, but the other four do not, pointing to the mediation of classical forms possibly through more localized forms. This is also affirmed by the fact that the spell is addressed to Bhogoboti, the benign and benevolent Mother Goddess, instead of Rati, the seductress whom curative spells are classically meant to invoke. Bhagabati is the dominant form of the Mother Goddess in Bengal and the shift clearly seeks to align the spell to local beliefs. The most overt evidence of the influence of the market however, comes from the seemingly meaningless syllables such as '*Hring*', '*Hrang*', '*Noy*' and '*Poch*'. These are usually referred to, in Tantric lexicon, as *bij mantra*, or germinal phonemes. They symbolically represent other diverse divine powers and actions and are assembled in a strict and well-defined logic. However, the interesting twist to the classical readings of the spell comes in an introduction to the spell in one of the popular manuals that published it. In classical Tantric vocabulary, the word *Hring* (or *Hrim* in its more Sanskritized pronunciation) ought to stand for the goddess Sri or Lakshmi.[160] However, the introduction clarifies that the word is actually a *setu mantra*, or a 'bridging phoneme', which will allow non-Brahmins and laymen to recite the spell. The variations amply prove that not only had 'magical' cures for cholera survived in the market, but, indeed, they had found therein an arena for further development, innovation and expansion, which belied the usual narrative of marginalisation of these forms through the introduction of modernity.

In the hands of some enterprising entrepreneurs, these twin axes of innovation and appropriation could combine with potent force to undermine the very classicist framework that was seeking to marginalize them. Kaviraj Prasannachandra Maitreya wrote a lengthy essay entitled the *Demolition of the Pride of Homoeopathy and Allopathy*. In it he claimed that around 1878 he had to travel to a distant village. There he met two naked ascetics by the wayside. One was engaged in deep meditation, while the other was preparing cannabis to smoke. Maitreya got into a conversation with them. Apparently, they conversed in Sanskrit. Maitreya used to come and discuss spiritual matters with the two ascetics everyday where they sat under the roadside tree. At the time, a cholera epidemic had broken out in the area and the ascetics showed him a handwritten book called the *Aditya Samhita*. He learnt of four medicines from this book. Though he claimed that he had never been able to learn anything about the book, he did use the medicines and claimed that no patient who had been treated with the medicines had ever died in the fifteen years that elapsed between his meeting with the ascetics and the writing of the piece.[161] It need not overly concern us whether Maitreya's story was true or not. What is clear is that he is using both an alleged innovation and appropriation from a minor tradition to build a narrative where his own marginalized remedies are presented as part of an ancient, classical tradition, even when they are clearly not within the ayurvedic canon as such. Such stories underline how the market and its opportunities could be used to subvert certain forms of marginalization. It thus shows the medical market to be, above all, was an arena for contestation and competition.

It was this contestatory nature of the market that encouraged the development of claims of systemic superiority. In the medical market, especially when it came to cholera, the claims to superior efficacy of a system of treatment were far from settled and produced some of the bitterest exchanges between practitioners of different systems. From the 1880s there developed a forceful claim that in cases of cholera homoeopathy was more effective than allopathy or *kaviraji*.

These claims seem to have started initially due to the work of Dr Dwarkanath Ray. Dr Ray was born in a village called Shubhaddhya, outside of Dhaka, in 1854 in a family of Brahmo reformers. His elder brother, who was a lecturer at Dhaka College, raised Dwarkanath to be a devout rationalist. He was always expected to study medicine and, after finishing his schooling in Dhaka, studied at CMC. He recalled later that at the time, as medical students, they used to joke about the 'little balls of sugar' homoeopaths peddled. On finishing his medical studies in Calcutta, his brother wanted him to go to Britain to obtain the best medical education possible. After studying first at Glasgow, he later went to London to study at the London Hospital. It was at this time that he ended up one day, almost accidentally, at the Homoeopathic Hospital. The Resident Physician, noticing his cynicism, invited him over to observe the wards. This was in the 1880s, still some time before the discovery of antitoxins, and Ray was surprised to see homoeopathy curing cases of diphtheria and scarlet fever—diseases for which allopathy still had not found cures. It was then that he began to take homoeopathy seriously. His conversion was still slow, and he feared how his brother, who considered homoeopathy to be complete quackery, would receive the news. Eventually, however, he decided to pursue homoeopathy. His brother, who had raised him more like a son than a brother, disowned him for having turned his back on 'scientific rationality'. Dwarkanath's friends now advised him to go to America, since the London Homoeopathic Hospital did not yet have the power to give degrees. In 1883, armed only with a letter of introduction, he travelled to New York. In New York, he studied at the New York Homoeopathic College and wrote his dissertation on cholera. He later wrote that, as a boy in eastern Bengal, he had seen the ravages of cholera and had always wanted to study medicine, mainly to try to cure the scourge. After finishing his studies in New York, he returned to practice briefly in London and then in Bombay. Three years after returning to India, he married in 1888. His public stature grew through his successful treatment of well-known public figures such as Dadabhai Naoroji, B. M. Malabari and K. T. Telang.[162] His wife, who was a Bengali Brahmo as well, wanted him to return to Bengal. Eventually, they moved to Calcutta and established a highly successful homoeopathic hospital on Upper Circular Road. Dr Ray's thesis was, meanwhile, published as a book and became the homoeopathic textbook on cholera.[163]

By the 1890s homoeopathy's claims had crystallized and become something of a social prejudice. The editors of the *Chikitsha Sammilani*, for instance, mentioned as early as 1893 that it had become commonplace for homoeopaths to argue that they alone cured cholera, while in reality, said the editors, many patients continued to die.[164] Numerous books now appeared on the market on the subject of the homoeopathic cure of cholera.[165] So profitable was this trade in homoeopathic books on cholera that the market for the books themselves became highly competitive, and competition could be seen between rival homoeopathic books on the subject. G. K. Nag & Co, for instance, advertised that 'though there were several homoeopathic books on cholera', theirs was most useful.[166] Up to the 1920s this belief held sway and numerous Bengali books on the homoeopathic treatment of cholera were produced accordingly. It may well have been this very belief that led the Arrah municipality to hire a homoeopath when cholera broke out within their municipal limits.[167]

The thriving medical market, especially in the case of cholera—due both to its endemic nature in the region and the devastation caused by it—therefore encouraged innovation, competition and appropriation on a massive scale. On the one hand, the market appropriated the various 'marginalized' healing traditions and practices and provided them with a new arena of growth, while on the other, it reformatted these appropriated practices into forms more suitable for the specificities of the market. Most crucially, however, the systemic superiority of allopathic medicine—and by extension *daktari*—was subverted in the market and niches carved out by 'systems' like homoeopathy. The success of homoeopathy in the cholera market showed the potential for the medical market to invert the politics of state-sponsored medical hegemonization.

Conclusion

Cholera in the Bengali language archive is distinct in every way from its presence in the governmental archive. The subjects of the discourses are different ('population' and 'individuals in affective networks') just as the controversies are distinct ('modes of transmission' and 'ethics of self-care').

In terms of the treatment, there were a number of overlaps between *daktari* treatment and other treatment regimes. These overlaps cannot be conceptualized as straightforward borrowings. Instead, as the use of substances like opiates and camphor alongside contraptions like the 'cholera belt', showed that, faced with a medical crisis that none of the approaches could yet fully solve, they all sought legitimacy by aligning their praxes with each other. In this continuous process of realignments, there was no authentic original that all the regimes drew upon; only a series of mimetic gestures that tied them together.

The devastation caused and the endemic nature of the disease created a long-term crisis of medical authority, which, in turn, created an opportunity for all kinds of 'marginal' healings methods to thrive—albeit after being suitably reformatted. Innovation and appropriation of 'marginal' traditions and practices, however, did not rule out contest and competition. It was within this competitive medical market that, in the case of cholera, allopathy's state-sponsored superiority was successfully—albeit briefly—challenged by homoeopathy, and ascriptions of 'marginality' came undone.

Table I.* Tables Indicating Deployment of 'Native' Physicians in the Treatment of Cholera in 1818–19 in Nadia

Names of Physicians	Where Deputed	When Deputed	When Recalled	Period of Service	Monthly Allowance in Rupees
Ramprasad	Thana Meherpur	20/9/1818	22/2/1819	5 months 3 days	8
Maheshchandra	Thana Meherpur	20/9/1818	22/2/1819	Ditto	8
Teencowrie	Amjhupi	18/11/1818	22/2/1819	3 months 5 days	8
Ramchandra	Amjhupi	18/11/1818	22/2/1819	Ditto	8
Gobinda	Hardi	27/12/18	26/1/1819	1 month	8
Parvati	Hardi	27/12/18	26/1/1819	Ditto	8
Ramtanu	Daulatganj	15/11/18	22/2/1819	3 months 8 days	8
Bykuntha	Daulatganj	15/11/18	22/2/1819	Ditto	8
Jagannath	Raal Boalia	1/8/18	11/9/1818	1 month 11 days	8
Jagannath	Raal Boalia	18/11/18	22/2/1819	3 months 5 days	8
Bykuntha	Dalimtola	20/11/18	22/2/1819	3 months 3 days	8
Debiprasanna	Chitrasali	20/11/18	22/2/1819	Ditto	8
Ramchandra	Thana Santipur	23/11/18	22/2/1819	3 months	8

Signed: J. Mellis, Surgeon, 2nd March 1819, Krishnanagar.

* ΣΟΥΡΧΕ: Ρεπορτσ οφ αν Επιδεμιχ οφ Χηολερα ιν Μεδινιπυρ,Ναδια, Βιηαρ ανδ ιν Χαλχυττα, Μαρ 1819–Νοϖ1820, Α&ΑΧ Χαλλ Νο. Φ/4/746. Αλλ σπελλινγσ οφ προπερ νουνσ ηαϖε βεεν μοδερνισεδ ωηερεϖερ ποσσιβλε. Συχη ναμεσ ασ τηοσε ωηιχη ελυδε ρεχογνιτιον βψ μοδε ρν σπελλινγσ ηαϖε βεεν ρεταινεδ ιν τηε οριγιναλ ανδ ινδιχατεδ βψ σινγλε ινϖερτεδ χομμασ.

Table II. [ϒ]

Names of Physician	Thana Where Deployed	Total Attacked	Cured	Deaths
Kashiram Dutt	Kotwali	34	29	5
Ramtaran	Kotwali	14	12	2
Nausher	Kotwali	109	85	24
Sasticharan	Kotwali	28	23	5
Sreenath	Kotwali	19	15	4
Raghab	Kotwali	17	14	3
Rammohan	Kotwali	34	27	7
Kali 'Nudithee'	Kotwali	38	29	9
Ramshankar	Kotwali	31	24	7
Ramprasad	Kotwali	35	30	5
Ramsundar	Kotwali	71	61	10
Swarup	Kotwali	28	23	5
Kali Das	'Maunpore'	14	8	6
Keshab	Shantipur	37	29	8
Bykuntha	Shantipur	150	97	53
Ramjoy	Shantipur	148	98	57
Ramkumar	Shantipur	10	7	3
Bholanath	Shantipur	22	12	10
Madanmohun	'Maunpore'	23	16	7
Ramjoy	'Maunpore'	25	17	8
Sasti	'Maunpore'	16	10	6
Radhamohun	'Maunpore'	14	8	6
Ramkantha	'Maunpore'	17	11	6
Pitambar	'Maunpore'	21	14	7
Kalu	Mominpur	39	30	--

Signed: J Mellis, Surgeon, dated 20th June 1819, Krishnanagar.

[ϒ] The Surgeon J Mellis, recommended a compensation of 2 annas per cured case for every physician mentioned in this table.

Chapter VI

DHATU DOURBALYA: DIAGNOSING THE RHIZOID PATHOLOGIES OF WEAKNESS

Nowhere is the biomoral character of Bengali medical discourses and their shaping within a cosmopolitan medical market more clearly marked out than in the texts on what has come to be called the *dhat* syndrome in psychiatric literature. Most available histories of this affliction, however, have been framed by the debate amongst psychiatrists over whether it can be called a 'Culture Bound Syndrome' (hereafter CBS) or not. These histories, therefore, follow contemporary medical practice in assuming *dhat* to be a single, unified, pathological reality, be it an independent category or part of some larger denomination. This means that the phenomenon is thought to have a fixed set of symptoms located in the human physiology, and a clearly defined vocabulary to distinguish these.

We will argue, however, that the Bengali physicians in the late nineteenth and early twentieth centuries had not conceptualized it as a unitary pathological reality. We will argue that they had conceptualized it as a shifting cluster of ideas. The specific form the cluster took and the vocabulary that was deployed to describe it could often vary. What were described as symptoms in one text could be described as a related illness in another. Moreover, words and categories used could change—slightly or more drastically. New categories could be added or old ones discarded. Following Deleuze and Guattari thus, we suggest that the reality of the *dhat* complaints in these texts should be conceptualized as a rhizoid reality.[1]

Rhizomes are, of course, a class of plants that could be anything from a grass to a ginger. Their usefulness as a conceptual metaphor lies primarily in their shape. They are marked by a series of random connections and disconnections. Furthermore, the places where different radial networks connect are widely varied. Finally, a rhizome can be broken off at any point and can commence another network of connections from that point, while the broken section might also carry on expanding. Using such a model to understand a pathological category has the potential for radically reorienting both the way popular pathological understanding has been conceptualized and the relationship betwixt the popular and the erudite levels of medicine.

The approach de-centres the meaning of the pathological category by refusing to look for a single *authentic* meaning. Instead it accepts the 'superficial' form in which the category appears in lay usage, alongside numerous other overlapping designations of the pathology. By refusing to look for a single, *authentic* meaning, it resists the temptation to impose categories derived from erudite texts upon popular understandings of an affliction. In the case of *dhatu dourbalya*, what is most interesting, however, is that a popular, de-centred understanding was actually adopted by erudite *daktari* authors. Here then, we find a telling example of not only the ways in which the popular and erudite world of medicine often overlapped amongst *daktari* authors, but also of how intellectual categories and arguments could flow from the popular to the erudite levels (instead of the reverse, which is more common).

The History of Culture in Debates on the *Dhat* Syndrome

Before developing the idea of *dhat* complaints as a rhizoid reality, we need to first investigate why available histories of the disease have been unable to locate its rhizoid structure and continue to speak of it as a homogenized unitary category. This blind spot, we will argue, is a consequence of the way the terms 'history' and 'culture' have been used in the CBS debate, of which the histories form a part.

CBS, along with a variety of similar but slightly different designations, was first proposed in the 1960s by authors such as Wig and Yap.[2] Littlewood and Lipsedge have defined them as 'episodic and dramatic reactions specific to a particular community—locally defined as discrete patterns of behaviour'.[3] The label CBS has since had a chequered career in psychiatric literature. However their very existence, the precise designation for them as well as their nosological status have all been the subjects of much debate, especially since the 1980s. Scholars such as Hughes have pointed out that the existence of alternative titles such as 'atypical psychosis' and 'exotic syndrome' clearly demonstrated how European experience was considered the baseline, while experiences of people in the 'majority world' were portrayed as 'deviant' and not normal.[4] At the same time, scholars such as Littlewood have described CBSs that were only found in the 'West', thereby attacking the conception that CBS was always something associated with 'non-Western' societies.[5] The obvious validity of such critiques eventually forced the leading international diagnostic classificatory systems to change the status of CBS in a conscious bid for neutrality. Both the ICD-10 of WHO and the DSM-IV of the American Psychiatric Association have thus incorporated 'culture' as a diagnostic factor.[6]

Perhaps the most debated South Asian CBS is the *dhat syndrome. Dhat* was first described by Wig in 1960 and has since then, like the other CBSs, had a chequered intellectual career. The syndrome is associated almost exclusively with South Asian populations, in South Asia itself as well as amongst diasporic communities originating in South Asia, though similar syndromes such as *shen k'uei* and *shen-kui* are also known to exist in Southeast Asia. Sufferers are usually young males, between 20 and 38 years of age, complaining of weakness, fatigue, palpitations and sleeplessness. 'Most significantly [however], patients attribute these symptoms to a white discharge in their urine (which they claim is a 'vital substance'—semen).'[7] At its most generalized level, it is an anxiety over the physiological effects of semen loss and has included in various contexts not only loss of semen with the urine, but also involuntary emissions, deliberate ejaculation, etc. The term '*dhat*' itself has been described by Sushrut Jadhav as an 'English corruption of the Sanskrit word *dhatu* and erroneously equated with either "semen" or "semen-loss" in modern psychiatric literature'. Jadhav, who dismisses the idea of *dhat* being a CBS, calling it a 'cultural misunderstanding', goes on to draw upon the *Charak Samhita*—an important ayurvedic text often considered to be canonical—to explain the culturally specific meanings of *dhatu.* He also draws upon the writings of Galen and Aristotle to show that similar anxieties have been found in the 'west' as well. While calling for greater cultural awareness and sensitivity on the part of 'European transcultural psychiatrists' and those inspired by the 'the general climate of post-Independence India (emphasising Gandhian [*sic*] self-reliance)',[8] Jadhav does not stop to consider his own selection of sources through which to describe this 'Indian culture'.[9] He finds no contradictions in using an ancient Sanskrit text and Gandhi to define a unitary 'Indian culture'. The same derivation from ancient Sanskrit texts, despite the absence in them of any direct reference to a specific malady caused from the loss of semen, is found in a number of authors on the subject, such as Bhugra and Buchanan; Chadha, Ahuja and Sumathipala; and Siribaddana and Bhugra.[10] The last mentioned also attempt a tabular presentation of the history of semen-loss anxieties to prove their universalism. The table lists all historical authors who have allegedly contributed to the development of an almost 'global' anxiety about semen loss. It starts tellingly with Agnivesa's redaction of Charak which is dated to '1500 BC', going on to Susruta, for whom no date is ascribed, followed by Hippocrates, Aristotle, Galen, Celsus, Esquirol, Tissot, Maudsley, Beard and Freud before concluding with *The Lancet* in the nineteenth century. Ironically, then, by incorporating 'culture' into psychiatric theory, it (i.e., culture) has not only been universalized, but, in fact, has in effect come to lose any real historical location. It no longer matters whether any clear genealogy can be drawn at all between Charak and Tissot, or if such a genealogy ever did exist, in what form or way were they connected. Were there any real routes—textual or oral—through which Tissot may have picked up on Charak's writings? If Tissot did indeed pick up Charak's writings—given that the two were separated by a huge swathe of time—what were the exact channels of communication and how had these intermediaries represented Charak's ideas? Most of all, it does not matter whether the patients—who more often than not have no medical training at all—ever read these texts. Thus there is no seeming incongruence between asserting that it is the 'lower' and 'least educated' rungs of Indian society who are most concerned with semen loss and offering Charak's erudite Sanskrit treatise on the number of blood drops needed to make up a drop of semen as the source of their anxieties.

'Culture' becomes a mere spatial signpost devoid of any lived reality in these writings. Its only identity derives from a geographic suffix (i.e., 'Indian culture', 'European culture', etc.) which otherwise does not seem to bequeath any particularity other than in name alone. The chronologies and geographies of *dhat*'s origins coincide, perhaps more dangerously, with those of the imaginations of a Hindu Indian nation state. 'Indian culture', in this imagination, must derive from an ancient Sanskrit, 'Hindu' (Jadhav, for instance, refers to ayurveda's connections to Hinduism) past. All that is not Sanskrit, not textualized, regionally specific or brought to India by migrants, merchants, conquerors and preachers does not find a place in this account of 'culture'. All those messy areas where power, gender, culture, society, economy, literature, etc., came together and overlapped to create not only texts, but performances, praxes and also—let us not forget—*versions* of texts, are exiled from the domain of culture. None ask if all the various forms of '*dhat*' in South Asia do indeed derive from the Sanskrit canon? What kind of authorities did writers in different regions themselves quote in establishing this pathological category?

'Culture', in this reading, lacks its own history. History is a global, linear scale—which in effect is pure chronology—on which the contributions of distinct 'cultures' can be mapped at fixed points. These 'cultures' themselves are unchanging and static. Most importantly, these 'cultures' can be understood with reference to a handful of well-known texts. These iconic texts themselves are also devoid of history. They do not mutate with time or function within social contexts which influence their reading.

Having thus committed itself to geographically and chronologically stable, abstract and classically derived categories, it is not surprising that this discourse fails to notice the actuality of the rhizoid reality of *dhat* complaints.

Defining *Dhatu Dourbalya*

The most popular designation, though by no means the only one, for such complaints in late-colonial Bengal was *dhatu dourbalya.* Between 1890 and 1920, newspapers in Bengal were covered with advertisements of specifics claiming to cure *dhatu dourbalya.* One author, writing in 1896 wrote, 'Anyone who makes a survey of the number of patent medicines being sold for this malady and the extent of the sales of such medicines will not think any discussion of this subject exaggerated…We have looked into the matter and can say this with confidence that there are no patent medicine sellers who do not trade in at least one or two remedies for this affliction. Some offer it openly while others do it clandestinely, over and above all these are the classical remedies, the remedies of the hakims, remedies of divine origin and so many more.'[11] The visibility of the affliction in the daily lives of the turn-of-the-century Bengalis was beyond question, but what exactly was this disease? Does it resemble the *dhat syndrome* of today? If so, how close is the resemblance?

Dr Lalitmohan Chattopadhyay, who wrote one of the most detailed series of essays on the affliction appearing in the Bengali medical press regularly between 1896 and 1905, clarified that the term '*dhatu*' signified a number of a different things in lay Bengali usage. Pace Jadhav et al., we observe, that, of all the various meanings of the term, as Chattopadhyay used it, many clearly did not derive from the writings of Charak. The first meaning that sprung to Dr Chattopadhyay's mind was the grammarian use of *dhatu* to signify the basic semantic units of sound. The 'pulse', which was the iconic diagnostic tool of 'indigenous' medicine in Bengal, was also often known as '*dhatu*'. Its lay usage in this last context, however, was significantly often shortened to '*dhat*'. The word *dhat* also referred to what the author described as the '*secretions* of the body'. The use of the English word 'secretions' in the Bengali text was, in all probability, deliberately designed to show the essays proximity to allopathic rather than any 'ancient ayurvedic' tradition. Dr Chattopadhyay further clarified that to speak of 'dhatu loss usually meant losing semen'. All 'necessary and prime parts of the body' (*prayajaniya o pradhan, pradhan ongsho*) are also said to be called *dhatu.* A final meaning derives from the lay designation of gonorrhoea, which was referred to as '*dhat-er pirha*', or the illness of *dhat* or the 'constitution'. Another possible meaning that Dr Chattopadhyay missed, but is often used by other authors and continues to be found in everyday linguistic usage, is *dhat* as 'constitution' or 'nature' of a person. Lay Bengalis thus, for example, often refer to people having a constitution prone to common colds as *shordi-r dhat*, or, indeed, while referring to obstinate character traits—*kotha shona or dhat-e nei* (it is not in his nature to ever listen to others). The word *dhatu* further referred to metals and sometimes synecdochally to 'mercury'.[12] Innumerable Bengali medical texts thus refer to *dhatu-ghatita aushadh* (metal or, indeed, mercury-made medicines). The treatment of the word by the first Bengali encyclopaedia—*Biswakosh*—published in 1885 is instructive. While it discussed numerous meanings of the word ranging from the linguistic to the physiological, it did take up the physiological register for extensive discussion in its own right. Significantly, however, it assiduously refused to reduce *dhatu* to semen. Despite quoting from Susruta about the seven *dhatus,* its discussions of pathological states caused by *dhatu* insisted on the need for balance amongst all of the *dhatus.* An excess or diminution of any one was said to be pathogenic. Theoretically, therefore, according to the *Biswakosh,* the loss of semen could actually be good in some cases, i.e., where there is a relative excess of *sukra dhatu.*[13]

As Michael Foucault amongst many others has pointed out, our knowledge of our bodies is not independent of the vocabularies that name it and the institutional praxes through which it becomes 'known'. The discontinuities, limits and multiple possibilities of these vocabularies cannot be flattened out by a spurious assumption of a linear continuity stretching from distant Charak to the local GP. One of the earliest detailed comments on the disease is found in Dr Hur Chunder Sen's manual from 1882. Dr Sen was the Medical Officer-in-Charge of the Sherpur Dispensary and worked consciously within the 'western' medical tradition. His work was conspicuous in its trenchant use of English pathological designations throughout. His account of what looks very similar to *dhatu dourbalya* is to be found under the designation of 'Spermatorrhoea'. He listed all the complaints usually found associated with *dhatu dourbalya*, such as mental and physical weakness and fatigue, the passing of chalky fluids thought to be semen with urine and, he adds, sometimes also stools, involuntary discharges of semen, general weakness, impotency etc.[14] Dr Sen made no reference to any ayurvedic texts and did not use the term *dhatu* at all in his descriptions. Yet his description of 'spermatorrhoea' clearly articulated the same cluster of ideas. Sen's description very closely resembles that of Radhagobinda Kar in his canonical *daktari* work, the *Bhisak Suhrid.* Kar uses a range of 'indigenous' terms such as *swapnadosh* and *sukrameha* but equates them with 'spermatorrhoea'.[15] Bill Bynum has pointed out that the Victorian preoccupation with 'Spermatorrhoea' derived principally from the writings of the English sexologist William Acton.[16] The continued use of this

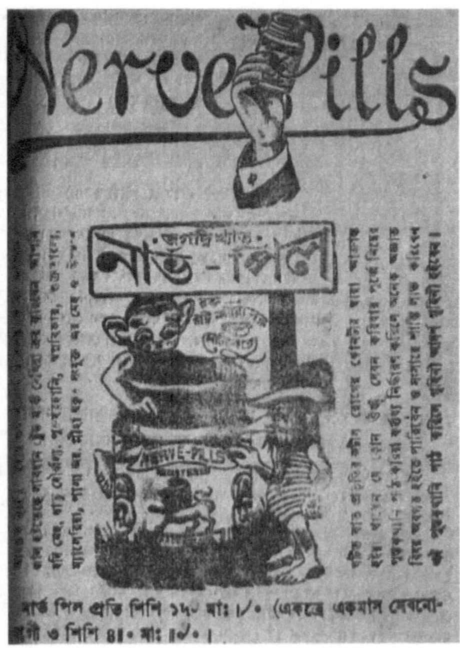

Fig. IX. Advertisement for Nerve Pills, Gupta Press Dairektari Panjika for 1322 BS.

category in numerous *dhat* texts even today clearly proves that this Victorian malady had a crucial impact upon the Bengali pathological designation.

Further attention to the actual categories being used in the texts and their arrangement reveals another striking feature about this malady. It was seldom imagined as a unitary pathology. Doctors often thought of it as a composite of multiple complaints. Writers like the prolific Dr Chattopadhyay framed the category as a composite category comprised of a network of several minor symptoms and independent maladies. He wrote that 'it would not be unfair to describe the mechanical and active (*jantrik o kriyagata*) dissonance' between the principal parts of the body as '*dhatu dourbalya*'. 'Thereby', he continued, 'different afflictions could be described together'. The list of diseases he gave as being caused due to such 'dissonance' were both those, for which only English names were available—such as "entic dyspepsia", "sexual debility", "impotency" and "spermatorrhoea"—as well as those which were described by Bengali names—such as '*snayubik pirha*' (nervous affliction, '*swapna-bikar*' (dream distortion) and '*sadharan dourbalya*' (normal weakness). Similarly Kar, while writing about the causes of this disease, mentioned that it might arise out of a range of other afflictions (some of which were only known by their

English names whilst other could only be described by Bengali names) like, '*amashay yukta atisar*' (diarrhoea with mucous), worms, piles, fistula, simple constipation, 'nervous phymosis' (*snayabik faimosis*), 'prostrate' secretions, blisters, internal application of 'cantharidise', etc. Similarly, amongst the symptoms of the disease, according to Kar, were, 'monomania', 'dementia', epilepsy, impotence (*dhwajabhanga*), paralysis, 'strabismus', nervous 'asthma', and so on. Many of these symptoms, debilities and complaints had, of course, medical careers of their own. '*Dourbalya*' or 'weakness' in itself, for instance, was often used as an independent pathological category as well. Similarly, '*snayubik pirha*', '*swapna-bikar*', 'dyspepsia', 'impotency', etc., were all known to exist as independent complaints as well, with their own sets of symptoms. [Fig. XII.] What was important was that together they came to signify *dhatu dourbalya*. The latter malady was thus a composite created out of these several constituents. The constituents, moreover, were not wholly subsumed within the composite. Chattopadhyay did not want to deny the existence of the constituent ailments. They, too, existed at a subordinate, but independent, level.

The list of actual 'symptoms' that were included under *dhatu dourbalya* was quite extensive. Dr Chattopadhyay lists a total of 23 'physical' and 14 'mental' symptoms of *dhatu dourbalya*. The physical symptoms range from sunken eyes and roughness of skin to cracked voice and balding, while the mental symptoms range from disorganized thinking and sighing to cowardliness, sleeplessness and 'hypochondriasis'.[17] The symptoms, however, could also vary from one author to another. Dr Pulinchandra Sanyal and Kaviraj Avinashchandra Kabiratna, for instance, identified a burning sensation while passing urine as the main symptom associated with this affliction, though other symptoms, such as the passing of a chalky white substance with urine in the evening, were also mentioned. Kobirotno and Sanyal, significantly, also related the affliction they chose to call '*dhat-er pirha*' (a designation usually reserved for gonorrhoea) with the ayurvedic category of 'prameha'.[18]

The numerous advertisements of medicines claiming to cure the affliction also provide interesting clues to the way the disease was conceptualized by physicians of the time. As noted in Chapter II, advertisements appearing in *panjikas*, or almanacs, could stretch for several pages at a time, thereby constituting small treatises of a sort in their own right. A survey of these texts further complicates the symptomatology of *dhatu dourbalya*. Not only do the set of symptoms often vary widely, but even more interestingly, the relationship between symptom and disease itself seems to be variable. What is once referred to as a symptom of *dhatu dhourbolyo* might elsewhere become an independent but kindred disease in its own right. Kaviraj Prasannachandra Maitreya, for instance, advertised his specific *Jeeban Sahay* under the rubric of being a 'great cure' (*mahaushudh*) for diseases such as '*dhatu-kheen*' (weakness/slimness of '*dhatu*') and '*dhwajabhanga*' (usually translated as 'impotency'). In the text of the advertisement, he mentioned, 'taking the medicine regularly cures *sukrataralya* [dilution of the sperm], *swapnadosh* [dream-illness], *maithunashakti* [addiction to sexual intercourse], *shiraghurnon* [spinning of the head], *mandagni* [lit: perversion of the digestive fire] and the extremely painful *sukrameha* [lit: sweetening of sperm]'.[19] It is not clear if these various debilities and afflictions are component parts of *dhatu-kheenata* or whether they are independent diseases of a similar nature. Another advertisement for Dr Gavin's *Spermatone* mentioned *dhatu dourbalya*, *sukrotaralya* and *shaktiheenata* together as the three diseases that the remedy was effective against. In detailing its specific affects, however, the advertisement mentioned that 'it prolongs ejaculation, destroys *sukrataralya* [dilution of semen] and stops spermatorrhoea, *sukrameha* and *swapnadosh*. It nourishes the *dhatu*, augments memory, banishes mental fatigue, excites the appetite and cleanses the bowels'.[20] Yet another advertisement appearing in the *Amrita Bazar Patrika* in 1906 listed most of these complaints and some more as 'symptoms'. The *Sudhakar Batika* was said to be 'an infallible remedy for wet dreams, involuntary discharges, thinness of semen and other cognate ailments. If these diseases are not speedily cured they are followed by serious mental debility, general weakness, loss of appetite, giddiness and loss of cheerfulness. However obstinate the symptoms be, only a week's trial will work like magic on the patient…It makes the mind cheerful and brings in sound sleep'.[21] Though a cluster of ideas do seem to recur in these texts, their precise hierarchic arrangement in the form of symptoms and diseases seems to be rather confusing. Such lack of clarity is shared by both the advertising texts and the more didactic texts such as Dr Chattopadhyay's essays or the popular sexual manuals of the day such as the *Sukh Sombhog Rotnakor* or Surjyonarayon Ghosh's *Dampottyo Pronali*.

Such structural similarities once again point towards the constant blurring of the lines between medical 'orthodoxy' and 'quackery' in the domain of the medical market. In fact, when called upon to preside over a controversy about the 'immorality' of these advertisements, the Bengal Government found that for the majority of them, they could not distinguish 'quackery' from 'legitimate medicine' in legal terms due to the similarity of their idiom.[22] Dr Chattopadhyay, too, in arguing for the relevance of his treatise, pointed to the advertisements, thus drawing legitimacy from them. Such obvious evidence clearly undermines any suggestions that *dhatu dourbalya* was a culturally determined pathological category with roots in ancient Indian medical texts alone and alien to 'modern' medicine. It was, instead, very much a product of the late colonial history of Bengal and practitioners directly claiming affiliation to the allopathic/'modern'/'western' system of healing who were as active as the 'indigenous' practitioners in fashioning it as a conceptual category. The importance of Dr Sen's nomenclature lies in disabusing any lasting misconceptions about the roots of *dhat* lying solely in antique ayurvedic usage.

The Market and the Metaphorical Logic of *Dhatu Dourbalya*

The confusion in demarcating symptoms and maladies raises interesting questions about the nature of medical rationality that operated in these texts. The structure of the medical rationality used by doctors in nineteenth-century India has not really received any independent attention. Their rationality has been assumed to be derivative of contemporary European medical or clinical rationality.

This nineteenth-century clinical rationality, as pointed out by Bynum, was often represented as a process of thought by which the doctor translated 'symptoms' into 'causes'.[23] This form of rationality, however, did not act in a social vacuum. Instead, as Foucault has clarified in the case of France, this rationality was structured by 'establishing a relation, in medical discourse, between a number of distinct elements, some of which concerned the status of the doctors, others the institutional and technical site from which they spoke, others their position as subjects perceiving, observing, describing, teaching, etc.'[24] Both Bynum and Foucault have also elaborated upon the debt of this type of medical rationality to industrialization and the powerful emergent ideas about 'liberal government'.[25] In a society such as colonial India, where neither of these two factors were available—at least not to the same extent or form as in Europe—it is not surprising that medical rationality operated differently.

Jean Langford has therefore noticed a very different rationality at work amongst the ayurvedists she studied. She found that '[t]he ontological hierarchy wherein the symptom is simply an indicator and disease an objective entity, the focal point of treatment, is therefore not easily sustained. Diseases themselves are signs for aggravated *dosa*, while so-called symptoms like fever are treatable in themselves…[T]he binarism of symptom and disease, though invoked in clinical discourse, is nonetheless often irrelevant to clinical practice'.[26]

We have already seen in previous chapters that the pressures of the cosmopolitan medical market often blurred systemic boundaries. Moreover, as pointed out by Chattopadhyay amongst others, as *dhatu dourbalya* was by far the most commercially viable site in the medical market, it is not unreasonable to assume that allopathic medical rationality itself may have been influenced by this very different relationship between symptom and disease which is seen to exist amongst Langford's more recent clinical ayurvedists.

We will argue that the medical rationality which structured *dhatu dourbalya* is best described as a 'metaphorical rationality'.[27] The importance of metaphors in any kind of thinking, including 'hard' scientific theories, has been suggested since the early 1970s.[28] Scholars like George Lakoff and Mark Johnson forcefully argue that 'our ordinary conceptual system, in terms of which we both think and act, is fundamentally metaphorical in nature.'[29] However, what we are suggesting here is an even stronger and often conscious use of metaphors in medical thinking. Authors thereby deliberately urge medical rationality to be structured by metaphorical associations.

The need for this exaggerated use of metaphors in medical rationality, we will further argue, derived from the specific context of the medical market within which these texts circulated. The institutional matrix within which the Bengali *daktars* operated was very different from that which doctors Foucault or Bynum studied. Their pedagogical trajectories were different and so were their professional and social standings. The context of 'private consultation'—that 'great medical edifice of the nineteenth century'—was distinct and so was the power relation between them and their patients. It was, therefore, natural that the ways in which they themselves thought about disease and encouraged others to think would also be different.

It is with an eye to this distinct institutional context that we should interrogate the specifically pronounced metaphoricity of *daktari* medical rationality. Having to compete with a variety of other health professionals (such as *kavirajes* and *hakims* for one), their medical authority was far more tenuous than their European counterparts. Moreover, as we have seen in Chapter II, the social image of *daktars* in the late nineteenth century was not very high or positive. Furthermore, many of them had only received a rudimentary professional training and often had to supplement their meagre training with what they picked up from other medical traditions in the region. Finally, their livelihood often depended upon a fragile and highly competitive medical market where the patient's power to switch physicians was considerable and, hence, a successful physician had to be able to convince the layman of the efficacy of his cure. There was little opportunity to educate these laymen who were ultimately to decide upon whether they needed the medicine or not. The *daktars* hence had to eschew complicated medical syllogisms in favour of easily understandable rationales. As we recall from Chapter II, Rajsekhar Basu, writing in the 1920s, mentioned that whenever anyone fell ill in his average middle-class extended family, it fell upon him in his capacity as the head of the family to decide which *type* of physician (i.e., *daktar*, *kaviraj*, shaman, etc.) to turn to. If the *daktar* was to successfully attract custom, it would not do to speak only in the language of complicated medical arguments. It is another matter that given their pedagogical and social backgrounds, they may themselves have avoided a strictly 'western' clinical rationality. In sexual matters, considerations of delicacy that many *daktari* authors explicitly cite would have further confounded their problems and encouraged the use of metaphors. Metaphor, which has been described as a linguistic act that renders an unfamiliar idea familiar by invoking an already familiar idea, emerged, therefore, as the major vehicle for medical thinking and expression about *dhatu dourbalya*.[30]

Since it involved the expression of the unfamiliar in terms of the familiar and since the *daktars* sought to communicate with the middle-class medical consumers, predictably, most of the ideas invoked as part of the description of *dhatu dourbalya* were replete with images drawn from the middle-class milieu. It was especially the Gogolesque world of the *keranis* that Sumit Sarkar has so ably described that was visible in the metaphors of *dhatu dourbalya*.[31] The repeated references to 'hard study', or the pressures of education, in causing *dhatu dourbalya*, for instance, are clearly aimed at the *keranis*.[32] Unlike the handful of upper-class *bhodrolok* reformers who had hailed the colonial education system for its 'modernizing' role, the majority of the lower-middle class looked upon the years of toil through school and college to be a singular burden. An education system which stressed memorization rather than independent thinking and whose eventual aim was an intellectually stultifying clerical job, obviously failed to appeal to those who were forced to take it up in the hopes of a job. Similarly, the repeated references to digestive discomforts (*ajirna, agnimanda, dyspepsia*) also make perfect sense if we recall that the water supply of urban Calcutta remained highly problematic throughout the late nineteenth century, making cholera and regular stomach problems chronic for most of the urban lower andmiddle classes.[33] The general ideas about debility, weakness and even racial decline were all too common in the Bengali middle-class milieu in the late nineteenth century, though they would predictably have been much more poignant in the lower and middle classes who increasingly came to identify the period as *Kaliyug*, or the last apocalyptic age of Hindu mythology where everything of value and virtue was already diminished and waning.[34]

Sexual anxieties, too, would have no doubt proliferated in an age when the majority of lower-middle class men could not afford to live with their families in the city. They usually lived in 'messing' houses throughout the week and returned home for the weekends. Sexual transgressions and recourse to prostitutes to satisfy their carnal appetites had thus become a prominent feature of the *kerani* lifestyle. So widespread was the cultural visibility of such transgressions that Durgacharan Sanyal, writing a racy 'social history of

Bengal' in the 1890s, spent nearly five pages arguing that Hindu men had throughout history had recourse to prostitutes when they lived away from their families for employment. Sanyal wanted to argue that there was nothing novel or particularly reprehensible about this, for as long as men needed to live away from their families, they would also need other sources of sexual gratification.[35]

Sometimes the metaphorical rationality went beyond merely references to specific lifestyles and its attendant anxieties. Quite a few advertisements even sought to explain curative claims through metaphors. Particularly popular were claims in which the metaphors also reverberated with the above-noted polyvalence of the term '*dhatu*'. One seller, for instance, claimed that 'it is well known that diseases of *dhatu* [here he meant 'semen'] can only be cured by medicines made of *dhatu* [here he meant 'metals'], that is why our medicine made from [gold] cures *sukrodosh* quickly and effectively'.[36]

The most crucial deployment of metaphor came in the form of 'concept metaphors'. The concept metaphors were those thought-images that organized the symptoms recounted into a recognizable pathological reality. Bynum, though he does not quite use these words, has hinted at the concept metaphor of a 'spermatic economy' informing Victorian notions of spermatorrhoea.[37] The concept metaphor that organizes *dhatu dourbalya* is explicitly one of a 'spermatic economy'. What could, after all, be the most readily remembered thought-image for the *kerani* than having to run a household on a meagre salary? Dr D. D. Gupta thus explained in an essay titled *Bodily Income and Expenditure* that just as it was not good for one who earned Rs 10/- a month to be spending Rs 15/-, similarly, one had to budget the income and expenditure of the body as well. Moreover, the English, claimed Dr Gupta, were much better at budgeting—be it to do with money or the body. 'From the king to even the most common of householder, every Englishman,' the author claimed, 'produces a list of income and expenditure at the beginning of every year, whereas many a Bengali householder does not even know the exact monthly expenditure in his home'.[38] Though Dr Gupta made no direct mention of *dhatu dourbalya*, his insinuation could hardly have been lost on his readers. Moreover, he referred to the classical seven *dhatus*. Since none of the other six, such as blood, flesh, bone and marrow could be *consciously* 'expended', and since his article was explicitly aimed at dissuading the *conscious* 'expenditure' of *dhatu*, his advice could only have been directed at 'semen'. Authors such as Dr Chattopadhyay, who had written in serious periodicals on the subject, had remained apologetic for the indelicacy of the topic, and Dr Gupta's reticence to explicitly mention 'semen' was almost certainly motivated by similar considerations of delicacy.[39] He did, however, make explicit claims about the exact amounts of *dhatu* transaction that the body daily undertook. Gupta claimed that it had been determined by tests that the human body 'expended' 1.5 to 2 *seers* of material in an average day. Even whilst obviously not elaborating at such length, most advertisements referring to *dhatu dourbalya* explicitly use the terms *aye* and *byaye* ('income' and 'expenditure') in reference to the loss of 'semen'. Apart from obviously helping to convey his ideas to lay readers, the concept metaphor is also crucial in delineating the malady from earlier, pre-nineteenth century maladies, to which it often bore a family resemblance. Bhab Misra's influential text from the sixteenth century, the *Bhabprakash*, for instance, using the conceptual metaphor of churning milk to produce *ghee* (clarified butter), stated that those who ejaculate semen easily or with slight effort have a surfeit of it and are therefore more healthy than those who do not do so.[40]

This positive perspective had already shifted by the eighteenth century. Gobinda Das' *Bhesaja Ratnavali*, written in the period, had introduced a pathological category already exhibiting some resemblance to *dhatu dourbalya*, but known as *sukrameha*. The concept metaphor, however, was still very different and suggested a very different intellectual genealogy for *sukrameha*. The Sanskrit text read: '*Sukramehe prathamatah kriya shangshadhani hita/Retasha rakshanang tatra karjanchati prajatnatah*' (In *sukrameha*, firstly, the correction of actions is good/ Persevere to end the action [and] in that place preserve the sperm).[41] The conceptual metaphors here are of preservation and nurture (*rakshanang*) of what is already depleted through illness. The metaphor of preserving and nurturing sperm has obvious resonances with the Siddha, Marfati Sufi and Nathpanthi Tantric traditions. The eighteenth century had seen a particularly marked rise of numerous peasant religions influenced by these traditions. These traditions and the large number of sects influenced by them all over Bengal sought physical perfection or spiritual liberation through religio-physical rites involving semen retention. However, the transition from the churning of milk metaphors to that of preservation was still incomplete, and some influential authors continued to speak of preserving semen while using the metaphor of churning. The peasant prophet Lalan Fakir, therefore, wrote in his characteristically allusive language that:

Even if you always mix milk and butter
The churning rod will still separate them
O Heart! Such is the way to a drop of the Elixir
It is not at all simple to achieve[42]

Here Lalan deploys what is known amongst Baul and Fakir sects as *Sondhya Bhasha* (The Language of the Evening): a coded language. Through a series of phrases with double meanings, Lalan argues that just as the semen is produced by a process allegorical to the churning of the butter from the milk within the body, so, too, should it be preserved during sexual intercourse. The Baul–Fakir traditions have ritualized rites that require sexual union without ejaculation. Some sects go so far as to claim that it is even possible to reabsorb ejaculated semen during such ritual sexual acts.[43]

So ubiquitous, however, was the knowledge of their rites and their metaphors that even orthodox (*ba shara*) Sufis who were opposed to such heterodox (*be shara*) practices came to frame their opposition by the same conceptual metaphor. Shukur Mohammed thus wrote in his epic medieval poem *Gopichander Sannyas* that:

> There are women in the market, women on the riverside, women everywhere
> All the men you see are imprisoned by women
> From a thousand drops of menstrual blood is a drop of love-juice [*rati maharas*] formed
> When that wealth is exhausted, men become the slaves of women[44]

Clearly, Mohammed's opposition to the waste of semen is not due to any perceived medical reasons. He merely feels that such wastage would render men the slaves of women. Interestingly, Mohammed's text also gives a radically different interpretation of the oft-quoted ideas about a 'thousand drops of blood' being needed to produce a single drop of semen. Irrespective of their agendas and interpretations, however, the shared eighteenth-century concept metaphor is that of *preserving* resources already depleted by disease, not that of bringing on disease through failing to balance income and expenditure.

Hugh Urban has described the widespread use of mercantile metaphors in eighteenth-century Bengali popular religious songs, owing to the new and increased exposure of rural Bengali society to the market. The alteration of the concept metaphors amongst eighteenth century authors like Das and Mohammed might also have been influenced by this growing exposure of rural Bengal to the 'market' (which Mohammed clearly mentions) and 'commerce'.[45] Their distance from the nineteenth century texts, however, is still significant. The extent of the divergence can be gauged by Binodlal Sen's Bengali gloss on Das's passage in a nineteenth-century critical edition of the latter's text. Where Das had spoken of 'preservation', Sen translated it as 'not spending' (*jahatey sukrer byay na hoy*).[46]

It was this altered metaphorical structure that was energetically popularized in the nineteenth-century texts on *dhatu dourbalya*. This new metaphorical framework undoubtedly drew upon earlier ideas, but its structure was undeniably framed by the metaphors and images of the nineteenth-century world of the *keranis*.

Partial Genealogies of a Modern Disease

Despite the obvious differences then, we can see in *sukrameha* one of the forebears of *dhatu dourbalya* in the eighteenth century. Alongside a host of other terms such as spermatorrhoea or *Prameha*, it formed a web of related terms that were often found associated with *dhatu dourbalya*. Though its occurrence proper preceded that of *dhatu dourbalya*, it did not simply form a part of the genealogy of the latter category. It continued to be used as an associated term in the *dhatu dourbalya* texts in varying capacities as symptom, synonym, related disease or simply as an independent category appearing side by side. Its precise relationship to *dhatu dourbalya* cannot, therefore, be discussed without some discussion of the entire web of associated terms with which it appeared conjointly in its usual usage. The question of *dhatu dourbalya*'s actual derivation, too, must depend upon an understanding of the role of terms like *Sukrameha* that appear as both preceding and associated terms.

As already suggested, conceptualizing *dhatu dourbalya* as a rhizoid reality allows us to explain how parts of one pathological reality—be it a disease or a symptom or any other related phenomenon—can get transferred to another pathological reality without necessarily meaning a wholesale derivation. Such an approach is particularly useful for us because the 'associated terms' that appear together in *dhatu dourbalya* texts are themselves entangled and heterogeneous terms. Terms such as *swapna-dosh*, *dourbalya*, *agnimanda*, *nervous debility*, *dhwajabhanga*, *na-mardangi* and even *hysteria* appear with varying regularity and in varying roles in these texts, thus suggesting that their meanings, too, are shifting and unstable.[47] Given the range and variability of the terms it would be impossible to attempt to trace the histories of all of them. We shall therefore confine ourselves to tracing only the most regularly appearing terms and their interrelationships.

<u>*Sukrameha*</u>: Radhagobinda Kar used this designation to describe a pathological reality very akin to *dhatu dourbalya*. To Kar, it included a wide range of symptoms ranging from the 'usual', i.e., 'seminal discharges from the genital organs during sleep, urination, defecation, or after long periods of horse-riding, travel by a vehicle or sitting or immediately following such activity', to the more unusual symptoms like 'constantly feeling cold water dripping down or tiny ants crawling on one's back'.[48] The causes of the disease, too, were wide-ranging. They included on the one hand, excessive sexual intercourse and masturbation, and on the other, 'going to sleep on one's stomach'.[49]

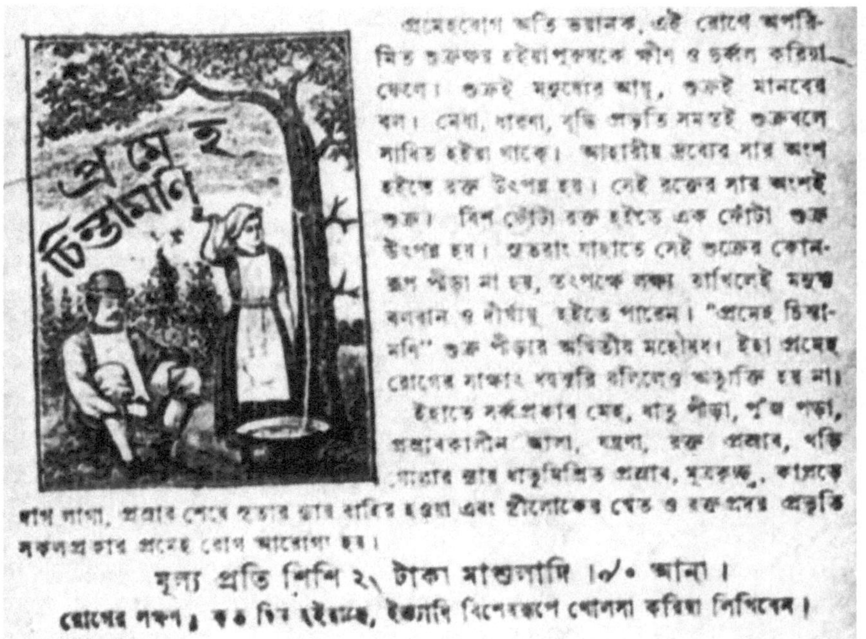

Fig. X. Advertisement for Prameha Chintamani, Nutan Panjika (1896).

We have already seen that *sukrameha* was described by Gobinda Das' eighteenth-century text. Significantly, Das did not discuss what caused the disease or what the main symptoms of the affliction were. However, in the closing remarks to the section on it, Das did mention that, once afflicted, one ought to avoid 'foods which produced *kaaph*, foods with strong tastes, heat from a fire, strong sun, addiction to women, stopping the urge to urinate or defecate, staying up at night, anger, deep sorrow, sleeping during the day, fasting, too much thinking, extreme laziness and keeping bad company'.[50] Though no details of the malady are given, two of the medicines in the section are said to stop the ejaculation of semen while dreaming. Once again, significantly, Das avoids calling it by a proper name, while his nineteenth-century editor Sen's gloss on the passage uses the term *swapna-dosh*. In Radhagobinda Kar's text, on the other hand, *swapnadosh* and *sukrameha* are treated as synonyms and equated to spermatorrhoea.[51] Prior to the eighteenth century, however, the genealogy of *sukrameha* is inextricably linked to the narrative of *Prameha*.

Prameha: A related category that appears independently in the *Bhesaja Ratnavali*, but is also one of the prominent 'associated terms' in the *dhatu dourbalya* texts, is *Prameha*. Like *Sukrameha*, Das' text does not describe the malady in detail. However, it does mention, while discussing one of the remedies, that taking the remedy would cure '*Prameha, Prameha-jata pirha* [diseases arising out of *Prameha*], *Klaiba* [one of the several types of impotency mentioned in earlier texts], *dhatu-khaye* [lit: *dhatu*-erosion], *kash* [cough], ...*jirna* [wasting] and *bisham-jwar* [a type of fever]'.[52] It , seems, therefore, to have, in the eighteenth century, its own set of 'associated terms'. Interestingly, some of these associated terms are common or closely resemble the terms later found to be associated with *dhatu dourbalya*. In this regard it is worth noting that Gananath Obeysekere, in his now classical account of this particular illness, had pointed out that the ayurvedists in Kandy, whom he had studied, used to conflate the symptoms of various sexual complaints—originally discussed as part of other diseases in the Sanskrit canon—with anxieties over semen loss which were possibly of vernacular vintage under the category *prameha*.[53] In the Bengali popular usage of the designation such conflation often resulted in the hoary ayurvedic genealogy of the word itself being juxtaposed with visibly European images. (Fig. XIII.)

In the texts of the *Charak Samhita* as well as the *Susruta Samhita* available in Bengal, *Prameha* was said to be of forty distinct types.[54] Of these, ten were caused through forms of derangements of *kaaph*, another six through the derangements of *pitta*, four by derangements of *bath*, and the final twenty forms resulted from the combined derangements of all three *doshes*. Of these, *sukrameha* was one of the ten types of *kaaphoj Prameha*. However, all that the *Charak* or *Susruta Samhitas* mentioned about it was that it caused semen to be passed along with urine. It did not further elaborate about this and did not mention if such outflow of semen had any bad effects. Significantly, the *Charak Samhita*, while describing another category, i.e., that of *pittoj Prameha*, did mention the same list of forbidden actions for the afflicted (avoiding heat from the fire, the strong sun, sleeping during the day, etc.) as Das had done for *Sukrameha*. The *Sukrameha* described in the *Bhesaj Ratnavali* is, therefore, created by the narration of a subcategory of *Prameha* as an independent category. Moreover, it comes to acquire some of characteristics of another subcategory, viz., *pittojo Prameha*. Equally importantly, other characteristics such as *dhatu-khoy*—which are found in descriptions of *Prameha* in the *Bhesaja Ratnavali*—are absent in the classical texts. This is a perfect example of a rhizoid development in which chains of signification have been broken and reconnected. These reconnections, however, should not be seen merely as a linguistic phenomenon. The redescriptions are not merely a copyist's error. Their renegotiation hints at an attempt to fit available intellectual categories to new experiences.

We have already hinted at the growing importance of semen in medieval Bengali religious traditions. The reasons behind this growth in the importance of semen cannot be understood without some reference to the social and political history of medieval Bengal. Though Hinduism did become the royal religion in Bengal in around AD 1067, when the Hindu Sena dynasty managed to displace the Buddhist Pala dynasty, this Hinduism was itself not a seamless tradition. Kunal Chakrabarti has argued that it was in the medieval period that pre-Brahmanic cultural and religious elements were fused with the incipient Brahmanic culture to create a uniquely Bengali cultural identity.[55] This fusion was neither smooth nor free of conflict. Legends collected towards the end of the nineteenth century suggested that Tantrics had even briefly managed to dominate the Sena court and evicted the orthodox pundits from it.[56] The Sena rulers were, moreover, originally from the Karnataka country in the Deccan. As devout Shaivites, they may also have introduced Shaivite Siddha ideas into Bengal.[57] Not only did some of the Siddhas attach great importance to semen retention, but their view of mercury as the 'divine semen' of Shiva also contributed to the growth of ritual uses of the semen.[58]

With the advent of Islam in the thirteenth century, heterodox Sufi ideas engaged in a dialogue with Tantric and Tantric-influenced cults such as the Nathpanthis. The importance of semen and the ritual uses of its retention can be gauged by the fact that one of the first and best known Tantric texts to be translated into Arabic and Persian and to have been circulated all over the Islamic world, even reaching Egypt and Istanbul, the *Amritakund*, devoted one of its ten chapters to *bindudharan* (Lit: holding back the drop). Sufi Yoga thereby came to develop its own version of the Tantric idea of *chakras* from the fourteenth century onwards.[59] In Sufi lore, these became known as *mokams*. Medieval Bengali texts from the sixteenth century onwards are replete with exegeses on *mokam tatwa*. The basic idea behind the *chakra/mokam* system is that through breathing exercises, the retained semen can be made to rise up the central nerve (*susumna nadi*) in the spinal column arriving at and 'awakening' each of the *chakras/mokams*, or stages of spiritual consciousness on the path to spiritual and physical liberation. The difference between Islamic Yoga and Nath Yoga is merely that while the last stage in most Islamic texts such as the *Jog-Kalandar* or the *Chari Mokam Bhed* tends to be located in the heart, in the Nath texts such as the *Gorakh Bijay*, it is located in the head.[60]

Given the widespread influence of these ideas in medieval Bengal and Bihar, it is but natural that such ideas began finding their way into medical texts of the region as well around the same period. The fourteenth-century text written by *Sharangadhar*, which was almost certainly influenced by Yogic ideas—which it most visibly incorporated through an extensive section of sphygmology (pulse diagnosis)—described eight different types of spermatic disorders—*sukradosh*. Each of these had their individual names.[61] Interestingly however, none were called *sukrameha*. By the sixteenth century, Bhab Misra's text was even more elaborate. The *Bhabprokash* went so far as to state that 'though life [*jeeb*] is resident in every part of the body, it is semen, blood and excreta which are the main stays [*sic*] of it. Therefore, if semen, etc., are eroded, he who lives is also eroded'.[62] Once again, close attention to the actual linguistic formulation clearly suggests its proximity to Nath-Yogic and Sufi-Yogic ideas. The '*jeeb*', for instance, is often found in the heterodox *dehatattwa* (Lit: Body-Wisdom) texts. It is usually depicted as an anthropomorphic embodiment of life itself that lives in a clearly localizable part of the body. Further ritual practice involving the use of blood, semen and excreta—together known as the *chari-chandra sadhana* (worship of the four moons)—is a defining facet of many of Bengal's Tantric-influenced heterodox cults. Upendranath Bhattacharya, a leading authority on the subject, has suggested that the popularity of these *chari-chandra* practices dates from around the twelfth century, a date that, interestingly, coincides roughly with the references available in legends about the dominance of Tantrism in the Sena court.[63] Clearly distinguishing itself from the use of these ideas in the later *dhatu dourbalya* texts, however, the *Bhabprakash* includes a fairly extensive discussion on foods which produce sperm (*sukrol*), and foods and women that weaken or absorb sperm (*lekhon* or *rechok*).[64] The metaphor of budgeting a household on a small salary or medical consequences of prodigality is clearly alien to it. It does, however, show the context within which the redefinition of the relationship of *Prameha* and *Sukrameha* were taking place. It demonstrates clearly that the renegotiations of the categories were happening within a wider context in which these categorical changes reverberated with other realms of social experience and change. The new rhizoid networks that were being formed were, therefore, not purely linguistic networks defined by texts alone. They also connected to other chains of signification in society.

Swapna-dosh: This was one of the seemingly most curious of the 'associated terms'. Kar's early textbook had used it as one of the synonyms for the affliction he described. By 1915 it also occasionally occurred as an independent category that subsumed the other associated terms including *dhatu dourbalya*.[65] It remains in use even today. Its rhizoid roots, too, stretch beyond the strictly medical domain.

Both Hindu and Islamic traditions have a long history of writing on dreams and refuse to see them as purely illusory or fantastical events. As Wendy Doniger O'Flaherty has pointed out, 'Indian dream theory not only blurs the lines between dreaming and waking but emphasize the importance of dreaming as a kind of mediator between two relatively rare extremes—

waking and dreamless sleep.'[66] As O'Flaherty's reading of the myth of the rape of Usa by Aniruddha—which is repeated in several Sanskrit texts—shows, sexual congress in dreams has consequences in real life in the Sanskrit lore. Thus love bites exchanged during a rape in a dream, for instance, are, in some versions of the myth, still visible on Usa's body upon waking.[67] The semen on the male dreamer's bed upon awakening, however, O'Flaherty points out, was ambiguous physical evidence of the reality of the dream. While on the one hand, its presence proved the reality of the orgasm 'inside and outside the body of the dreamer', on the other hand, unlike the love bites, it did not prove the actual existence of a real sexual partner. It is thus, suggests O'Flaherty, that in classical Sanskrit philosophy, both the dream and the emission of semen come to signify 'the basic process of illusory creation'. While O'Flaherty is preeminently concerned with Sanskrit texts, it cannot be overlooked that classical Islam also had a rich tradition of dream theory. Nile Green points out that Islamic traditions had picked up many of its dream-related ideas from the pre-Islamic heritage of the Near East. However, the importance of dreams in Islam was further enhanced by their being a medium for communication between divines and humans. Thus, the Holy Quran itself was revealed in part through 'visions'. Later Sufis further developed the relationship between dreams and visions.[68] In parallel with this 'visionary' import of dreams, the older pre-Islamic heritage of oneiromancy, or dream reading, spread, along with Islam. In places like Bengal, these varied traditions combined and overlapped to create a strong current of belief in not only the reality of events seen in dreams, but also in the use of dreams as a way of prognosticating the future. Particularly, Tantric and Marfati traditions did much to develop dream theory in the region.

In the nineteenth century there were signs to suggest that the demand for dream interpretation was burgeoning in certain sections of urban Calcutta as well. Many cheap tracts on dreams and dream reading were produced as a proof of this growing demand. Mohammed Khater, a prolific Bengali writer of popular literature, written especially within a broadly Islamic tradition, produced such popular texts as the two volumes of *Asrar al-Khwabnama* and the *Solemani Talenama*.[69] Innumerable popular legends about divine commands given in a dream (*swapnadesh*), medicines revealed in a dream (*swapna-dutta aushadh*) and 'poetic inspiration received in a dream' abound in the region.[70] These exchanges while dreaming were accepted by all concerned as a valid and real experience. Dream commands were immediately honoured, dream medicines were considered fruits of divine grace and thankfully taken by many and dream inspiration was said to have inspired many a great medieval Bengali text. Dreams were not creatures of the imagination, but rather a dimension of space: a dimension within which meaningful actions and exchanges could take place. Things that happened in the dream did not thus lose their reality upon waking. Bengali allopathic doctors in the nineteenth century tried to adapt this belief in the reality of dreams into their medical rationality. Dr Kunjabihari Das, writing in 1897, argued that nightmares, which he called '*bukchapa*' (Lit: pressing one's chest) or its more extreme form '*bibhishika-darshan*' (Lit: witnessing scary things), were both *diseases*.[71] It is perhaps significant that Dr Das' essay appeared in the same year and in the same periodical as the bulk of Dr Chattopadhyay's writings on *dhatu dourbalya*.

Dr Chattopadhyay himself, however, equated *swapna-bikar* with the English designation of 'night pollution'.[72] He defined this condition as the ejaculation of semen while one is asleep.[73] The proper noun 'night pollution' had been in use in Puritan circles in Britain and America since at least the middle of the seventeenth century. It appears repeatedly, for instance, in the diary of the American apocalyptic poet Michael Wigglesworth.[74] The usage did also refer to morally troubling dreams and the consequent loss of semen, though, not surprisingly, authors like Wigglesworth mourned their effect upon the destiny of the soul rather than the health of the body. Though the use of 'night pollution' as a compound proper noun seems to still be emergent in the writings of Wigglesworth—for in only a single case of the three references he makes to the general idea does he use it as a proper noun—the general idea of morally reprehensible involuntary nocturnal emissions has a much older history in Judeo-Christian theological traditions.

The main concern of early Christian authors on the subject had been the moral culpability of such nocturnal emissions and dreams. As early as in the fourth century, St. Augustine and John Cassian had sought to distinguish between the ritual impurity caused by it and *sin*. Augustine had held them to be caused by a superfluity of humours that the body necessarily ejected, while Cassian had mentioned three main causes for such emissions: excess of food and drink, a wandering mind and the devil's machinations. Only the deliberate overindulgence in either food and drink or sexual fantasies was morally culpable. Subsequent authors also tended to look upon it as an involuntary and necessary bodily function, assigning only slight penitence for them. From the twelfth century onwards, a more rigorous regime was invoked. In the thirteenth century, as theological distaste for non-marital sexuality increased in orthodox Christian circles, the moral culpability of nocturnal emissions was also made stricter. However, even in the writings of Thomas Aquinas, who is often considered the most authoritative commentator on sexual morality of the day, nocturnal emissions themselves were thought reprehensible only if associated with sinful thoughts or actions.[75]

Though such religio-moral implications of the subject had no doubt kept it in the public domain for long, as noted above, until the seventeenth century these anxieties were more moral than medical. Even if medical arguments had been made about this, it was not part of the orthodox medical literature of the day. It was only in the eighteenth century that the situation changed through the publication of Samuel-Auguste Tissot's popular treatise *L' Onanisme.* Tissot was Swiss, and his work appeared in print in 1760 in French and was based upon data collected in Lausanne. Though an earlier anonymous English pamphlet called *Onania* had appeared in 1710, it was after Tissot's work that the idea was adopted by the European intellectuals of the day.[76] Tissot argued that semen was an 'essential oil' and when lost from the body in great amounts, would cause 'a perceptible reduction of strength, of memory and even of reason, blurred vision, all the nervous disorders, all types of gout and rheumatism, weakening of the organs of generation, blood in the urine, disturbance of the appetite, headaches and a great number of other disorders'.[77]

Tissot's writings were quickly translated into English and went into five editions by 1781.[78] Tissot's impact on nineteenth-century British sexologists remained quite widespread and *Onanism* was copiously quoted by William Acton—possibly the foremost sexologist of his day. Developing Tissot's views on the matter, Acton's influential book *The Functions and Disorders of the Reproductive Organs* related nocturnal emissions directly to 'lascivious dreams'. However, Acton's writings also retained an Augustinian element and thus asserted that 'emissions occurring once in every ten or fifteen days, [were] in the nature of a safety valve and even conducive to health' in certain people.[79] Acton, nevertheless, spent considerable space in proving that the dreams, and through them, emissions, could be controlled by an active will. Disabusing any notions of a homogenous 'western' view on the matter, however, he also highlighted the extent to which lay opinion on the matter differed from medical opinion, stating that it was popularly believed that it was wrong to check the emissions.[80]

Chattopadhyay's extensive use of English and Latin terms, especially in his description of the physiology of sperm production and penile erection, clearly attests to his familiarity with the 'western' sexual medicine of his day. Yet his awareness of this 'western' science was not through erudite editions of Acton or any other major sexologist. Instead, his awareness was most likely through an obscure sexual manual published by a merchant in Bombay. He explicitly acknowledged his debt to a book called *Sexual Science* for the basic descriptions of the disease.[81] Though he does not mention the author of this treatise, and there are several books of the title, the book referred to in all likelihood was John Balfour's pamphlet entitled *Sexual Science: A Guidebook for Married and Single Men*, a second, revised edition of which had been published from Bombay in

1894, just two years before the publication of Chattopadhyay's first essay.[82] The difference between Chattopadhyay's descriptions and those of Acton's are thus both slight and total. On the one hand, he mentioned the Augustinian ideas that had come down through Acton that nocturnal emissions were necessary bodily evacuations of surfeit matter, while on the other, he calls this 'surfeit' matter the product of bodily erosion. Moreover, the erosion itself was said to be the result of the corrosive effect of lascivious fantasies and thoughts of fulfilling them.[83] While Chattopadhyay followed Acton in saying that the emissions were the result of the body's urge to rid itself of unnecessary products, he differed on the 'safety valve' theory of Acton.

By so equating the two terms 'night pollution' and *swapnadosh*, two dissimilar terms with different genealogies and conceptual background were being brought together. This combination not only mimetically legitimized ideas in both traditions but also altered them. Thus, authors like Kar and Chattopadhyay accepted capacity of an active will to control the dreams. Kar wrote, 'To treat *swapnadosh*...give up the reprehensible thoughts and actions which cause it...' He further clarified that *swapnadosh* was the 'discharge of semen through the imagination (*anuman*) of sexual activity'.[84] The dreams, therefore, are not completely real phenomenon any longer, but rather works of the imagination that can be controlled by an active will, and yet, like real objects, they can have real 'corrosive' consequences.

Na-mardangi: This category is perhaps one of the rarest in our sources, though it is to be found more frequently in present day commercial texts on *dhatu dourbalya*.[85] The word literally means 'not-man-hood' and is of Hindustani origin not usually used in Bengali texts. Occasionally it also appears in its shortened form as *na-mardi*. It appears especially in advertisements in the *Muhammadiya Panjikas* (Islamic Almanacs) of the day and there, too, parenthetically in relation to other associated terms.[86]

Though the term is frequently translated into English as 'impotency', it is actually not identical to it. The lay usage of both *na-mardangi* and *na-mardi* in Hindustani usually implies cowardice. The word *na-mardi* as a common noun also refers to *Hijras*—the third gender recognized in most South Asian cultures.[87] As is well known, the *Hijras* are not just 'impotent men' but constitute an alternate gender identity. Gayatri Reddy has argued that the *Hijra* gender identity is only meaningful if we adopt a 'performative' definition of gender, i.e.. a conceptual scheme in which genders are not identified by fixed, immutable genital characteristics, but rather through the performance of specifically gendered acts.[88] *Na-mardi*, therefore, is akin to a gender identity rather than merely meaning an 'impotent male'. Moreover, most classical and medieval texts speak of multiple neuter genders and not a single 'impotent male' gender.[89]

In most of the advertisements where this term appears, it does so with another word—*dhwajabhanga*—in parenthesis. This related term, *dhwajabhanga,* bears out the contention that *na-mardi* is not wholly akin to impotency in a person of definite male gender. Gobinda Das' eighteenth-century text devotes an entire chapter to *dhwajabhanga,* but significantly the word itself appears only once in the chapter after the heading. For the rest of the chapter the term *dhwajabhanga* is used again as a synonym to *klaibya.* About *klaibya* it is mentioned that, 'The subject devoid of the capacity for sex [*rotishaktiheen*] is considered a *kleeb.* Addiction to this is called *klaibya*'.[90] *Klaibya* moreover is of seven different types. Some of these seven types of *klaibya* are indeed related to specifically semen-related problems. However, the mere presence of semen does not in Indian medical literature signify a 'male' gender. The *Bhabprakash,* for example, recognized four distinct types of sperm-carrying neuter genders.[91] More recently LGBT (lesbian, gay, bisexual, transgender) scholars such as Ruth Vanita have shown that even high-classical texts such as the Susruta Samhita saw women as possessing a kind of seminal fluid akin to semen and capable of causing conception.[92] Clearly then, both the common usages of the word *na-mardi* itself and its equation with *dhwajabhanga* suggest a very different usage than the usual understanding of 'impotency' in the English language.

The translation of *na-mardi* as impotency, in the present case at least, tends to normalize heterosexual, reproductively oriented sexuality. Placing the word back within its multiple etymological chains, however, shows it to be better described as an anxiety over particular types of sexual performance rather than fixed to a biologically male subject's incapacity to produce seminal fluids capable of reproduction.

Durbalata: The term *durbalata,* or 'weakness', as it came to be known in the late nineteenth century, was one with absolutely no previous history in Indian medicine. Trying to describe the disease, Dr D. D. Gupta wrote, 'The term *dourbalya* is not used to refer to a specific complaint. It refers to a combination of certain ordinary not-wellnesses (*sadharon ashusthota*)'.[93] Its main symptom was a general feeling of ennui and dreariness without any specific physically locatable malady. The patients felt jaded and felt incapable of doing any work at all, though they could not pinpoint what was wrong with them, and neither could physicians find anything specifically wrong with them. It was said to be capable of afflicting anybody from the richest of the rich to the poorest of the poor. Once afflicted, it ought to be attended to immediately, as any delay would, in Dr Gupta's view, render the patient permanently incapable of any work.

It was said to have two diametrically opposite causes.[94] On the one hand, overwork was said to lead to *dubalata,* while on the other hand, too little work was also said to produce the same effect. For the overworked, rest was advocated and for the underworked compulsory heavy work was prescribed. It seemed to be the consummate medical expression of the work ethic of an urban salaried middle class.

Suggested remedial measures left little doubt that it was also a disease born of the novelty of the urban lower-middle-class lifestyle. Dr Gupta advocated early morning baths in the river as the prime cure for this ailment. He also advocated going for walks in open gardens and parks. Regularly meeting with friends and family and enjoying the time spent with them was also said to help. Other more specific prescriptions included for men going away on short trips to 'see new sights', without one's family and for housewives occasionally not getting up early in the morning and staying in bed till later in the day.[95]

Clearly, these prescriptions were directly connected to the problems of adjusting to a new lower-middle-class urban lifestyle. In the world of the Bengali *kerani,* the men and women, uprooted from their village homes, were chained to the drudgery of routine urban life. Baths, which in any Bengali village is a social act where people meet, talk and gossip at the village pond or rivulet under open skies in leisured relaxation, were transformed into hurried individual acts squeezed in between the timings of the municipal water supply and the sirens sounded around the city to signal the opening of the offices and performed in cramped bathrooms or under municipal taps. Opportunity for walks in open spaces were reserved for the city's elite, while the *kerani* spent their time trying to get to the office and getting back from there. The larger social contexts with extended families and friends in the village had also, in most cases, been shrunk to small nuclear families. Some women had been uprooted from their rural contexts and extended social networks. As urban wives, their lives revolved around domestic work with little help or support from other women of an extended family network. Moreover, their days were as regulated as those of their husbands and children, but begun much earlier in order to cook lunch, which was now—breaking with tradition—taken before the husband left for office. All these were profound changes. The bodies and minds of people were being wrenched from routines and cycles they had grown up with and inserted into completely new routines of space and time.[96] It was the initial strains of this radical transformation that received a medical name as *durbalata.*

Yet, it is doubtful that the complaint would have become such a potent metaphor of the condition of the urban *keranis,* had it not been for the needs of the medical market and the consequent popularity of specifics offered to cure it. So huge was the market for these specifics and so ludicrous their advertising claims, that the early-twentieth-century Bengali satirist, Rajsekhar Basu, included a fictional account of a cook at the palace of a small princely state who claimed to have developed a sherbet for removing *durbalata* known as the *Changayani Sudha* (Re-invigorating Elixir). It was, claimed the cook, made from 'twenty *kaviraji* herbs, twenty types of *daktari* wines, twenty *hakimi* medicines, ashes of diamond, ashes of gold, ashes of pearls, all possible "vitamins" and a quarter of a *seer* of electricity'.[97] Basu's sketch aptly highlights the exoticism of the remedies being offered as well as the range of sources from which they sought legitimacy.[98] The exaggeration in Basu's sketch, given even a cursory survey of the advertisements of the day, is but slight.

Durbalata also, of course, resonated with the registers of Bengali racial effeminacy and was often combined with still other pathologies such as 'dyspepsia', '*snayubik durbalata*' (nervous debility), *dhatu dourbalya*, etc., to generate further semantic and connotative expansions. Thus, both as an independent term and appearing in a compound form with other terms, it proliferated into different registers and appealed to an ever-wider group of people, though what crucially motivated this massive proliferation was its utility in the medical market as well as its descriptive proximity to the world of the *kerani* consumers of that market.

Hysteria: The inclusion of *hysteria* is perhaps the most curious feature of the associative networks within which *dhatu dourbalya* is textually constructed. *Dhatu dourbalya* is usually depicted as a quintessentially male malady, while, of course, *hysteria* is often thought of as an overwhelmingly female malady. Its introduction into the advertising texts of *dhatu dourbalya* thus posits a certain correspondence between the two diseases which allows us to explore the ways in which these texts framed male and female bodies.[99] In fact, contemporary investigators have found that complaints very similar to *dhat* are found to be widely prevalent amongst South Asian women, too.[100]

Most of the medicines such as the *Amritashakti Rasayan* or the *Mahashakti Rasayan* which equate hysteria with *dhatu dourbalya* suggest that the remedy's curative action in hysteric women was the equivalent to its curative action in men plagued with *dhatu dourbalya*. The rationale for this equivalence is said to lie in the way that both *dhatu dourbalya* and hysteria disrupt happy domesticity by preventing the birth of children. The remedy, by removing this obstacle and making the birth of children possible, restores domestic bliss. The *Mahashakti Rasayan* advertisements wrote under the picture of a happy couple with a small boy and a girl on their laps that 'Be it diseases of the *dhatu* in men or *badhok*, hysteria or [illegible], etc., in women, whatever it is, if they are childless, or have sickly or short-lived children or if after one or two children they have not had any more, for such men and women the *Mahashakti Rasayan* is the only medicine'.[101] Similarly, the *Amritashakti Rasayan*, after detailing the symptoms of *dhatu dourbalya* and hysteria, went on to add that 'those whose children do not live or are short-lived, for them this is medicine is [*sic*] *Dhanwantari* [the mythic god of medicine]'.[102] Such equivalences premised upon the respective roles of happy conjugality were also reflected in the theoretical elaborations of the concept of *dhatu* in more erudite texts of the time. According to the *Biswakosh* (Bengali encyclopaedia), apart from the seven traditional ayurvedic *dhatus*—blood, flesh, marrow, bone, chyle, skin and semen—there were two other '*dhatus*', which were created out of substances inhering within the seven main *dhatus*. The first of these, known as *oja-dhatu*, or *bal*, was responsible for a range of actions from keeping the body rigid and energetic, maintaining the humoural balance and general vigour. Its erosion caused lassitude, improper sensory functioning, feelings of guilt, drowsiness and even fainting. The erosion of this important type of *dhatu*, however, was not related explicitly to sexual actions. Instead, it was clarified that such erosion could happen from 'mental or physical stress, anger, sorrow, too much worrying over one thing and labour'. Symmetrically with the *bal dhatu*, however, was the *basha dhatu*. Where *bal* was born out of the vigorous and powerful essence of the seven *dhatus*, the *basha* was born out of the soft, slippery and butter-like substance inherent in the seven *dhatus*. Just as *bal* was responsible for power and vigour in every aspect of human life, the *basha* was responsible for beauty and 'softness' (*komalata*). It was found in greater quantities amongst women and was responsible for their beauty, lack of body hair, their tender feelings, etc.[103]

The lifestyle changes in the late nineteenth century saw the first cracks develop in the joint family structure, and a new ideal of conjugal partnership between men and women began emerging. However, men and women were still not seen as identical. Equality was framed in terms of complementary roles. Innumerable men and women wrote about this complementary ideal and many more articulated it through their daily lives. As Sambuddha Chakrabarti has shown, this new idea of a complementary domestic partnership between a man and a woman—as distinct from a woman or man's incorporation into a large kinship network—can even be observed in the way modes of address changed between husbands and wives at the time.[104] The expansion of the concepts of *dhatu* seems to mirror this new emergent idea of men and women as complementing partners in a happy domestic unit. The complementary articulations of *dhatu dourbalya* and *hysteria* stem from this reimagination of the domestic ideal itself.

The fundamental equivalence of *dhatu dourbalya* and *hysteria* on the basis of both being thought to obstruct (in their own ways) the basic generative functions—production of children—in itself, however, was not novel to the Bengali situation. The unani tradition looked upon hysteria as a disease caused due to the 'floating of the womb' within the body.[105] The 'western' medical tradition had also tended to relate hysteria to women's reproductive faculties.[106] The symmetry proposed in the Bengali texts however was more direct. It was not merely a functional equivalence. It was more an idea of there being different kinds of specific *dhatus* in male and female bodies whose impairments were comparable.

Each of these 'associated terms' thus have varied and patchy histories. Their histories and chronologies connect them with diverse other chains of texts and meanings. Sometimes they appear as part of the descriptions of other terms, such as the case of *sukrameha* and *prameha*. Sometimes the terms appear as parts of compound terms such as *snayubik durbalata*. They often lose some parts of their meanings through their incorporation into new semantic networks or, indeed, come to acquire new elements. This is best in evidence in the case of the terms *na-mardi* and *dhwajabhanga*.

That there was some vague awareness of the misfit between some of these terms that were being presented as equivalents can be observed through the efforts in some texts to reconcile the different terms by representing them as 'different types' of a single pathology such as *prameha*. The *Prameha Kalyan Bati*, for instance, informed its possible consumers that 'On taking *Prameha Bati*, all twenty types of *Prameha* are very easily and permanently cured. *Swapnadosh*, burning sensation during urination, emission of sperm during or after urination, involuntary emissions…for all these *Prameha Kalyan Bati* is a sure remedy'.[107] Others reconciled the contradiction by positing a linear process where an independent disease could mutate into other independent diseases. Advertisements for the *Mahashakti Rasayan*, for instance, suggested that 'Causing semen to be ejaculated unnaturally due to bad influences in one's youth or at the beginning of youth or by excessive sexual contact with women leads to sperm *dhatu* being depleted or become diseased. This leads to fundamental diseases such as *prameha*, urinary complaints, *swapnadosh*, etc. In time, *dhatu dourbalya*, *sukrotarolyo* and *indriyo shoithilyo* [sensory slackness] arise. In time, these lead to *dhwajabhanga*'.[108]

Substantiation of Bengali Racial Weakness

What provided the overarching framework for these texts was the immense visibility of the discourse on Bengali racial effeminacy.[109] Susan Sontag points out that the 'promotion of the self as an image' is a 'distinctively modern activity' and such promotion draws generously upon disease metaphors.[110] Certain diseases, therefore, become pregnant metaphors for the articulation of a number of portent and socially redolent images of the self under various conditions. Such metaphors are not merely external glosses put upon the intimate experiences of bodily illness. Instead, these metaphorical images allow the body to function within a single system that makes it (the body) the site of the most intimate experiences of the self, the main text for the social perception of the self and the object of control and domination by power, all together.[111] Metaphors allow a circularity that permits, on the one hand, social experiences to be experienced as bodily states, and bodily states, on the other, to becoming ways of articulating the self's relationship with society and power. Just as the social experience of lower-middle-class urban life on a stretched budget became the organizing *topos* for *dhatu dourbalya*, at another level the affliction itself articulated the angst of the political, social and economic 'impotence' of the Bengali *bhodrolok*. It was this perception of racial/national weakness that allowed the feelings of individual frustration, social perceptions of the powerlessness of the colonised and the body politic to come together. Such a consensus was impossible without the metaphoric quality of the affliction, which allowed it to slip with ease between the registers of psychology, sociology, political economy and biology. It was hardly surprising then—given the peculiar exigencies of colonial South Asia—that the perceptions of physiological debility, though usually couched in the language of race were usually mapped almost exclusively onto the bodies of *bhodrolok*.[112] Various discourses, ideas, political rivalries, social anxieties, etc., were articulated through the image of the weakened, impotent *bhodrolok*.[113] As we have seen in Chapter III, ideas about 'national' and 'racial' weakness continued to inform *daktari* discourse about a variety of contagious diseases even into the twentieth century.

The concern about sexual debility was yet another somaticized expression of this general idea of weakness and emasculation. Frequently, *dhatu dourbalya* texts mentioned 'mental' states such as 'feelings of heart-wrenching guilt/anxiety' (*sarbada marmapirhay nipirita*), 'lack of cheerfulness', 'lack of happiness', etc.[114] Yet, significantly, they were presented as somatic complaints ascribable to specific somatic, rather than social, causes. Such feelings were undoubtedly produced largely by the strains of lower-middle-class life in the urban sprawl (and the repeated feelings of powerlessness that accompanied it) and its mismatch with the social and psychological rhythms of tighter-knit rural communities. Yet, what allowed these individuated perceptions of inadequacy to be recoded as a feeling of national/racial inadequacy was the specific colonial context and the powerful ideological influence of the effeminacy discourse. What was crucial was that these 'feelings' or 'perceptions' were localized in a specific bodily substance that, in turn, by its inheritable character was capable of affecting the entire 'race'. One advertisement for a medicine claiming to cure *dhatu dourbalya* mentioned that the problem with afflictions like these was that it 'remained in the system, for not one, nor two, but up to seven generations'. It went on to state how Bengalis were 'aged in their youth; by twenty-five or thirty, the limbs of many had gone limp, by forty many are truly diseased (*jaragrastha*)'.[115] Such assertions allowed the individual perceptions of inadequacy to be reformatted as a national/racial problem which was capable of affecting innumerable future generations. The *dhatu dourbalya* discourse combined both the range of generative disorders and a variety of common psychological states into a narrative and experiential economy structured by a framework of racial/national impotence and weakness. Some mid-twentieth century 'western' doctors working with South Asian patients observed a tendency amongst the latter to express 'emotional' or 'mental' states as somatic complaints.[116] As Sushrut Jadhav and others point out, however, this tendency should not be essentialized as something peculiar South Asian cultures. Jadhav et al. argue that this essentialization is premised upon an assumption that the 'western' subject is somehow 'culture free'. They go on to show that white British men have equally culturally specific ways of expressing emotionally depressive states.[117] Instead, for cross-cultural psychiatrists like Jadhav, the existence of such 'local' categories highlights the need to engage with the narrative and imaginative strategies through which situated subjects everywhere articulate emotional and bodily states.

As we have seen in Chapter III, from the end of the first decade of the twentieth century, there was an increasing tendency to find a substantive basis for racial 'weakness' and an attempt to correct it by techno-scientific solutions. In the case of *dhatu dourbalya*, too, we see both these tendencies at work. The 'weakness' was variously localized in the pseudo-substantive *dhatu*, semen, 'nervous system', blood, urine, etc. *Dhatu*, blood and the 'nervous system' were particularly popular substances in which debility was located. Once identified in a particular substance, it was to be neutralized by a host of therapeutic substances.

We have already mentioned, in Chapter II, the characteristic trait of Bengali *bigyapans* to advertise a whole range of commodities in the form of minor texts inserted into other texts. Medicines dealings with *dhatu dourbalya* were frequently advertised through such *bigyapans*. Significantly, specifics for *dhatu dourbalya* immediately preceded or followed general virilificants known as *salsas* or *sarsas*. G. K. Nag & Co., for example, advertised their specific for *dhatu dourbalya*—*Nervigor*—immediately following the *Swarna-ghatita Sarsa-Vito*.[118] D. Gupta & Co.'s specific *Balkarak Sera* also immediately followed their *Essence of Jamaica Sarsaparilla*.[119] Similarly in, Navashakti Aushadhalaya's advertisements, their specific for *dhatu dourbalya*—*Shakti Sindhu Rasayan*—immediately preceded the *Amrita Bindu Swarna-ghatita Salsa*.[120] (Figs. IX & XI.)

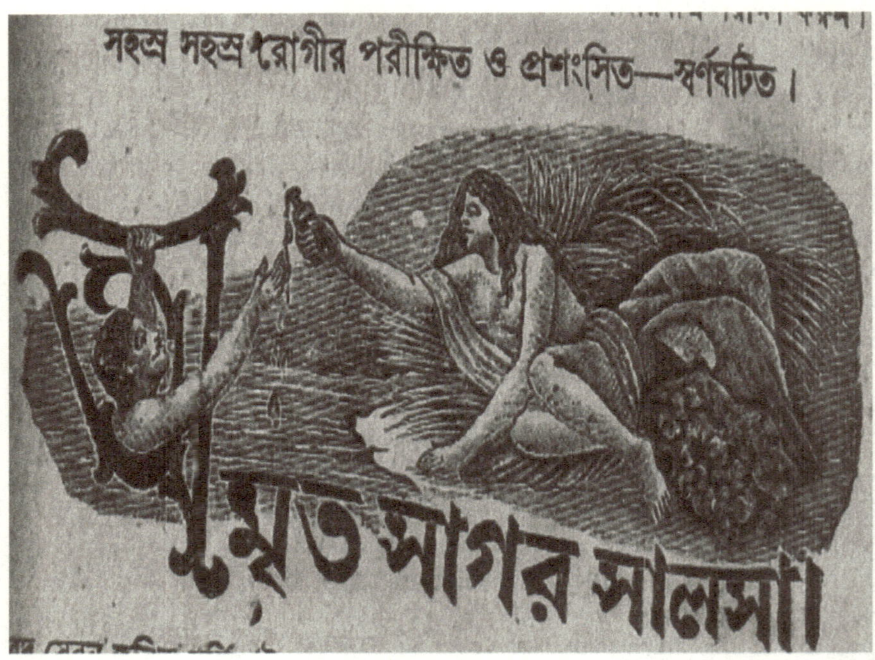

Fig. XI. Advertisement for Amritasagar Salsa, Gupta Press Dairektari Panjika for 1322 BS.

The two words *salsa* and *sarsa* were often used within a very similar narrative framework and seemed to refer to medicinal substances with very similar qualities. They were supposed to remove old impurities from the blood—often thought to be caused by chronic ailments or powerful medicines—and 'strengthen' the system. (Fig. X.) Their actions, therefore, were complementary to the specifics which neutralised *dhatu dourbalya*. The advertisement for the *Amrita Bindu Swarna-ghatita Salsa* explained its action: 'British (*bilati*) and other local (*deshiya*) *salsas* cure disease but the poisons stay back in the body…Later these poisons express themselves in particular *dhatus* during slight variations of routine (*sadharan aniyam*). Taking the *salsas* regularly also makes them lose their effect. But thousands of contented patients vouch for the efficacy of the *Amrita Bindu Salsa*'.[121]

Originally the word *sarsa* was a shortened form of *sarsaparilla*. The *sarsaparilla* is usually identified with Central American plant used medicinally by local populations, and which were later globalized by Europeans.[122] There is, however, also an Indian variety of the plant, the *Hemidesmus Indicus*.[123] *Salsa*, on the other hand, was a word which meant 'sauce' in Arabic, Spanish and Italian,

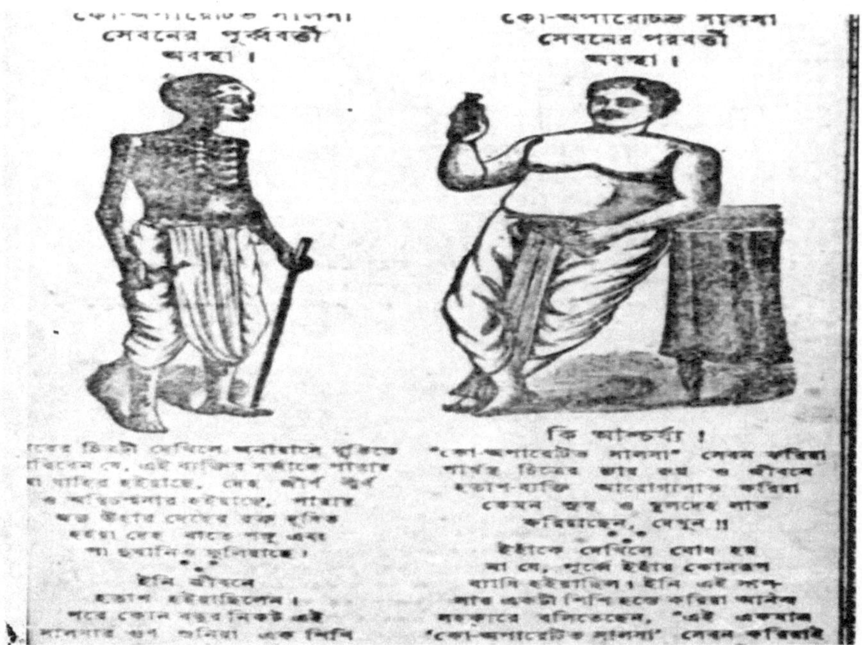

Fig. XII. Advertisement for HD Manna Co-operative Salsa, Nutan Panjika (1901).

but later came to designate any spicy foods with sauce, in some English uses. American English identifies it with Mexican foods, while British English identifies it with Indian chutneys. In the hands of Bengali pharmaceutical entrepreneurs, however, these differences were collapsed, and *sarsas* and *salsas* came to occupy very similar socio-medical valences. *Sarsaparilla,* alongside rhubarb, potassium iodide, tamarind, purges, 'rest and general cleanliness', had, since the 1860s and 1870s, come to replace Mercury bichloride and arsenate as the main treatment for congenital syphilis.[124] Some of the medical advertising aimed at *dhatu dourbalya* drew upon this connection with congenital syphilis, but at the same time, also repositioned the medicine within a framework of *dhatu* and general debility.[125] One conspicuous example of how this repositioning worked was through the frequent claims that the *salsa/sarsa* being advertised was '*swarna ghatita*' (made from gold).[126] This ascription drew upon older associations which used alchemy as a model for rejuvenation therapies.[127] This modelling in turn depended upon the play of the word *dhatu*, which—as already pointed out above—meant both 'metal' and bodily substrates.

The popularity of the *sarsas* and *salsas* were also stoked by the rampant fear about mercury poisoning as a consequence of prolonged treatment of venereal

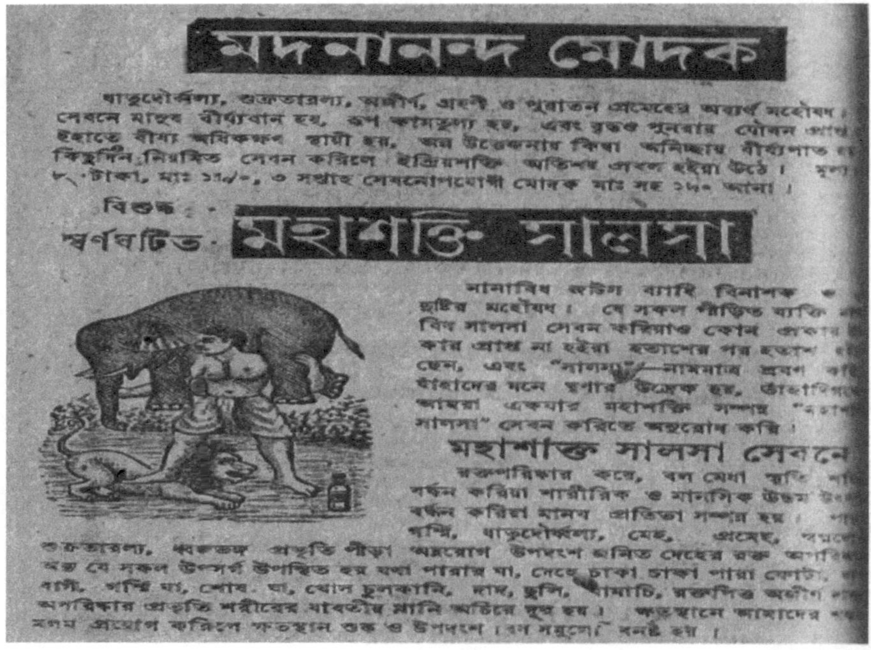

Fig. XIII. Advertisement for Mahashakti Salsa, Gupta Press Dairektari Panjika for 1322 BS.

and other diseases pertaining to the genital organs or reproduction.[128] The confusion of *sarsa* and *salsa* also led to a slight popular preference for drugs made from 'American' herbs as effective remedies for long-term *dourbalya.* The existence of numerous medical advertisements claiming that the medicines advertised therein were made from herbs from the Americas (most popularly from Jamaica) attested to the popularity of this belief. Some enterprising American patent-medicine sellers, such as a certain Ms Mulford Company, sought to capitalize on this. Mulford Company sold a medicine called *Ferarson*—which was supposed to have contained, apart from a very powerful 'American [herb] known to be a great medicine for *dhatu dourbalya*' called 'Condureng', along with Coca and Cinchona. Alongside these valuable American herbs, *Ferarson* also contained, however, arsenic, phosphorous, strychnine, etc.[129] Even well-known American firms such as *Parke-Davis* were selling medicines for *dhatu dourbalya* by the 1920s. *Parke-Davis'* medicines were called, perhaps rather unimaginatively, *Aphrodisiac Tablets.*[130]

Dhatu dourbalya was, from the very beginning, driven by a medical market that sought to objectify and substantiate racial weakness. Substantiation occurred on two sites. On the one hand, it was localized in a substance within the body, therefore giving it a material basis, while on the other hand, it was sought to be 'corrected' by specific medicinal substances. Studying contemporary patterns of usage of antidepressant medication by urban middle-class Bengalis in Calcutta, Stefan Ecks has argued that, for contemporary patients, consumption of antidepressants is presented by the pharmaceutical companies as a way of overcoming social marginality.[131] In the contemporary advertising rhetoric, its emphasis on self-diagnosis and its tendency to perpetually broaden the scope of 'depression' bears strong continuities with the *dhatu dourbalya* discourse from over a hundred years ago. Two observations of Ecks, therefore, are worth reiterating in our present study. First, that the impetus for this discourse is driven by the medical market, and second, that consumption of the medicines might itself be a seen by some consumers as a way of overcoming marginalization. Both these points are relevant for the market in *dhatu dourbalya* cures. Ecks' work in contemporary Calcutta also shows that while by the 1920s the market in weakness-neutralizing drugs had been globalized with American companies becoming increasingly popular, this expansion has not yet wholly displaced other categories for perceiving inadequacy, which continue to resist substantiation.[132]

Conclusion

The psychiatric debate that has raged over the existence of *dhat* syndrome as a Culture Bound Syndrome has obscured the actual character of this pathological category by seeking to represent it as a unitary category. It is, in effect, composed of numerous shifting names, designations and anxieties. It is a rhizoid reality comprising an unstable association of shifting terms appearing together. It is informed, moreover, by a medical rationality that has marked points of difference from the clinical rationality of nineteenth-century European medicine. Developed as it was in the cosmopolitan atmosphere of the medical market, rather than in learned teaching hospitals, its rationality operated by metaphorical associations and self-prescription. *Dhatu dourbalya* substantiated the complex set of experiences, prejudices, anxieties and discourses on Bengali racial weakness in bodily substances capable of being corrected by therapeutic substances.

It can in no way be seen to be an ahistorical product of long-standing cultural proclivities or a universally shared pathological belief. Its specific contours in late colonial Bengal, instead developed through contingent historically specific entanglements of several medical ideas from different traditions, the market-driven pressure towards substantiation, metaphorical medical rationality, etc. In short, it was a creature both specific and contingent to its historical context.

CONCLUSION

The term *daktar* used as a designation to particularly and solely describe practitioners of a separate system of medicine had not caught on in printed Bengali texts till the second half of the nineteenth century. Yet, there is no doubt that a significant number of Bengalis had come into contact with 'western' medicine well before that. The eighteenth-century 'Black Doctors' and 'Compounders', and later, in the nineteenth century, the many physicians employed temporarily during the cholera epidemic of the 1820s, all had a chance to practice some form of 'western' medicine or other. The lack of detailed archival evidence, however, makes it, as yet, difficult to reconstruct what sort of medicine these early pioneers practised or how significant their role was within the extant economy of healing.

A relatively more detailed picture of the actual practice of early Bengali practice of 'western' medicine emerges from the 1840s. This picture presents a highly diverse and heterogeneous world. The men involved came from a wide range of backgrounds and had a wide variety of skills. They also occupied very different positions within the world of *daktari* medicine. The historiographic recovery of this plurality, however, is often confounded by an uneven archival record and the codes through which texts preserve biographical information. Some medical lives such as those of lowly Compounders or locally entertained native doctors retain only fragmentary traces in the archive, while those such as the relatively well-placed mid-century Sub-Assistant Surgeons, whose lives are more accessible through the governmental archives, are preserved through textual codes that hide as much as they reveal. A juxtaposition of biographies and methods of recovery allow us to access some of the rich plurality of the world of *daktari* medicine. The archival and representational 'limitations', however, do not necessarily detract or impede the understanding of *daktari* medicine as such. Instead, as suggested in the Introduction, the nature of the sources are in themselves shaped by the very processes that we have unpacked in this book and are, therefore, an integral part of the argument.

The world of *daktars*, however, did not remain unchanged throughout our period of study. We have seen how the social roles, educational routes and professional designations changed over time. Yet, since the *daktars* were not a homogenous professional group, but rather a heterogeneous social designation, the long-term changes affected different sections amongst them differently. This makes any general conclusions about the *daktars* as a whole difficult to draw. Changes—though varied in their chronologies—were significant and wide-ranging. Most visibly the self-image of *daktars* as being the upholders of an aggressive rational critique of popular religiosity in time gave way to their role as mediators of a complex cultural realignment which repositioned popular religiosity and *daktari* rationality in mutually reinforcing positions.

These developments were overdetermined by the developments in the sphere of medical publishing. This domain of Bengali medical publishing was itself heterogeneous and plural. The use of the term *daktari* in its various registers since the 1860s, however, served to constitute a surface identity of *daktari* medicine as a distinct 'system' of medicine marked out from other similar and comparable systems like *kaviraji* and *hakimi*.

Amongst the ruder publications of the *Bot-tola* genre, *daktari* came to signify a 'meta-system' that included within it all other 'systems'. These other 'systems', in turn, were primarily the more prominent genres of medical publication that had developed since the 1850s. Amongst the more polite forms of *daktari* writing—both in books and more prominently in medical periodicals—a dual accent on 'lay' (nonmedical) readership and an onus on intersystemic dialogue led to a deeper, structural impact on the intellectual milieu of *daktari* medicine. The lay readership acted as a weight towards a constant engagement with things the patients themselves could do to cure or prevent disease. This in turn led to a long-term engagement with the sovereign preventive or curative power of the body itself without recourse to overt medical intervention. Its emphasis on intersystemic dialogue, on the other hand, while strengthening the perceptions of *daktari* being a 'system' that was comparable but distinct from *kaviraji*, *hakimi*, etc., also served to position *daktari* medicine in line for complex renegotiations of its diagnostic and therapeutic strategies.

The insistence on the 'powers' or 'forces' innate in the body drew upon both intellectual resources in the 'West' and in the 'East' and realigned them within a complex politics of identities. Such intellectual processes cannot be described simply as 'hybrid', for they were not born out of the combination of two distinct but different medical traditions. Instead, they were fashioned through the complex and political entanglements of multiple internally diverse and multistranded traditions.

The dialogic engagement with 'indigenous' medicine ensured a degree of 'provincialization' of 'western medicine', even in the domain of polite medical writing. Though most of the college-educated *daktars* who wrote in this domain, were—to some degree—partisans of the superiority of 'western' medicine, none could deny that *daktari* was but *one* treatment option amongst others. This led them to engage, often deeply and regularly, with the theoretical and practical actualities of *ayurvedic* medicine.

The market also mediated the production of some of the most prolific *daktari* texts in the form of *bigyapans*. The Bengali *bigyapans*, or advertisements, were conspicuous in establishing a vernacular surface identity for *daktari* medicine. These texts, which were distinct from the English genre of print advertising, functioned as minor texts in their own right and did much to frame the popular social image of *daktari* identity. *Daktari* medicine was created, therefore, through a complex process whereby material conditions of the print industry and the medical market entangled with sundry political, professional and social aspirations of diverse physician groups collectively described as *daktars*. As a heterogeneous group, they had access to various intellectual and practical resources and the logic of the combination of these resources was often a matter of situational circumstance and the politics of identities.

In conceptualizing the transference of disease from a healthy to a diseased individual, *daktari* authors found one of the most productive sites on which to actualize the nation. Whereas imperial ideas about disease transference had tended to express the governmental logic of control and order, the *daktari* authors tended to focus on the technologies of selfhood that would develop the self and its environment in ways that prevented contagious diseases.

Instead of seeing contagion negatively as an incitement to control, demarcate and separate, they operationalized its productive potential to articulate a multifarious project for national development. This multidimensional project was a 'nationalist project' to the extent that it actualized the nation through its identification of specific bodies, spaces and practices as *national* and its subsequent attempts to develop these (bodies, spaces and practices) as part of an overall national development. It did not derive, hence, from any pre-given programmatic exposition of *nationalism*, but it produced the materialities which programmatic nationalism would seek to cultivate and manipulate.

Intellectually, the roots of these concepts and practices drew upon both 'western' and 'eastern' resources. Any search for a *pure* genealogy of any of the various ideas and practices used in articulating the nation is, therefore, a futile project. What is important to notice is how these entangled practices—such as those of concerning *naitrojen guna*—were actualized in a specific historical situation as a *daktari* reality. These *daktari* realities were neither simply 'ideas' nor 'misunderstandings' without a basis in reality. They were instead what Latour has described as 'factishes'.

The word in Latour's usage is a composite of the words 'fact' and 'fetish' and gets beyond the binarism of belief and knowledge. It is defined by Latour as a 'robust centrality which allows action without having to believe in the difference between constructionism and empiricism…'. Latour is equally unconvinced of both the claim that reality exists wholly independently of our perceptions of it and that reality is wholly a matter of ideational constructs. It is this dichotomy that Latour argues, which drives us to distinguish between 'constructionism', i.e., the relativist claim that reality is socially constructed, and 'empericism', i.e., the belief that reality exists 'out there' independently of our consciousness of it. None of these two positions are capable of convincingly explaining human actions that always assume, involve and are constrained by certain nonhuman elements (or 'actors'). 'Germs' are a good example to illustrate Latour's point. The 'constuctionists', in holding that 'germs' are wholly a human 'construction' of reality—something that ultimately exists only in the mind—cannot successfully explain why the discovery of 'germs' and its subsequent medical manipulation has led to a massive reduction in certain deadly diseases. On the other hand, those who believe that 'germs' are a 'reality-out-there', wholly independent of human perception, are incapable of explaining how pre-germ theories of disease causation, such as those about miasmas, animated human actions and decisions and how these, too, were occasionally quite successful in controlling the spread of disease. It becomes, for the empericists, then, a mere wager about what was relatively more successful. It can explain neither why nor how humans, before the discovery of germs, were still capable of obtaining some medical success. They also ignore the fact that many such 'theories', such as that about 'germs', actually developed from those very older debates, which they would not reject as wholly incorrect. The factish combines these two spheres in a dynamic materialist model based on mutual mediations of capacities to act. Humans and non-humans are, in Latour's scheme, 'actors', who in particular collectivitities or networks are capable of allowing each other to act in certain ways.[1] Thus, a *naitrojen guna* or '*jeebanu*' ('germs') allows a *daktar* to act in certain ways: to say and do certain things involving it. In this sense it has an operative material reality and stands outside of the binaries of (misplaced) *belief* and (true) *knowledge.*

Since factishes such as *naitrojen* or *jeebanu* operate within different (though no doubt partially overlapping) operational networks than 'nitrogen' and 'germs', their material realities are not identical.

It was through these vernacular, entangled realities that specific *national* bodies, practices and spaces were identified and framed. The very description of Bengali bodies as being deficient in *naitrojen guna* and the specific agendas elaborated according to it or, indeed, the identification of *pana* as a source of national physical decline (despite assertions by British doctors denying the influence of *pana* on health) allowed the articulation of both specific *national* 'substances' and specific *national* programmes in relation to those *substances.* In other words, it was the 'factishes' like *naitrojen guna* and *pana* that showed very literally what the *nation* was 'made of' and precisely what needed to be done to improve/develop it.

For Latour, 'articulations' are where 'actors' (human or non-human) animate each other, connect with each other and allow them to do or say certain things. The larger the 'collectivities' or 'networks', the greater the operational reality of the factish concerned. The successful factishes, therefore, were connected to the longest 'networks' of articulation. This also means that they were capable of articulating with other significant networks which made up their immediate context. These 'other significant networks' comprised psychological networks (such as those of rural nostalgia and urban angst), ideological networks (such as those of neo-Hinduism, various contending nationalisms, etc.), economic networks (such as those of middle-class Bengali employment patterns, the medical market, etc.), practical and ethical networks (such as those of dietary practice, bathing in the morning, etc.) and so forth. The successful 'articulations' of concepts like *naitrojen guna* with these significant networks gave them their reality. As operative concepts, these in turn materialized the reality of the nation itself.

The relationship between factishes and the nation, however, is not a unidirectional, causal one. Just as the 'factishes' materialized the *nation,* the nation in turn actualized the 'factishes'. The entire science of hygiene and sanitation thus came to be reframed as 'ancient Hindu culture'. Through what was a classic example of 'double articulation', the *form* actualized the *substance* and the *substance* materialized the *form.*[2] The vernacularization of 'western' medicine and the actualization of the nation were produced through a process of double articulation in which both processes enabled the unravelling of the other.

These articulations that gave *daktari* medicine itself its unique vernacular identity came to a crisis during the plague epidemic in the 1890s. As medical judgement itself became politicized, it became clear that the categories that the *daktars* and British doctors employed in visualizing pathological reality did not match. It was not a question of who was right and who was wrong. It was merely that at this period of supreme crisis, the affective communities within which physicians functioned and operational networks of their factishes articulated diverged dramatically. This divergence, in turn, made their factishes impel them to very different forms of action. A sense of reality organized as a factish is, as stated above, a dynamic state. Since European doctors and Bengali *daktars* acted very differently at the time of the plague, it shows the emergence of very different diagnostic and therapeutic factishes. But these different diagnoses and therapies did not preexist; they were produced in the course of the very actions which were informed by them. It is partly because of this double articulation of the actions and the reasons for the actions, that it is not exhaustive to explain the differences between Kishori Mukherjee and William Simpson merely in terms of 'domination' and 'resistance'.

The wider 'articulations' of medical factishes becomes most conspicuous when 'medical' projects get taken up by religious ideologues. The 'vernacularization' of 'western medical science', therefore, became a wider project of cultural translation, where *daktars* were no longer the sole mediators. The reinscription of medical duty as religious performance showed the operation of a complex cultural realignment whereby elements of a 'cosmopolitan' (in Pollock's sense of the term) science are negotiated into vernacular registers. This realignment was framed by a very different mode and locus of power. Instead of relying on either the state or the Civil Society, the power through which these *daktari* antiplague measures were to be implemented came to be located in the religio-social community. The community itself was in turn visualized as a large extended Bengali family, at the head of which were the Bengali Hindu *bhodrolok*. This vision of a socio-religious community was hierarchic, communal (in the South Asian sense of the word) and unegalitarian, nonetheless altruistic. The ties of love held this community together and structured the mutual obligations of its members. It allowed, also, a particular specie of sanitary intervention. Crucially, the agent of such intervention was not the state or the Civil Society, but the socio-religious community as a whole. This communitarian framework of sanitary work, being as hierarchic and unegalitarian as it was, represented the 'lower' classes as being gullible, irrational subjects in need of sanitary salvation. A survey of the medical responses of these classes to the plague crisis, however, amply shows that their medical rationality was not very different from that of the *bhodrolok*. Like the *daktari* efforts to 'empower' the potential patients themselves through the invigoration of inner powers of disease prevention and cure, the spells and simples of the subaltern orders also sought to bolster the body's defences. The medicinal agents they used for effecting such empowerment, however, were very different from those of the *daktars*, yet within the totality of their experiential worlds these substances had roles which bear comparison with those of the *daktars*.

While plague was an epidemic that appeared briefly in the mindscape of the *bhodrolok*, cholera was an endemic that had haunted Bengal more or less throughout the nineteenth century, occasionally breaking out into virulent epidemics and even pandemics. Thus, whereas the 'politics' of plague was foremost in the *daktari* writings on the topic, it was 'commerce' that often dominated the writings on cholera.

The origins of the *daktari* discourse on cholera predate the evolution of the label *daktari* itself. Faced with one of the most massive epidemic outbreaks of the disease in the early nineteenth century, the newly established British Raj had employed a large number of 'indigenous' physicians to distribute cholera medicines. These physicians had also been encouraged to write on the topic. The only printed book from that period, though, was Peter Breton's *Olauthar Vivaran*—one of the first Bengali printed books on *daktari* medicine. Confronted with what many Europeans came to believe was a distinctively Indian disease as well as the sheer scale of its devastations, the European doctors were much more open to collaborating with South Asian physicians. The narrative structure of the cholera texts produced by European doctors and their Bengali subordinates were significantly different. Instead of focussing upon its character as a 'disease of disorder' and crowds narrated through statistical tables, the *daktars* focussed on emotional context and familial suffering of individual patients to develop their ideas about cholera. The representation and structure of the text—especially in their emotional language, the details and importance of the patient's familial environment and the repetition of certain preferred tropes (such as the death of the young rather than the old)—bore witness to the very different relationship between *daktars* and their patients from that of the British doctors, as well as to the influence on *daktari* writing of contemporary Bengali literary conventions.

The long acquaintance with the disease in the region also meant that, unlike plague, there were many social memories and meanings ascribed to the disease. The plurality of meanings and memories can be gauged by the wide variety of names the disease was known to have in the region. Later authors, therefore, had to first choose by which name to call the disease when they spoke of it. The names, however, were not mere shells to be fitted onto a preexisting pathological reality. Each name articulated slightly different networks of meanings and therefore framed a slightly distinct pathological 'factish'. The choice of the name used, therefore, was part of the arguments made in the body of the text and often pithily encapsulated the politics of the text itself.

The cholera ethics espoused by the *daktars* was more akin to their response during the plague or, indeed, to contagious diseases in general. They accented the capacity of the individual, through his/her actions, thoughts and conduct, to influence the incidence and course of the disease. This insistence on an ethico-moral aspect of cholera management was also exported to Britain when the disease arrived in the colonial metropole through the experience of British doctors like James Adair Lawrie, Geoffrey Hamilton Bell and others who had served in India. The content of these ethico-moral interdictions, however, reflected the different moral contexts within which they operated. The complete consensus over the ill effects of drunkenness in India, for instance, contrasted with a more ambiguous position of the issue in British cholera practice.

In the absence of any particularly effective remedy for cholera, patients and their families were willing to try almost any remedy. This made the market for cholera treatment and medicine one of the most robust and competitive. Numerous treatments—old and new—abounded. In this voluminous market, however, there was evidence of both similarity and difference. Many of the actual medicinal substances used by *Ayuvedists,* homoeopaths and *daktars* were, in fact, the same. Though their precise usage—especially the timing—often differed widely, their use and importance no doubt gained from the fact that they were known as effective remedies in other 'systems' of treatment.

More interestingly, the cholera market also showed how the privileges of the *daktari*/'western system' of treatment in relation to the state and its archives, came undone in the medical market. Since the 1880s, there emerged a powerful idea that the homoeopathic system of treating cholera was the most effective. For nearly the next three decades—in the domain of the medical market—the homoeopaths in Bengal enjoyed a privileged position and it was indeed *daktari* medicine which was marginalized.

The cholera market also showed how, instead of the increasing marginalization of 'magical' or 'faith-based' cures under the onslaught of modernity, the emergence of a modern medical market—shaped by such modern developments as rapid urbanization, printing, advertising, etc.—actually provided these 'magical' remedies with a new context for development and survival. Spells and magic squares to cure cholera proliferated and were circulated widely through cheap medico-magical recipe books. Though these publications gave a wider circulation to these recipes and ensured their archival survival, their very insertion into the market introduced certain changes in them. The sacral contexts within which they were to be recited and performed were altered and reformatted in order to enhance their marketability. These texts, therefore, are not mere anachronistic survivors, but, indeed, historically contingent texts that themselves bear the impress of both the market itself and the history of the market.

If the importance of the market in the *daktari* writings on cholera was significant, they were paramount in the writings on *dhatu dourbalya.* The history of this syndrome helps to highlight several important historiographic concerns.

Syndromes such as *dhatu dourbalya* have all too frequently been described under the common label of *dhat* or *jiryan.* These, along with a few other comparable syndromes, have come to be labelled as Culture Bound Syndromes (CBS). The debate on CBS has been rich and varied. Though recent writing has done much to challenge the earlier cultural prejudices inherent in the frameworks used to describe CBS, their understanding of the relationship between history and culture remains problematic. In most recent writing, culture had indeed lost all value, becoming mere empty signs ranged over a uniform, linear and homogenous history. CBS has thus been shown to be present in both the 'East' and the 'West' and has been said to derive from such ancient 'Indian' authors as Charak. The actual specificities of this syndrome in their actual historical contexts and the actual historical connections—if any—that connect such disparate authors as Charak and Tissot have been left unexplored. By exploring the specificities of *dhatu dourbalya* as it came to be used amongst the nineteenth-century *daktari* authors, we hope to reorient this debate by reanimating the relationship between culture and history, specifically through the mediation of the market.

Those *daktars* who chose to write on *dhatu dourbalya* pointed out that the greatest visibility of the disease was in the numerous advertisements that were peddled for it. Confessedly then, the disease proved that the world of the medical market and that of the polite *daktari* writing—despite differences—were not unrelated. *Dhatu dourbalya* was a classic example of a disease framed principally in the market and taken up thereafter by the polite authors.

This formative influence of the market was visible in the very rationality that framed the pathological reality of the disease. The affliction came to be described most often by recourse to analogies and metaphors. Of course, part of the reason for this lay in concerns about overstepping the norms of decency, but here, too, it was the market that had forced the *daktars* to write for a mixed audience of physicians and laymen where considerations of decency would not be as perfunctory as they might have been if the texts were written solely for physicians. More importantly, the analogical structure of reasoning suited the medical market better than the didactic rationality of the medical colleges. Since the syndrome was developed mainly through advertisements, they sought to convince a lay reader with no particular medical experience. Here, the use of analogies and images from the day-to-day lives of the primary target consumers were worth much more than complex medical theory.

This metaphorical rationality, however, produced a distinct type of pathological reality. It was not a unified and clearly defined affliction with a relatively fixed set of symptoms. Instead, it was an assemblage of a number of terms which usually appeared together. There was no certainty as to how these terms related to each other. Sometimes they appeared as symptoms, sometimes as related diseases and sometimes merely as synonyms. In order to understand the pathology of *dhatu dourbalya*, therefore, it is crucial to theorize this rhizoid structure.

Each of these terms had several and distinct histories of its own. Some went back centuries though their usage had changed over time, others were of recent vintage. They drew upon multiple traditions of healing, from both the 'West' and the 'East', and constituted together a pathological reality that medicalized the numerous ascriptions of Bengali racial weakness that had come to mark late-colonial Bengal. At this level, the pathology itself became a metaphor. This multilayered metaphoric deployment allowed *dhatu dourbalya* to slip easily between individuated perceptions of bodily weakness, social ascriptions of *bhodrolok* impotence and body-political projects and debates over political empowerment of the *bhodrolok*.

It also resulted in a progressive substantiation of 'weakness' whereby it came first to be located in bodily substances like '*dhatu*', 'blood', etc., and finally to be manipulated by pharmaceutical substances. Most significantly, rather than Charak—or even Tissot—its immediate frame derived from the peculiarities of *daktari* medicine's own location within history, culture and market.

There are some general shifts that might be noticed to hold true across our various case studies. One important shift was the increasing tendency to use techno-scientific solutions. While the onus on the body's capacity to resist disease remains vibrant even in the 1930s, after the 1920s, the means to bolster this capacity to resist is increasingly sought in pills, injections, etc., instead of the earlier accent upon the patient's own will and lifestyle. A popular *daktari* author from the 1920s, Kiranchandra Ghosh, for example, produced a book titled *E Myanual obh Injekshan Chikitsa* (A Manual for Treatment with Injections) in 1921.[3] Some idea of its popularity can be had from the fact that, in the five years following its publication, it went through as many as three editions. This trend is enabled by a greater substantiation—i.e., location in particular 'substances'—of bodily capacities. The trends were already in motion by the beginning of the twentieth century, but it is doubtful that without the professional ascent of the *daktars* within the medical establishment in the period following WWI, these trends would have become as pronounced. The epistemological configuration of these changes must be located as much in a history of abstract concepts as well as the changing power relations between *daktars* and their patients. What had preempted earlier objectifying technologies such as medical statistics from taking hold of *daktari* medicine had been a combination of the low bureaucratic position of the *daktars* as well as their proximity to their patients. As *daktars* came to occupy high bureaucratic positions, the administrative apparatus at their disposal as well as their distance from the patients—augmented by the increased social status, administrative power, etc.—led to the growing popularity of objectifying technologies. Even relatively low-ranking medical officers in the 1920s, such as Dr M. Shamsuddin, who was a Sub-Assistant Surgeon (the post-1910 designation for Hospital Assistants), revealed the extent to which his practice depended upon complex gadgetry and pharmaceutical intervention. In a short piece on the 'Influenza Heart', in the section on diagnosis, where his predecessors had usually listed a host of symptoms, he explained how to use a 'sphygmomanometer', an 'electrocardiogram' and a 'stethoscope'. In the section on treatment, too, he spelt out his reasoning for giving particular medicines in a syllogism with numbered steps, each outlining the physiological actions that needed to be corrected and the drugs necessary to bring about such correction. Even upon the patient's recovery, he advised a course of pills aimed at helping the process of recuperation—even specifying the company that sold such pills.[4] Clearly, *daktari* medicine was beginning its techno-scientific fascination with diagnostic gadgets and pharmaceutical interventions, which increasingly objectified the patient by marginalising his/her will and accenting the mechanical logic of biomedicine. It was this alienation through gadgets and pills that Rajsekhar Basu's short story, *Chikitsa Sankat,* satirized.[5] A short satirical drama by the well-known *daktar* Sundarimohan Das amply brings out this shift. In the drama, Das criticized the physicians who encouraged their wealthy patients to lead profligate lives and then prescribed expensive (and in Das' story, harmful) medicines to cure them. Though *daktars* persisted in the faith in the capacity of the patient to resist falling ill, while the newer *daktars* increasingly trusted medicines to help the patient do so, those of Das' generation espoused the importance of healthy lifestyles to promote the body's capacities to resist disease.[6] These trends, already visible in the 1920s, became more pronounced in the 1930s. It would indeed be an intriguing question to investigate whether *daktari* medicine, as a vernacularized form of 'western' medicine, survived the changes ushered in by the appropriation of the state by the nation it had helped actualize in 1947. Such questions and the changes to *daktari* medicine in the last two decades of colonialism will, however, have to await another occasion.

NOTES

Introduction

1. Iliffe, *East African Doctors,* 25.
2. Kumar, *Disease and Medicine,* xvi.
3. Kumar, *Disease and Medicine,* xvii.
4. Crawford, *A History of the Indian Medical Service, Vol. II,* 101.
5. Crawford, *A History of the Indian Medical Service, Vol. II,* 101.
6. Crawford, *A History of the Indian Medical Service, Vol. II,* 103.
7. Wade, *Select Evidences of a Successful Method of Treating Fever and Dysentery,* 5, 7.
8. Pahari, *Unish Sataker Banglaye Sanatani Chikitsa Vyavasthyar Swarup,* 33.
9. Crawford, *A History of the Indian Medical Service, Vol. II,* 106–7.
10. For an excellent description of the NMI see Alavi, *Islam and Healing:* 54–69.
11. Crawford, *A History of the Indian Medical Service. Vol. II,* 434.
12. Crawford, *A History of the Indian Medical Service, Vol. II,* 113.
13. Palit ed. *Science and Nationalism in Bengal 1876–1947,* 10.
14. Government Order No. 28 of 28 January, 1835, reproduced in full in Crawford, *A History of the Indian Medical Service, Vol. II,* 438.
15. Kumar, "Emergence of Western Medical Institutions in India 1822–1911", 162–3.
16. I am indebted to Mrs Ceridwen Harris for information on the life of Edward John Lazarus, who was born to a Jewish family in Calcutta in 1825. Lazarus converted to Christianity and was baptised twice; in 1843 at Fort William and again in 1845 at the Lalbazar Church. In later life he was based in Benares and became a leading orientalist and Sanskritist. Personal email from Ceridwen Harris dated 18[t] January 2008.
17. Alavi, *Islam and Healing:* 188–96.
18. Kumar, "Emergence of Western Medical Institutions in India 1822–1911", 163–5.
19. Crawford, *A History of the Indian Medical Service Vol. II,* 115.

20. Crawford, *A History of the Indian Medical Service Vol. II,* 116.
21. Crawford, *A History of the Indian Medical Service Vol. II,* 117.
22. Sinha, *Public Health Policy and the Indian Public, Bengal 1850–1920*, 36–8.
23. Crawford, *A History of the Indian Medical Service Vol. II,* 121 & 123.
24. Anonymous, "Prize Essay on Plague Prevention", *Indian Medical Gazette,* XLII, 1907, 303–04.
25. Kumar, "Emergence of Western Medical Institutions in India 1822–1911", 168.
26. O'Donnell, *Census of India: Bengal Vol. III*, 510–12.
27. Gait, *Census of India: Bengal Vol. IV,* 322–23.
28. Sinha, *Public Health Policy and the Indian Public, Bengal 1850–1920,* 38; Kumar, "Emergence of Western Medical Institutions in India 1822–1911", 167–70.
29. Gait, *Census of India: Bengal Vol. IV,* 322–23.
30. Risley, *The Tribes and Castes of Bengal,* 362.
31. Kumar, "Emergence of Western Medical Institutions in India 1822–1911", 172.
32. Ernst, "Beyond East and West."
33. See Kumar, "Medical Encounters in British India, 1820–1920"; Palit et al., eds, *History of Medicine in India: The Medical Encounter*
34. It is cogent to add that some authors who, while remaining within the intellectual tradition which framed colonial medical exchanges as an 'encounter', have sought to transcend it by speaking of such an 'encounter' in the plural, i.e., 'encounters'. The difference in this usage and those of Palit or Kumar reside in the differential mappings of the site of the encounter. Instead of mapping the encounter on to the abstract spaces of 'cultures' or 'medical systems', these authors map the plural 'encounters' onto the intimate and numerous spaces of the 'body'. See Das, "Medical Knowledge of the Body: Colonial Encounters"; Bhattacharya, "Anatomical Knowledge and the East West Exchange".
35. 'Encounters' have been the subject of several recent Hindi films which are a good guide to how the word is used in popular lexicon. See for instance *Ab Tak Chhappan, Encounter: The Killing, Kaagar, Risk, Shootout at Lokhandwala,* etc. Vikram Chandra's recent novel *Sacred Games* also describes an 'encounter' in detail.
36. Arnold, *Colonizing*; Harrison *Public Health.*
37. Gupta, "Indigenous Medicine"; Bala, *Imperialism and Medicine.*
38. Buckingham, "Patient Welfare Vs. Health of the Nation"; Hodges, "Governmentality, Population and the Reproductive Family".
39. Sivaramakrishnan, *Old Potions, New Bottles*; Alavi, *Islam and Healing.*

40. Attewell, *Refiguring Unani Tibb : Plural Healing in Late Colonial India.*
41. Vaughan, *Curing their Ills*; Anderson, "Postcolonial Technoscience".
42. Anderson, "Postcolonial Technoscience", 647.
43. Anderson, "Postcolonial Technoscience", 646.
44. Anderson, "Postcolonial Technoscience", 643.
45. Anderson, "Postcolonial Technoscience", 644.
46. Vaughan *Curing their Ills*, 25.
47. Vaughan, *Curing their Ills*, x.
48. It is cogent to note that there are two broad channels along which the process of 'provincialization' has been observed by scholars. First, the ways in which 'western' medicine was deployed and developed differently in the colonies than in the metropole. Vaughan's work is a good example of this approach. Second, the way in which 'western' medicine was appropriated by members of the colonized society. Iliffe's work is an excellent example of this approach. The distinction between these two is not always clear and it may not be advisable to insist on the distinction in all cases (for peculiarities of colonial deployment often mediated the specificities of appropriation), yet it remains a useful shorthand to organizing the growing literature on 'appropriation' of 'western' science.
49. Anderson, "Postcolonial Technoscience", 646; See Kumar, *Science and the Raj.*
50. Raj, *Relocating Modern Science*; Habib et al., *Domesticating Modern Science.*
51. Ramanna, "Ranchodlal Chotalal"; Ray, "Voluntary Associations"; Dutta, "Upendranath Brahmachari".
52. The work of Kapil Raj is an exception to this general trend, but it does not engage with medicine. Raj, *Relocating Modern Science.*
53. Iliffe, *East African Doctors.*
54. Patton, *Physicians, Colonial Racism and Diaspora in West Africa*; Bruchhausen, "Medicine by Non-Doctors"?
55. Vaughan's comments in this particular case have, in part, been influenced by the fact that her material has very little on how Africans themselves came to see 'western' medicine. Here Iliffe's work provides a partial supplement.
56. Anderson, "Postcolonial Technoscience", 647; See Cooper, "Conflict and Connection".
57. Anderson, "Postcolonial Technoscience", 643.
58. Scheper-Hughes, "Culture, Scarcity and Maternal Thinking"; Cohen "The Other Kidney". For a more 'historical deployment' of this approach, see, Anderson, "The Possession of Kuru: Medical Science and Biocolonial Exchange" and Scheper-Hughes, "Ishi's Brains, Ishi's Ashes".

59. It is nowhere our wish to represent colonialism itself as 'shifting'—though it was unquestionably complex. Instead, we are seeking to open up an analytical window into the complexity, heterogeneity and hierarchy of the South Asian response to colonial repression and dislocation.
60. Kumar, *Disease and Medicine*, xix. Also see Kumar "Medical Encounters in British India, 1820–1920".
61. Guha, *Dominance without Hegemony*.
62. Indeed, there is enough evidence that even the limited interest the colonial state took in the health of its subjects often necessitated the employment of 'indigenous' healers on local administrative initiatives during periods of crisis. See Hume Jr., "Rival Traditions: Western Medicine and *Yunan-i-tibb* in the Punjab".
63. Ramasubban, "Imperial Health".
64. Arnold himself does not suggest a complete hegemony as Kumar does.
65. See Porter, *Quacks*; Cook, "Good Advice and Little Medicine".
66. Jenner et al. ed., *Medicine and the Market in England and its Colonies*.
67. Bode, "Taking Traditional Knowledge to the Market"; Banerjee, "The Long Road to Khari Baloi"; Sharma, "Creating a Medical Consumer".
68. Chakrabarti, "Medical Marketplaces Beyond the West".
69. Hodges, "Chennai's Biotrash Chronicles: Chasing the Neo-Liberal Syringe".
70. Burnham, *How the Idea of Profession Changed in the Writing of Medical History*.
71. Johnson, "Imperialism and the Professions". For a refutation of this argument see, Iliffe, *East African Doctors*, 3–4.
72. It is a common feature to find medical advertisements selling self-treatment books or medicines, where the author/proprietor has given details of his own qualifications as a mark of his professional identity. Some even highlight their having been in government employment at some time or other, further cementing their identification with the profession. In effect—whether these claims are true or not—the touting of this professional identity is an attempt to get competitive edge in a medical market.
73. Alavi, *Islam and Healing*, 30–31.
74. Letter from the Secretary, Home Department, Government of India to the Secretary, Financial (Medical) Department, Government of Bengal dated 23[d] May, 1913 in File 2M/13 Proceeding No. 40 A, Bengal Municipal (Medical Branch) Proceedings, 1913. A&AC Call No. P/9145.

75. Apart from the numerous advertisements for specifics 'discovered' by *daktars* in government employ (some of which we shall discuss in Chapter V), there were also numerous instances of medical officers writing testimonials for particular drugs which were later included in advertisements.
76. File 3M/13, Proceedings No. 227–29 B, Bengal Municipal (Medical Branch) Proceedings. A&AC Call No. P/7037.
77. File 2M/2, Proceeding No. 135–37 B, Bengal Municipal (Medical Branch) Proceedings. A&AC Call No. P/7037.
78. For uses of the idea of Medical Pluralism See Feierman, "Change in African Therapeutic Systems"; Janzen, *The Quest for Therapy in Lower Zaire*; Prins, "'But What Was the Disease'"; For uses by historians of South Asia See Ernst, *Plural Medicine*, 1–18.
79. Nichter, "The Layperson's Perception of Medicine as Perspective into the Utilization of Multiple Therapy Systems in the Indian Context". Also see Khare, "*Dava, Daktar* and *Dua*: Anthropology of Practised Medicine in India".
80. The same point is made at the level of epistemology by Anirban Das. See Das, "Medical Knowledge of the Body: Colonial Encounters".
81. Shapin, "Nibbling at the 'Teats of Science'".
82. The term 'macroparasites' is used by Deepak Kumar to designate the colonizers. Disease and Medicine, xix.
83. Basalla, "The Spread of Western Science".
84. Ernst, *Mad Tales from the Raj.*
85. Arnold, *Colonizing*, 17.
86. Harrison, *Public Health.*
87. Kumar, *Science and Empire*; Sangwan, *Science, Technology and Colonization.*
88. Kumar, *Science and the Raj.*
89. Kumar, *Medicine and the Raj*; Harrison, "Book Reviews: Anil Kumar, Medicine and the Raj", 360.
90. See Gupta, "Indigenous Medicine".
91. Arnold, *Warm Climates and Western Medicine*; Harrison, *Climates and Constitutions*; Worboys, "Germs, Malaria and the Invention of Mansonian Tropical Medicine".
92. Hardiman, *Healing Bodies, Saving Souls*; Hodges, "Indian Eugenics in an Age of Reform".
93. Ramanna, *Western Medicine and Public Health*; Bhattacharya, *Expunging Variola.*
94. Pati et al., ed., *Health, Medicine, Empire.*
95. Sinha, *Public Health Policy and the Indian Public: Bengal 1850–1920*, 5.

96. Palit, *Science and Nationalism in Bengal 1876–1947*, 11.
97. Palit, *Science and Nationalism in Bengal 1876–1947*, 1–2.
98. Lourdusamy, *Science and National Consciousness in Bengal 1870–1930*, 236.
99. On forced sterilization see, Blair, "Mrs Gandhi's Emergency"; for Narmada Valley displacements see Sangvai, "Narmada Displacement"; for Indo-Pak Nuclear race see Tarkunde, "Nuclear Tests and 'Nation'".
100. Nandy ed., *Science, Hegemony and Violence* also see Sardar, *The Revenge of Athena: Science, Exploitation and the Third World.*
101. Kothari et al., "Violence and Modern Medicine".
102. Nandy, "Introduction: Science as a Reason of State".
103. Nandy, *Alternative Sciences.*
104. Chakrabarty, "*Shareer, Samaj O Rashtra: Oupanibeshik Bharatey Mahamari O Janasanskriti*".
105. Prakash, "A Different Modernity".
106. See Chatterjee, *Our Modernity & Nation and Its Fragments.*
107. Chakrabarti, "Science, Nationalism and Colonial Contestations"; Also see *Western Science in Modern India.* For Skinner's comments see, "Meaning and Understanding in the History of Ideas".
108. Goswami, *Producing India;* Zachariah, *Developing India*; Roy, *Beyond Belief.*
109. Latour, *Pandora's Hope*; De Landa, *Intensive Science.*
110. Scheper-Hughes, "Ishi's Brain, Ishi's Ashes".
111. Scheper-Hughes, "The Globalization of Organ Stealing Rumours"; Morgan, "'Properly Disposed of'".
112. Anderson, "Kuru: Medical Science and Biocolonial Exchange"; Bhattacharya et al., "Medical Garbage and the Limits of Global Governance"; Hodges, "Chennai's Biotrash Chronicles".
113. Mills, *Cannabis Britannica: A Social and Political History of Cannabis and the British Government*; Osseo-Asare, "Bioprospecting and Resistance: Transforming Poison Arrows into Strophantin Pills in Colonial Gold Coast, 1885–1922".
114. Ray, *Felt Community.*
115. Sinha, *Public Health Policy and the Indian Public, Bengal 1850–1920*, 36–37.
116. Bayly, *Empire and Information*, 55.
117. Nandy, "Defiance and Conformity in Science", 33.
118. Tagore, "*Nation Ki?*"
119. Kaviraj et al., *Civil Society*; Chatterjee, "Modernity, Democracy and a Political Negotiation of Death".
120. Foucault, *History of Sexuality Volume I*, 141.
121. See Cohen, "Other Kidney"; Alter, "Gandhi's Body, Gandhi's Truth".
122. Marriott, "Hindu Transactions".

123. Interestingly, in a slightly different context, Cohen's work has sought to develop a framework within which to understand different kinds of calculations of self-interest. He has for this purpose developed philosopher Giorgio Agamben's distinction between two types of life *bios* and *zoe*. The distinction might also be fruitfully applied to our material, but developing it here as a theoretical model would be outside the remit of the present study. See Cohen, "Other Kidney"; Agamben, *Homo Sacer*.
124. See Rose, *Inventing Our Selves*.
125. For an account of the anxieties and precautions of the local police as well as the muted distaste of the propertied classes to the festivities of *Chodok*, see Singha, *Hutom*. For *daktari* support of the festivities, see Bagchi, *Bagher Baccha*.
126. Kumar, *Disease and Medicine*, xix.
127. Palit, *History of Medicine in India*, 15.
128. Arnold, *Science, Technology and Medicine in Colonial India*, 176–77.
129. Berger, *Ayurveda, State and Society*, 5–6; See also the classic Leslie, Asian Medical Systems.
130. See Wise, *Review*.
131. Attewell, *Refiguring*, 24.
132. Arnold, "Plurality and Transition".
133. Derrida, *Archive Fever*, 3.
134. Greenblatt, *Learning to Curse*.
135. Eisenstadt, "Multiple Modernities"; Gole, "Snapshots"; Chakrabarty, "Difference-Deferral"; Robinson, "Islamic Reform"; Kaviraj, "An Outline".
136. Kaviraj, "An Outline".
137. Arnold has, with some justice, argued that Pollock's model is itself premised on the tendency to see South Asia as a 'system'. Pollock's comments about the *longue duree* difference in the historical experience of South Asian communities with Europe and the capacity of such experience to effect attitudes and practices towards modernity, can, we believe, be recuperated within a more historicist analytical framework, without subscribing to the more 'systemic' elements of Pollock's model. See Arnold, "Plurality and Transition".
138. Pollock, "Cosmopolitan and Vernacular in History".
139. See Taavitsainen et al., "Vernacularisation of Medical Writing in English"; Cifuentes, "Vernacularisation as an Intellectual and Social Bridge".

140. Crossgrove, "The Vernacularization of Science, Medicine and Technology", 50.
141. Alavi, *Islam and Healing.*

Chapter I. Healers in Context: Forgotten Pioneers

1. Ginzburg et al., "Microhistory".
2. Foot, "House"; Darnton, *Cat Massacre*; Stewart, *Pickett's Charge.*
3. The search for repeated events which will reveal a macrohistorical pattern was led by those associated with the French journal *Annales.* See Le Goff, *Medieval Imagination.* For the most determined assertion of the opposite position that held historical events to be unique and denied the possibility of repetitions, see Cobb, *Sense of Place.*
4. Bloch, *Feudal Society.*
5. Bhadra, *Protapchand*; Amin, *Event.*
6. Stone, "Prosopography".
7. Lepore, "Historians".
8. Chattopadhyay, *Science and Society*: 99–100; Sen Gupta, "Soorjo".
9. Rai Kanailal Dey Bahadur (usually spelt as Kanny Lall Dey) was the son of Rai Radhanath Dey Bahadur. He graduated from the Calcutta Medical College in 1854 and subsequently taught Chemistry at the Presidency College and the Medical College. He was a lifelong champion for the greater use of 'indigenous drugs', wrote several books on the subject and put together several displays for various international exhibitions. Lethbridge *Golden Book*, 229–30.
10. All biographic information on Tamiz Khan used here, unless otherwise indicated, is to be found in Anonymous, "Obituary".
11. See for example, Calcutta University, *Minutes*, 124, 128.
12. Alam et al., "Munshi".
13. Sen Gupta, "Soorjo".
14. Quoted in Anonymous, "Obituary".
15. Bernutz et al., "Members," 55.
16. See Transactions of the Epidemiological Society of London, 12: 1893 and Australian Medical Journal, 8: 1880.
17. Kar, "*Bhumika*", *Bhisak Suhrid.*
18. Basu, *Charitabhidhan*, 173; File 1A/22 Proceedings B 35–40, Bengal Municipal Proceedings (May–October) 1897: 32, A&AC Call No. P/5172. Some measure of his popularity amongst students and his personal endeavour in the popularity of the *Bhisak Darpan* can be had from an acrostic poem—possibly written by one of his students—published in the first issue

of the sixth volume of the journal in which the first letter of each line spelt out Dr Ahmed's name. The gist of the acrostic roughly translates thus: 'The victor, victorious Lord of the World, life in this world/ It was his desire that made *Bhisak Darpan* a reality/The ailing go to him to find a way/O Compassionate One you show them the way/With the new year comes new life/In delight I call to all my friends/Come join in with compassionate hearts/Give evidence of your compassion to our Doctor/On thus working together even the impossible shall be possible.' Some of the adjectives used, such as the 'Compassionate One' (*Deen Doyamoy*) or the Lord of the World (*Jogodeesh*), are usually used to referred to God; the acrostic format of the poem—whereby the first letter of the each line spells out 'Zahiruddin Ahmed'—proves how high a position Dr Ahmed occupied amongst his students. Anonymous, "Zahiruddin Ahmed".

19. Basu ed., *Samoyiki*, 687.
20. Alam et al., "Munshi".
21. Chatterjee, "History as Self-Representation".
22. All information on Annadacharan's life used here, unless otherwise stated, is taken from Kaviratna, "*Daktar* Annadacharan".
23. Such a mismatch between the Indian doctors' status within 'native' and 'white' society and the trenchant belief that the 'government' and 'British justice' will eventually recognize the talents of a man are reminiscent of another Indian doctor who served in British Burma slightly later than Khastagir—George Orwell's Dr Veeraswami in *Burmese Days*.
24. Much has been made of the conflict between homoeopathy and allopathy, particularly through appraisals of the life of the celebrated doctor Mahendralal Sircar's switch and the attendant hostility this caused him to face from professional colleagues. Within the world of *daktari* medicine, however, the relationship between homoeopathy and allopathy was much less confrontational. Many dispensary-level *daktars* openly used both systems and many of the leading *daktari* periodicals published articles on allopathy and homoeopathy. The framework of conflict might have been limited to the upper echelons of the medical bureaucracy. Its narrative importance undoubtedly derives from the attempt by many Bengali authors to use Mahendralal Sircar's life as a model for showing the need to stand up for one's convictions. For the openness towards homoeopathy at the local level, see the Arrah dispensary episode mentioned later in this chapter. Also see the writings of Saradaprasad Chakrabarty, particularly *Bishuchika Chikitsa Sar* and *Saral Chikitsa Tattwa*. For use of Sircar's travails as a didactic model see, Shastri, "Mahendralal Sircar".

25. Kaviratna, himself an orthodox Hindu, interestingly avoids all but the most scant mention of Khastagir's involvement with Brahmoism. The details of his involvement in the splits of the Brahmo Samaj are mentioned by Shibnath Shastri in Shastri, *Ramtonu*, 225.
26. Singha, *Hutom*.
27. Much has been written on the rational tendencies unleashed among certain sections by the Bengal Renaissance, but no work—to our knowledge—looks at the immensely important performative aspects of this clash of reason and unreason described by Singha, for one, as yet another *hujug*, or sensation.
28. Singha, *Hutom*, 180–85.
29. Singha, *Hutom*, 185–92.
30. Kipling, *Kim*, 234–38.
31. Amin, *Muslim Women*, 148.
32. All information used here about Nabinchandra Datta's life, unless otherwise stated, is taken from Datta, "Rai Nabinchandra".
33. For a contemporary account of this resurgence of Hinduism at the expense of Brahmoism, see Shastri, "*Brahmo Samajer Prabhaber Hrash*". For a good critical reappraisal of these developments, see Chakrabarty, "*Hindu Punerutthyan*".
34. Choudhury, "*Chikitshokgoner Sochchoritro*".
35. Bagchi, *Bagher Baccha*, 50–54.
36. Mukhopadhyay, "*Pnajite Swasthya Charcha*". Also see Sengupta et al., *Charitabhidhan*, 107.
37. All information about the life of Capt. Narendranath Dutta used here, unless otherwise stated, is taken from Chakrabarty, *Captain Narendranath*.
38. Sen Gupta, "Soorjo".
39. Sengupta et al., *Charitabhidhan*, 261.
40. Sengupta et al., *Charitabhidhan*, 53.
41. For a clear description of who the Local Native Doctors were, see Report on the Endemic Dispensaries in Beerbhoom District for the Year 1873, Bengal (Medical Dept) Proceedings, 1874, A&AC Call No. P/175.
42. Half Yearly Dispensary Reports, 1840, A&AC Call No. V/24/732: 12.
43. We have discussed this early history of Native Doctors and the Dispensary System in Mukharji, 'Structuring Plurality'; Also see Alavi, *Islam and Healing*: 154–204.
44. Half Yearly Dispensary Reports, 1842, A&AC Call No. V/24/733: 82.
45. Half Yearly Dispensary Reports, 1842, A&AC Call No. V/24/733: 178.
46. Half Yearly Dispensary Reports, 1842, A&AC Call No. V/24/733: 196.
47. Wise, "Preface", *Review*.

48. Half Yearly Dispensary Reports, 1844, A&AC Call No. V/24/734: 33–34.
49. Half Yearly Dispensary Reports, 1840, A&AC Call No. V/24/732: 14.
50. Half Yearly Dispensary Reports, 1845, A&AC Call No. V/24/734: 41.
51. Report of the Charitable Dispensaries under the Govt of Bengal, Bengal Medical Consultations 1874, A&AC Call No. P/175.
52. File 35 dated January 1876, Bengal Medical Consultations 1876–77, A&AC Call No. P/873: 1–2.
53. Half Yearly Dispensary Reports, 1845, A&AC Call No. V/24/735: 28.
54. File 346 dated 5 September 1876, Bengal Medical Consultations, A&AC Call No. P/873: 191.
55. Ibid: 276.
56. File 10 dated January 1876 ('B' Proceedings 2–3), Bengal Medical Consultations 1876–77, A&AC Call No. P/873.
57. File 121 dated 29 November 1876 ('B' Proceedings 196–197) Bengal Medical Consultations 1876–77, A&AC Call No. P/873.
58. File 352 dated 13 October 1876 ('B' Proceedings 118–119), Bengal Medical Consultations 1876–77, A&AC Call No. P/873.
59. File 255 dated 31 December 1875 ('B' Proceedings 166–167) Bengal Medical Consultations 1876–77, A&AC Call No. P/873.
60. File 107 dated 26 February 1877 ('B' Proceedings 126–127) Bengal Medical Consultations, A&AC Call No. P/873.
61. File 3C/21 dated December 1897 ('B' Proceedings 148–49), Bengal Municipal (Medical Branch) Proceedings (November–December) 1897, A&AC Call No. P/5173: 30.
62. *Nizamat-Tibb* DUMC Call No. DU/73 & DU/360; *Risala Quanuncha* DUMC Call No. HR/1; *Kitab-i-Daktari* DUMC Call No. DU/189; *Nushkhajat* DUMC Call No. DU/437. The use of the Arakanese Era in a medical manuscript in the *Nushkhajat* is specially interesting as it points to the strong possibility of persistent Southeast Asian influences on medicine in the Chittagong region.
63. File 203A dated 15 September 1876 ('B' Proceedings 160–161) Bengal Medical Consultations 1876–77, A&AC Call No. P/873.
64. File 203A dated 2 December 1876 ('B' Proceedings 19–22) Bengal Medical Consultations 1876–77, A&AC Call No. P/873.
65. File 2 dated 6 January 1876 ('B' Proceedings 6–7) Bengal Medical Consultations 1876–77, A&AC Call No. P/873.
66. For the '*bayaaz*' see, Quaiser, "Unani"; for 'Taliqa Kobirajes' Risley, *Tribes and Castes*, 362.
67. Bandopadhyay, *Arogya Niketan*, 35–36. First published in 1952, the novel has been the recipient of the prestigious *Sahitya Akademi Puraskar* in 1956 and the *Rabindra Puraskar* in 1954–1955.

68. The 'enclavist' argument made by Radhika Ramasubban has been qualified by many scholars since. Its basic premise, however, which focuses solely on 'high western medicine' to the exclusion of vernacular forms and practitioners, continues to loom large. Ramasubban, "Imperial Health". For a critique of Ramasubban, see Arnold, *Colonizing*.
69. Basu, "*Jodu Daktarer Patient*," 183.
70. Mukherji, "*Bigyapan*" in *Chikitsa Darpan*.
71. Sanyal, "*Byakti Bishesher Math*" in *Chikitsa Kalpataru, Vol III*.
72. Ray, *Deb Ganer Marte Agaman*, 412.
73. File 215 n.d. ('B' Proceeding 74) Bengal Medical Consultations 1876–77, A&AC Call No. P/873.
74. Deb, *Thengapathic*, 90.
75. Deb, *Thengapathic*, 6–7.
76. Pinto "Development without Institutions: Ersatz Medicine and the Politics of Everyday Life in Rural North India".
77. See Datta, *Daktari Shikhya*.
78. Kar, *Bhisak Bandhu*.
79. Bandopadhyay, *Arogya Niketan*, 23.
80. Orwell, *Burmese Days*, 137–38.
81. Deb, *Thengapathic*, 86.
82. Both advertisements appeared regularly in the *Amrita Bazar Patrika* in and around 1900.
83. File Q/1 ('B' Proceedings 570–572) Municipal (Medical Branch) Dept., Government of Bengal, May 1905. Also see July 1905, File No. 28–29, WBSA.
84. For these private medical colleges, see, Arnold, *Colonizing*.
85. Guha, "*Ekti Rogir Vivaran*".
86. Mukherji, "*Hathurey Chikitsak*".
87. Sircar, "*Chikitsa Vyavsaya*".
88. Bagchi, *Bagher Baccha*, 85–86.
89. Roy, *Mayapuri*; Sengupta, *Narsin Hom*.
90. File 329 dated 12 September 1876 ('B' Proceedings 3–6) Bengal Medical Consultations 1876–77, A&AC Call No. P/873.
91. For Malda see, File 1 Collection 1 ('B' Proceedings 1–3) Bengal Municipal (Medical Branch) Proceedings (January–March) 1886, A&AC Call No. P2805; For Shahbad see, File 1P/20 n.d. ('B' Proceedings 383–384), Bengal Municipal (Medical Branch) Proceedings (November–December) 1897, A&AC Call No. P/5173.
92. File 35 dated January 1876, Bengal Medical Consultations 1876–77, A&AC Call No. P/873: 1–2.

93. File 1A/24 n.d. ('B' Proceedings 214–217) Bengal Municipal (Medical Branch) Proceedings (May–October) 1897, A&AC Call No. P/5172.

Chapter II. Daktari Prints: The World of Bengali Printing and the Multiple Inscriptions of *Daktari* Medicine

1. See Ogborn, *Indian Ink*; Das, *Sahibs and Munshis*; Ross, *Bengali Character*; Sripantha, *Chhapa Khana.*
2. Ghosh, *Power in Print* and "Revisiting the Bengal Renaissance".
3. Roy, "Disciplining the Printed Text"; Chakrabarty, "*Haridasher Guptakatha*"; Sripantha, *Bot-tola.* Of these, Roy and Sripantha provide very useful overviews of the world of early Bengali printing.
4. Recently Gautam Bhadra has argued that the 'high' and 'low' literatures cannot be distinguished simply by the presses or even the authors, as there were considerable overlaps between the two. Instead, argues Bhadra, the distinction between the 'high' and 'low' literatures was based on reading practices and the type of reader positions inscribed in the text's narrative structures. Bhadra "*Nera Bot-tolaye Jaye Kobar?*"
5. Sivaramakrishnan, *Old Potions.*
6. Alavi, "Unani Medicine".
7. Attewell, *Refiguring.*
8. Kar, *Bhisak Suhrid* and text titled "*Kar Samhita*" has been mentioned in Sengupta, *Charitabhidhan*, 464.
9. Alavi, *Islam and Healing:* 129–30.
10. Alavi, *Islam and Healing:* 65–9.
11. Between September 1829 and March 1833 alone, John Tytler was said to have received a whopping Rs 17,000/- above his salary for his translation of European medical texts into vernaculars. Alavi, *Islam and Healing*: 67.
12. These differences go to the very heart of the specificity of Bengali linguistic and regional history. Bengali had not been a court language enjoying elite patronage as Persian had been. Nor was it a liturgical language like Sanskrit or Arabic. The Bengali elite were usually Persianate. Its more orthodox religious literature existed in Arabic or Sanskrit. Leading men of the day like Raja Rammohun Roy, whose family had had minor connections to the court of the erstwhile Nawabs of Bengal, started his authorial career writing in Persian and not Bengali. In the absence of elite patronage or any specifically elite affiliations, Bengali emerged into preeminence only through the agency

of the emergent new elite which had come into being largely through contact and cooperation with the rising British power. Bengali was, therefore, less dependent initially on elite patronage and instead appropriated the new printing technology through early entrepreneurs.

13. Long, *Descriptive*, 32.
14. Ward writes that 'The Hindoo physician never prescribes to a patient without first receiving his fees…' Ward, *Hindoos*: 478; Bandopadhyay had one of the characters, Thakurdas Misra, tell his friend and eminent Kaviraj Jagatbandhu Moshai that, 'You cannot hide the fact that the Kavirajes make money from their patients. Simply by quoting Sanskrit verses from Yudishthira, the son of Dharma, you will not be able to conceal the account books of the Kavirajes'. Bandopadhyay, *Arogya Niketan*, 6.
15. Chakrabarty ed., *Dehatattwer*, 28.
16. Dutta, *Prankrishaushadhavali*; See Sengupta, *Charitabhidhan*, 311.
17. Long, *Catalogue*, 32–33; Also see, Sengupta, *Charitabhidhan*, 467.
18. Long, *Catalogue*, 33.
19. Breton, *Olauthar Vivaran.*
20. Pahari, *Chikitsa Vyavasthyar Swarup*, 165.
21. For an excellent description of the world of the NMI, see Alavi, *Islam and Healing*: 54–99.
22. Roy, *Chikitsa Vyavasthya*, 19–70.
23. Arnold, *Science, Technology and Medicine*, 62–63.
24. Mukharji "Structuring Plurality"; Also see Alavi, *Islam and Healing*, 154–204.
25. Burdett, *Hospitals and Asylums of the World:* 318.
26. Rameshwar Awasthi in fact had also been a teacher at the NMI and had made an unsuccessful plea to be allowed to join the newly formed CMC in 1835. See Alavi, *Islam and Healing*: 91, 96.
27. Wear, "Popularization of Medicine".
28. Long, *Catalogue*, 33, 35.
29. Though any references to the 'shastras' is usually taken to be a sign of classical influence, the term, in lay usage, did not always refer to any fixed or canonical set of texts. However, quotes from the 'shastras' were usually in Sanskrit. In Chapter VI we shall witness one such usage where medieval, locally composed Sanskrit poetical works are referred to as 'shastras' to validate particular comments about cholera.
30. Gupta, who had been trained at the erstwhile NMI and thereafter taught at Medical College, was one of the most significant points of contact between British doctors and 'indigenous' medical ideas.

Authors like T. A. Wise acknowledged his help in understanding the domain of 'indigenous' medicine.

31. Long, *Catalogue*, 32–36.
32. Royle, *Hindoo Medicine*; Wise, *Commentary*.
33. Mouat, "Hindu Medicine".
34. See Wilson, "Leprosy".
35. Wise *Review*.
36. For the Anglicist ascendancy, see Kopf, *Bengal Renaissance*; the introduction of the vernacular medical classes and the continued use of 'indigenous' medicines at dispensaries serve to qualify the linearity of the Anglicist triumph (at least in the case of medicine), which traditionally was thought to date from the establishment of the CMC in 1835.
37. Arnold, *Science, Technology and Medicine*: 62–63.
38. Ross, *General Report 1868*, A&AC Call No. V/24/664.
39. File 3C, Proceedings 186–88, dated 5 Sept 1876, Bengal Medical Consultations 1876–77, A&AC, Call No. P/873.
40. In order to get some idea of the intimate and encouraging relationship of the early Bengali surgeons and their immediate British superiors, see Half Yearly Dispensary Reports, A&AC Call No. V/24/732 to V/24/740. A good example of the alienation Bengali doctors increasingly felt even at the higher end of the medical bureaucracy can be gauged from the experiences and consequent resignation of Baman Das Basu from the IMS in 1907. See Arnold, *Science, Technology and Medicine*: 65.
41. Bhuttacharya, *Malarious Fevers*.
42. Quaiser, "Politics, Culture and Colonialism"
43 See for instance Attewell, *Refiguring*.
44. O'Donnell, *Census of India: Bengal*.
45. Gait, *Census of India: Bengal*.
46. Long, *Catalogue*, 35.
47. Mitra, *Homiopathic Chikitsa*; Chakrabarty, *Homiopathic Bhaisajyatattwa*.
48. Kar, *Bhaisajya Ratnavali*. For one of the best examples of this brief period when the vocabularies were incorporated into larger manuals and textbooks, see Raychaudhury, *Naradeha Nirnaya*.
49. Kar, *Bhaisajya Ratnavali*, 8. I am grateful to Gautam Bhadra for drawing my attention to the way the transliteration was actually worked out in the text.
50. For *quina*, see Kar, *Bhaisajya Ratnavali*:136; for *gallbladder* and *kidneys*, see Ray, *Bayu, Pittwa, Kaph*, 55–6.
51. Chattopadhyay, *"Paras-Bai"*.

52. File 1P/11 n.d. ('B' Proceeding 92), Bengal Municipal (Medical Branch) Proceedings (May–October) 1897, A&AC Call No. P/5172.
53. Mukhopadhyay, *Chikitsakosh*; Chakrabarty, *Daktari Abhidhan.*
54. Sen, *Venereal Diseases in Bengali.* For a full list of Khastagir's writings, refer to Chapter I. Numerous homoeopathic treatises written particularly on cholera would also fall into this category.
55. Jadunath Mukhopadhyay's books include *Chikitsa Darpan* (1880), *Dhatri Sikhya* (1867), *Saral Jwar Chikitsa* (1880), *Chikitsa Kalpadruma* (1882), *Kuinayn* (1892), *Palligram* (1892), *Shareer Palan* (1881) and *Bishuchika Roger Chikitsa* (1872).
56. We have discussed translations of ayurvedic texts at greater length elsewhere. See Mukharji, "Bangali Ayurbed".
57. Sen, *Ayurvediya Dravyabhidhan*; Gupta *Bhasabhidhan.*
58. Long, *Catalogue*, 32–33.
59. Datta, *Prankrishnaushadhavali*; Sobhan, *Elaj-e-Lokmani.*
60. Ghosh, *Sarpaghater Chikitsa.*
61. See Ghosh, *Bangiya Garhasthya Chikitsa*; Chaudhuri, *Garhasthyavigyan*; De, *Garhasthya Chikitsabhidhan*; Basak, *Grihamushtiyoga*; Gupta, *Mushtiyoga Samgraha*; Chakrabarty, *Totka.* Though there are some subtle differences between these three overlapping categories of *garhasthya chikitsa, mushtiyoga* and *totka*, for our present purposes, they may safely be considered as forming a single group.
62. Long, *Catalogue*, 35–36.
63. For chromopathy, see for example, Bandopadhyay, *Prakritik Chikitsa*; Ghosh, *Varna Chikitsa.* For mesmerism, see Anonymous, *Shokavijay*; Guha Thakurta, *Ashapradeep.*
64. Bhattacharya, *Dakini Vidya.*
65. Datta, *Daktari Shikhya.*
66. Bhattacharya, *Sentinels of Culture*, 72.
67. Advertisement of Bharat Pustakalay in *Gupta Press Dairektari Panjika* for 1322 BS.
68. Basu Barman, *Karyasadhak Aushadhgyan.*
69. Datta, *Daktari Shikhya.*
70. Kar, *Bhaisajya Ratnavali*; Mukherji, *Chikitsa Darpan.*
71. Attewell's fascinating account of conflicting models of authority in unani tibb in roughly the same period has interesting parallels with Bengali *daktari.* Though *daktari* was a new medical tradition in the region, it drew upon preexisting structures of medical authority at all levels of its practice. Just as Attewell finds the persistence of the biographic genre *tazkhirah* into the twentieth century, so, too, do we find the use of *daktari* biographies as biographical models well into the twentieth century.

These biographies generically accented certain virtues like idealism, extreme truthfulness, moral probity, philanthropy and broad intellectual interests, thereby proving that other paradigms of medical authority, besides the strictly professional ones, persisted. See. Attewell, *Refiguring*, 96–146. The biography of Mahendralal Sircar in Shibnath Shastri's history of the inception of Bengali modernity is a good example of the alternate models of authority that we speak of. See Shastri, *Ramtonu*, 193–99; also see the biography of Durgacharan Banerjee in Roy, *Deb Ganer Marte Agaman*, 366–69.

72. Bynum et al., "Periodical Knowledge".
73. Mentioned in the additional flyleaf inserted in the first issue of the journal.
74. Sen, *"Shesh Nivedan"*. The 'Value Payable' or VP post entailed the postman to collect the price of the item delivered in person. Since this implied a lack of reliability on the part of the recipient in his dealings with others, and as the postman's actions were usually easily observable by neighbours, especially in crowded neighbourhoods of old Calcutta, VP deliveries by the postman came to be seen as extremely socially embarrassing.
75. The *Chikitsak*, in its eighth issue, published the names of Prakashchandra Sheel, Compounder, Sylhet, Bhagabaticharan Das, Sub-Inspector of Schools, Cuttack and Bhairabchandra Bhattacharya, *Daktar*, Bardhaman for having 'requested the periodicals to be sent by VP post' and thereafter defaulting, thus causing the editors a loss of Rs. 0.50. The editors claimed they published the names in order to warn others of the unreliability of these buyers. The notice appeared on the unnumbered inside front cover.
76. This was by far the most popular strategy and can be seen in most journals. The most extensive lists however appeared in the *Chikitsa Sammilani*.
77. An editorial in the *Chikitsa Sammilani* at the commencement of its fourth volume lamented how not only were subscriptions not paid on time, but even reminders went unanswered. It mentioned that some debts had remained unpaid for over three years. It also mentioned an 'Inquiry Committee' which was investigating the 'popular' grievance that many people have been defrauded by dishonest editors who have not sent more than a few issues, even after subscribers had paid the entire subscription in advance. While the editorial did not deny such allegations altogether, it said that few such complaints were fuelling a paranoia that distracted from the plight of the editors at the hands of dishonest subscribers. Anonymous, *"Gata Varsha"*.

78. This claim was regularly printed on the inside front cover of the periodical.
79. Bagchi, *"Sampadak Paribartan"*.
80. Porter, *"Antrik Ajirna Rog"*; Rafdhar, *"Madhu Makkhika, Bolta ebam Bhimrul Dangshar"*; Sedgewick, *"Roganukrame Sambandhe Abhijattyer Adhitaptya"*; Vadley, *"Chikitsa Shastra Itihas"*. There is some confusion about whether 'Rafdhar' actually spelt his name in this fashion. Being an uncommon English name, the Bengali transliteration is not very helpful.
81. These were printed on the inside front cover of every issue.
82. The exchange started with the publication of Sanyal's "*Muley Bhul*". Replies and counter-replies followed from Maitreya and Sanyal over the following issues, despite the editor's repeated requests to settle the dispute amicably. The dispute dragged on for over three years and replies and counter replies from both disputers were still being published in the ninth volume of the CS. See also, Maitreya, *"Muley Bhul Boli Ki Kore?"*.
83. Gangopadhyay, "*Banglar Chikitsak Samaj*," 179.
84. Gangopadhyay, "*Banglar Chikitsak Samaj*," 179–80.
85. See Bagchi, "*Pet Bedana—Shul*".
86. Anonymous, "*Mulyaprapti*".
87. Anonymous, "*Mulyaprapti I*".
88. Kaviratna, "*Amader Katha*," 37.
89. Roy, "*Nivedan*".
90. Roy, "*Bhumika*," 1.
91. Unfortunately, the BD never published any subscription lists, and it is impossible to know if this trend towards nonmedical subscriptions held true for it as well. But there is some evidence to suggest that they, too, were trying to broaden their reach beyond the strict confines of the Subordinate Medical Service. The most overt evidence of the journal trying to broaden its appeal can be seen from the fact that from the twenty-first issue of the journal, it commenced publication of prescriptions for treating various diseases. This practice of using prewritten prescriptions, which was used by 'quacks' without institutional training or for self-prescription, had always been frowned upon by the 'professional' *daktars* and engaging in it clearly shows the journal trying to reach out to those beyond the professional pale.
92. File 408, Proceedings B 135–136, dated 19[t] December 1876, Bengal Medical Consultations 1876–77, A&AC Call No. P/873. The *Chikitsa Darpan* had been edited by Jadunath Mukherji and the *Chikitsa Kalpadruma* referred to here may well be a subsequent publication by the same editor, as he did later publish a book by that name in 1882. He also republished pieces from the *Chikitsa Darpan* in book form in 1880.

93. This short-lived and little-known journal edited by Hakim Majibar Rahman, only a few issues of which are available today, showed a clear attempt to engage with *daktari* medicine by trying to translate hakimi concepts into *daktari* registers. Part of the reason for the absence of a more voluminous engagement with hakimi traditions may have been due to the fact that the leading Bengali hakims like Saiful Mulk Hakim Habibur Rahman chose to write in Urdu rather than Bengali, thereby restricting the scope for the engagement with those writing in Bengali.
94. Articles by Rai Nibaranchandra Roy Bahadur particularly stand out for their Hindu revivalist flavour. See Roy, "*Vaigyanik Iswar*".
95. Sharma, "Creating a Medical Consumer". We are grateful to the author for allowing us to read this piece prior to publication.
96. Berger, *Ayurveda, State and Society*, 159–71.
97. Though Baudrillard's comments are particularly directed at 'consumer societies' and there may be some concern as to whether late nineteenth century Bengal might be described as such, there can be little doubt that advertising texts of the time did constitute a system of codified signs whose social exchanges were meaningful.
98. Ecks, "Pharmaceutical Citizenship: Antidepressant Marketing and the Promise of Demarginalization in India".
99. Bhadra, "*Boi-er Bigyapan*".
100. This is not, of course, to suggest that the more familiar format of advertisements limited to a page were also to be seen in Bengali, but merely to underline that *bigyapan* and 'advertisement' had certain generic dissimilarities as well. In the case of England, Elizabeth Furdell mentions that part of the reason that led to the shortened form of press advertisements familiar to us today was the imposition of advertising taxes by the Tory government in 1712. Furdell, *Publishing and Medicine in Early Modern England*, 136.
101. For an example of significantly smaller pages, see the advertisements of Sridhar Ayurvediya Aushadhalay inserted into the *Gupta Press Dairektari Panjika* for 1322 BS. The 16-page text also had individually and independently numbered pages from 1 to 16. For differently coloured advertising texts, see the eminent Kaviraj Bijayratna Sen's advertisements for his Ayurvediya Aushadhalay, also in the *Gupta Press Dairektari Panjika* for 1322 BS. This, too, had 16 independently numbered pages. The constant number 16 is due to the way printing presses worked. One impression comprised 16 pages at a time at most presses and, hence, printing 16 pages worked out cheaper than printing smaller numbers. It also proves amply that the advertising texts were printed independently of the text they were found in.

102. Gupta, *Sexuality, Obscenity and Community*.
103. Advertisement for Bharat Pustakalay in *Gupta Press Dairektari Panjika* for 1322 BS.
104. Advertisement for S. K. Roy & Co in *Gupta Press Dairektari Panjika* for 1322 BS.
105. See, for instance, advertisements of *Edwards' Tonic, Edwards' Liver and Spleen Ointment, Edwards Itches Ointment*, etc., in the *Brihat Mohammadiya Panjika* for 1318 BS. Ironically, Butto Kristo Paul, the founder's biographer, later portrayed him and his efforts to start the first South Asian-owned wholesale business in 'western' medicines, as an ardently nationalist gesture. Mukhopadhyay, *Sadhu Batakrista Pal.*
106. Advertisement for *Albert Powder* in *Lord Ripon's Panjika* for 1290 BS.
107. Advertisement for *Lytton Oil* in *Lord Ripon's Panjika* for 1290 BS.
108. See, for instance, advertisements of *Imperial Eye Drops* or *Imperial Itches Ointment* by GK Nag & Co, in the *Gupta Press Dairektari Panjika* for 1322 BS.
109. Advertisement for Napoleonic Tooth Powder in *Lord Ripon's Panjika* for 1290 BS.
110. It is cogent to reiterate that Hossain clearly espoused a *daktari* identity and his medicines as a consequence were also *daktari* medicines. He was also a leading personality in the world of lowbrow printing. He was referred to in advertisements of the *Mohammadiya Buk Agensi* as a 'great poet' (*mohakobi*). In these advertisements popularising his poetic works, too, however, he was consistently referred to as a *daktar* and an 'MD'. Advertisements for *Mohammadiya Buk Ajensi* in *Vrihat Mohammadiya Panjika* for 1318 BS.
111. Advertisements of Syed Abul Hossain in *Mahammadiya Panjika* for 1309 BS.
112. For an brilliant and fascinating exploration of the world of the *kerani*, see, Sarkar, *Writing Social History*.
113. Basu, "*Daktari O Kaviraji*".
114. Daeschel, *The Politics of Self Expression.*
115. We shall discuss many of these problems/anxieties within their *daktari* contexts in the following chapters.
116. See Mukherjee, *Calcutta Theatres.*
117. The *darpan*, or mirror plays, were usually very overtly political and had arisen towards the beginning of the nineteenth century to criticise social and political evils. Dinabandhu Mitra's vastly influential play, *Neel Darpan*, written in protest against the oppressive British indigo planters, was probably the best known drama of this genre.
118. Das, *Munisipal-Darpan.*

119. The *Prahasan* was an old Sanskrit genre that was revived with some changes for the Calcutta stage in the nineteenth century.
120. A detailed summary of the play is to be found in Goswami, *Prahasan*, 629–31.
121. Deb, *Thengapathik*.
122. Roy, *Daktarbabu*.
123. Quoted in Goswami, *Prahasan*, 630.
124. Basu, *Chikitsa Sankat*.
125. Anonymous cartoon appearing as plate 5 in the first (and perhaps only) issue of *Harbola Bhnar*.
126. For the Victorian debate on Wrongful Confinement see, McCandless, "Dangerous to Themselves and Others" .
127. Roy, *Mayapuri*; Sengupta, *Narsin Hom*.
128. The original incident and the furore caused by it are mentioned in Singha, *Hutom*.
129. Bagchi, *Bagher Baccha*.
130. Mukhopadhyay, "*Agni*".
131. Dasgupta, *Ledi Daktar*.
132. Raychaudhuri, "Translator's Note".

Chapter III. Contagious Nationalism: Contagion and the Actualization of the Nation

1. Bashford et al., *Contagion*, 1.
2. Conrad et al., *Contagion*, xvii.
3. Bashford et al., *Contagion*, 39.
4. Hamlin, "Predisposing Causes". See also, Pelling, *Cholera* and Pickstone, "Dearth, Dirt".
5. Gaudilliere et. al., *Disease Transmission*.
6. Gupta, "*Vividha Vishaya O Sambad*", 11.
7. Biswas, *Samsad Bengali-English Dictionary*, 243.
8. The biomoral qualities of the 'blood' and thereby, heredity, may have been particularly strong in the Bengal region due to the greater prevalence of Tantric traditions in the region, which had inherited the much older *Kaula* (of the *kul*) traditions that made extensive ritual use of blood as a inherited biomoral substance shared by the clan. See White, "Kamkala".
9. Mookerjee, *Medicine in Bengali*, 7.
10. Alavi, "Unani Medicine", 127; Berger, *Ayurveda*, 143–47.
11. Gupta, "*Bangali Saheb Nohe*".

12. Mookerjee, *Medicine in Bengali*, 6.
13. Ray, *Bhaisajya Sutra*, 4. While Ray was an ardent supporter of a Germ Theory of 'infection', he tried to reconcile this with older miasmatic theories as well. He described diseases as being either 'miasmatic' or 'contagious', but then went on to treat both types of 'poison' as being very similar. See for example *Bhasajya Sutra*,11.
14. The idea that there were multiple distinct *jeevanishaktis* or vital forces within one seems to have had some popular support as well. In 1915 the *Sulabh Ayurvediya Bhandar* was advertising a medicine called the *Amritakunda Salsa* in the *Gupta Press Dairektari Panjika*, which claimed that it could 'nourish all 64 *jeevanishaktis* discovered by the great sage Charak'.
15. Chakrabarty, "*Rog*", 212–13.
16. Guha, "*Shishuder Tiubarkel*".
17. Ray, "*Samkramak Shoth*", 52.
18. Prasad, "Crisis, Identity, and Social Distinction", 257.
19. Ali, "*Epidemik Dropsi ba Samkramak Shoth*", 329.
20. Ghoshal, "*Banglar Jwar Sambandhe Mantabya*", 245.
21. Mookerjee, *Medicine in Bengali*, 8–9.
22. See Thompson, *Cullen*.
23. Hamlin, "Predisposing Causes".
24. Mookerjee, *Medicine in Bengali*, 8.
25. Ray, *Bhasajya Sutra*, 5.
26. The main proponent of the Chill Theory in India was Dr C. F. Oldham who in 1871 published a treatise called *What is Malaria?* In introducing his theory, Oldham stated that he was going against the prevalent notions in the Anglo-Indian medical circles. In 1889, the Edinburgh Medical Journal, however, wrote confidently that it did not remember any serious attempt to uphold Dr Oldham's theory since then. Charles, 'Pelvic Floor', 931; Oldham *Malaria*.
27. Sen, "*Swasthya Rakshya*", 420.
28. Sedgewick, "*Roganukrome Sambandhe Abhijattyer Adhipatya*".
29. Buchanan, "*Samkramak Rog*", 243.
30. For foetal vital force, see Roy, "*Jeevanishakti*", 442–43; for cellular vital force, see Chakrabarty, "*Rog*", 213.
31 Roy, "*Jeevanishakti*", 445–46.
32 On 'governmentality', See Foucault, "Governmentality"; on 'ethics of care of self', See Foucault, "The Ethic of Care".
33. Livingstone, *Debility*, 1–26.
34. See Nandy, *Intimate Enemy*.

35. Here Vaughan's observations about how colonial medicine instigated the development of new collective rather than indivituated subjectivities are useful. Vaughan, *Curing their Ills*: 11.
36. Watson, *King's College*, 58–59.
37. Mookerjee, *Medicine in Bengali*, 8.
38. Guha, "*Shustha Shareere Vyamer Prayajaniyata o Karjya*".
39. Sen, "*Swasthya Rakshya o Swasthya Unnatir Upaya*", 415–16.
40. Sen, "*Swasthya Rakshya o Swasthya Unnatir Upaya*", 415–16.
41. Gupta, "*Vyam Charcha*".
42. Guha, "*Pratirodh Shakti*", 446–47.
43. Some of this discourse against intellectual over-exertion bore a striking resemblance to the European discourse that has come to be known academically as 'Muscular Christianity'. Even if the *daktars* drew on this discourse—as is very likely—their specific usage of it, together with their particular prescriptions of physical activity, as also the absence of any Christianity in their prescriptions, made their usage unique and not derivative. For 'Muscular Christianity' see Hall, *Muscular Christianity: Embodying the Victorian Age.*
44. Sen, "*Swasthya Rakshya o Swasthya Unnatir Upaya*", 415–16.
45. Sanyal, *Chikitsa Kalpataru IV*, 11.
46. Gupta, "*Vividha I*", 260.
47. Das, "*Gramer Sekal o Ekal*".
48. Mookerjee, *Medicine in Bengali*, 8.
49. Ray, "*Bangalir Shareer Poshan*", 60. Ray was himself a fairly well-placed and influential *daktar.* In June 1903 he was appointed Honorary Assistant Surgeon to the personal staff of the Viceroy. File 1A/16 Proceedings B 137–38 Bengal Municipal (Medical Branch) Proceedings 1903, A&AC Call No. P/6564.
50. See for instance, Ray, "*Shareer Poshane Chittenden*".
51. Basu, "Acetonuria"; Basu, "Indicanuria".
52. Ghosh, "*Bhakkhya Dravya*", 269–70.
53. Bhattacharya, *Bangalir Khadya*: 21; Gupta, "*Naitrojen Khadya*".
54. The intake amounts, however, were always relational to amounts prescribed for excretion. The operative numerical values assigned to the *naitrojen* discourse were actually about 'balance' between intake and output. The importance of numerical balances is something we shall discuss more fully in the next section.
55. This is not to suggest that *naitrojen* and nitrogen were mere 'representations' independent of a *reality-out-there*. For us this very

distinction between 'reality' and 'representation' is spurious. Both *naitrojen and nitrogen* are real substances which exist and have real consequences. They are different because they have different 'real' characteristics that and their role in the human body is different. The names do not exist merely in texts. They refer to actual real substances which have certain specific qualities. The form is not imposed on a pre-fixed reality, but substance and form mutually articulate each other. See Latour, *Pandora's Hope*; Deleuze et al., "The Geology of Morals".

56. Gupta, "*Naitrojen Khadya*", 81–82.
57. For a general discussion of the *gunas*, see Meulenbeld, 'Reflections on the Basic Concepts of Indian Pharmacology'".
58. Gupta, '*Pathya Nirdharan*", 174.
59. For *dhatus* see Wujastyk, *The Roots of Ayurveda*: xvii–xviii.
60. The classical work in South Asian history in this regard is, of course, Appadurai's *The Social Life of Things*. For more recent work with an interest in medicine and South Asia, see Attewell, "Crossing the Faultlines of Historiography". For an interesting similar work on China, see Nappi, "Winter Worm, Summer Grass".
61. Anonymous, "Nucleo-Poroteid Compound".
62. Anonymous, "Nuctarlin".
63. Basu, "*Bhaitameen Kichhu*"; Mukhopadhyay, "*Ekaler Bangali*".
64. Rima Apple's fascinating history of the embrace of vitamins by the American public since the 1920s has interesting parallels with the developments in Bengal. Apple, however, looks at the commercial and social lives of vitamins almost independently of the medical debates about their usefulness. In the case of the *daktari* writings of the 1920s and early 1930s, the commercial, social and the strictly medical often overlapped due to the closer links *daktari* medicine had traditionally developed with the medical market. As Palit has pointed out, by 1944—nearly 24 years since the official attempts to Indianize the IMS—of the 47,400 doctors in India, only 13,000 were in government medical institutions, the rest being in private practice. Palit et al. *History of Medicine in India*: 24; Apple, *Vitamania: Vitamins in American Culture*.
65. The discovery of vitamins was obviously not an unique episode affecting *daktars* and Bengal alone. The progressive discovery of micronutrients since the 1900s was a story of global proportions and went together with global links of medical science and pharmaceutical business. Many of the vitamins marketed in 1920s Bengal were actually sold by multinational pharmaceutical businesses, and many of the Bengali *daktars* quoted the researches of European and American scientists, but the peculiar valence

that vitamins came to acquire in Bengal also created a 'local' dimension to this global phenomenon by accenting prevalent beliefs about 'national weakness'. See Mukhopadhyay, *Ekaler Bangali.*

66. Prasad, "Crisis, Identity, and Social Distinction".
67. Chakrabarti, *Western Science in Modern India*, 284.
68. Johnson, *The Influence of Tropical Climates*: 433.
69. See Arnold, *Colonizing*: 42–3.
70. Benjamin Zachariah's insightful investigation into the history of *Development* in India argues that the search for mutual legitimation had resulted in the demarcation of a consensual space within which nationalist and liberal imperial administrative discourse operated. The limits of this consensual space however, Zachariah points out were usually set by the imperial discourse on *improvement.* Yet within this consensual space there was still enough scope for disagreement and manoeuvring. Zachariah, *Developing India.*
71. The *dravya-guna* literature was well-known even outside scholarly ayurvedic circles and related foods to bodies through a system of *gunas* and *doshas* (akin to 'humours'). Shankar et al, 'Ayurveda Today", 103.
72. Gupta, "*Shishuder Khadyer Pariman*".
73. Gupta, "*Aharer Pariman*", 49. In Chapter VI we shall see how this economistic logic of balancing income and expenditure was operationalized in thinking about other situations of bodily being as well.
74. Basu, *Village Sanitation and a Manual of Hygiene.*
75. In Foucaultian terms this also meant the internalisation of a certain technology of power.
76. Gupta, "*Anahar o Durbhikkhya*", 56; Bhattacharya, "*Bangalir Khadya*", 21.
77. Clinically, doctors tend to frame constipation as less than two bowel movements per week. The vast majority of cases the *daktars* would have had in mind were hardly likely to be as extreme. However, the perceptions of what constitutes a 'regular' bowel movement varies widely, not only within cultures, but also within individuals. Cf Whorton, *Inner Hygiene: Constipation and the Pursuit of Health in Modern Society*: 1–28.
78. Guha, "*Pratirodh Shakti*", 449.
79. Gupta, "*Vividha II*",191.
80. Gupta, "*Koshtabaddhata*"; also see, Gupta, "*Koshtabaddhata*".
81. Gupta, "*Beg Rodher Apakarita*". On the ayurvedic discourse on 'suppression of urges' see, Wujastyk, *The Roots of Ayurveda*: 15–21.
82. Advertisement in the *Gupta Press Dairektari Panjika* for 1322 BS.
83. Advertisement in the *Gupta Press Dairektari Panjika* for 1322 BS.
84. Sambuddha, "*Kaviraj*".

85. Smoult, "The Neilgherries", xvii; Waring "Aegle Marmelos", 199.
86. Whorton, *Inner Hygiene: Constipation and the Pursuit of Health in Modern Society:* 195–216.
87. Anderson, "Excremental Colonialism", 643. For a more sweeping theoretical exploration of the role of excrement in human history see, Laporte, *The History of Shit.*
88. Ishita Pande has recently begun a fascinating exploration of the history of excrement in colonial Calcutta linking it the emergence of a new sense of 'sanitary selfhood and citizenship'. See Pande, "Excrement, Class and Citizenship in a Sanitary City".
89. See Gupta, "*Beg Rodher Apakarita*".
90. See Gupta, "*Jalasaucha*".
91. For the traditions of sacralization of excrement in South Asia, see Barrett, *Aghor Medicine.* In Bengal proper these practices were popularised by folk-religions that adopted the practices of *chari-chandra-bheda*; for these, see Bhattacharya, *Banglar Baul.*
92. In this context it is interesting to note, however, that the *daktari* discourse never picked up the European interest in surgical cures for constipation that was fashionable around the 1910s. See Whorton, *Inner Hygiene: Constipation and the Pursuit of Health in Modern Society:* 55–80.
93. For a detailed account of the extent of the 'problem' and the attempts to control it, see Ray, *Food for Thought.* However, we do not feel that the importance of the problem can be adequately appreciated within a framework that notices merely the statistical narrations of the problem. Its import derived, in equal measure, from the huge symbolic investment in the 'adulteration' question.
94. Anonymous, "*Khadya-dravya Pariksha*": 21.
95. Gupta, "*Bajarer Khabar*", 175; also See Gupta, "*Dokaner Mithai*", 231.
96. Anonymous, "*Khadya-dravya Pariksha*".
97. Das, "*Gramer Sekal o Ekal*", 310–11.
98. Prasad, "Crisis, Identity, and Social Distinction", 255.
99. Anonymous, "*Khadya-dravya Pariksha*".
100. Guha, "*Pratirodh Shakti I*", 438; See Gupta, "*Saharer Dudh*"; "*Sambad*".
101. Anonymous, "*Gabsthrailokya-matarah*": 20.
102. By the decade of the 1920s some of the paranoia on adulterated milk also drew upon emergent discourses of Gandhian cow protection and *Gram Swaraj* (Village Autonomy) movements. The journal *Swasthya Samachar* for instance, prominently published a photograph of the editor giving a cow a bath during a *go-puja* (cow worship) festival

organized by the Gandhian *Swasthya-dharma Sangha*. See photograph published between pages 18 and 19 in *Swasthya Samachar*, 16:1, 1927.

103. Apart from the role played by milk in fortifying the body against contagion, the cow was also said to be effective against contagions in other ways. It was, for instance, said to be the source of cow dung and cow's urine, which allegedly 'Has [sic] Germ-Killing (*jeebanu-nashak*) powers according to Scientific opinion (*bigyaner mathe*)'. Anonymous, "*Gabsthrailokya-matarah*": 19.
104. Interestingly, some recent practitioners of alternative healing in the 'west' have sought to incorporate the symbolic and substantive values of milk into healing practices, and have consequently drawn upon some South Asian symbologies as well. See Ciccetti, *Dreams, Symbols and Homeopathy*: 168–80.
105. Das, "*Gramer Sekal o Ekal*".
106. Tragically, the same lament for the 'milk of one's cow' can be seen in many refugee narratives of those displaced by the Partition of India in 1947. Forced suddenly into an urban life of poverty, lacking both status and comfort, their voices again declaim the same refrain about the dangerous adulteration of milk. Cf, Basu, *Chhere Asha Gram.*
107. For the most insightful explorations of the history of the rural nostalgia and urban angst amongst Calcutta's lower middle classes, see Sarkar, *Writing Social History*.
108. Worboys, *Spreading Germs*: 109.
109. Ghosh, *Malaria*, 17.
110. Michael Worboys has pointed out that 'miasma' did not become a mere shrinking residuary category after 1860s. Instead, doctors using it developed well-articulated theories about the precise ways in which miasmatic or malarial poisons arose and affected individuals. Worboys, *Spreading Germs*: 39.
111. Mookerjee, *Medicine in Bengali*, 22, 25.
112. Mookerjee, *Medicine in Bengali*, 25–29.
113. Ray, *Bhaisajya Sutra*, 6.
114. Mookerjee, *Medicine in Bengali*, 25.
115. See Chakrabarty, *Habitations of Modernity*, 115–37; Basu Raychaudhury, "Nostalgia".
116. Gupta, "Samaj, Jati and Desh": 184.
117. Gupta, "Samaj, Jati and Desh".
118. Guha, "*Pratirodh Shakti I*", 429.
119. Sen, "*Banga Desher Swasthya*", 284.

120. For the arguments about the Hindus as a dying race see, Datta, "Dying Hindus".
121. Sarkar, *Swadeshi Movement in Bengal*, 47–62.
122. See Mookerjee, *Medicine in Bengali*, 22.
123. Shastri, *Ramtonu*, 201.
124. Sen, "*Swasthya Rakshya o Swasthya Unnatir Upaya*", 402.
125. Sen, "*Swasthya Rakshya o Swasthya Unnatir Upaya*", 418–19.
126. Sen, "*Smashan Kalkata*".
127. Shastri, *Ramtonu*, 35.
128. Singha, *Hutom*, 89.
129. Gupta, "*Bari Bhada*".
130. Gupta, "*Grihasthya o Janjal*".
131. Gupta, "*Streediger Swasthya*", 223.
132. Gupta, "*Palligramer Paniya Jal*", 244.
133. Gupta, "*Grishmakale Pallir Gram*", 265.
134. Basu, *Village Sanitation and a Manual of Hygiene*: 31–2.
135. Basu, *Palli Vasir Prati Nivedan.*
136. Das, *Palliseva; Dasgupta, Pallir Pran.* I am indebted to Dr Bipasha Raha for alerting me to these works.
137. We shall discuss this at greater length in Chapter IV.
138. See Chakrabarty, "Remembered Villages".
139. Alan Bewell's fascinating study provides a wonderful introduction into the complex nexus between colonialism, medicine and Romanticism in early modern Britain. By the second half of the nineteenth century, however, Romanticism was not a solely British—or even European—phenomenon. Other groups, such as the Bengali literati, had appropriated and reformatted its creative energies, and these in turn affected Bengali *daktars.* Unfortunately, this enthralling story cannot be pursued further in this book, but one of the most fertile sites on which this Bengali medical Romanticism actualized itself was that of village rectification. See Bewell, *Romanticism and Colonial Disease.*
140. Basu, *Chhere Asha Gram*, 28, see also 5.
141. Anonymous, "Committee".
142. Anonymous, "Bengal Water Hyacinth Bill".
143. Government of Bengal, *Provincial Autonomy*, 37–46.
144. Banerji, *At the Cross-roads*, 6.
145. Both Bentley and Sur's comments are quoted in Iqbal, "Environmental History". Iqbal gives a very good outline of the extent of the economic and environmental loss caused by *pana* in eastern Bengal. Chunilal Basu was another important adherent to the position that *pana*-infestation was

related to endemic diseases, though he qualified his assertion by stating that *pana* only became a cause of ill health when it was present in large quantities. See Basu, *Village Sanitation or a Manual of Hygiene*: 68.

146. Zachariah, *Developing India:* 15–16.
147. Basu, *Chhere Asha Gram*, 5.
148. Guha, "*Sustha Shareere Vyamer Prayajaniata*".
149. Nanda, "Hindu Nationalism and Vedic Science".
150. Gupta, "*Vividha III*", 238.
151. Gupta, "*Basagriha*".
152. Anonymous, "*Deshiya Swasthya Vigyan*", 101.
153. Under the heading of 'religious commitment', the author mentioned that there was 'clear evidence' that atheists (*nastik*) were unhealthier than believers.
154. Gupta, "*Samkramak Rog o Deshiya Pratha*".
155. See Shastri, "*Brahmo Dharmer Prabhaber Hrash O Hindu Dharmer Punarutthyaner Suchana*".
156. Mukhopadhyay, "*Pnajite Swasthya Charcha*".
157. Gupta, "*Ucchhistha Dosh*".
158. Gupta, "*Pratarutthan*".
159. Gupta, "*Basagriha*": 5. It is not our purpose to investigate whether these 'ancient' practices were indeed as close to sanitary concepts as the *daktari* authors said they were. To do so would not only implicate us in the very categories we seek to historicize, but would also entail the delineation of a specific set of practices as 'ancient Indian culture' and the ignoring others.
160. Quoted in Mukhopadhyay, "*Pnajite Swasthya Charcha*": 81.
161. Quoted in Mukhopadhyay, "*Pnajite Swasthya Charcha*": 82.
162. Haldar, "*Change ba Hawa Paribartan*", 213.
163. See Barrett, *Aghor Medicine.*
164. Quoted in Mukhopadhyay, "*Pnajite Swasthya Charcha*": 83.
165. Jyotirbhushan, "*Shuddhachar*", 348.

Chapter IV. Political Plague: Diagnosing a Neo-Hindu Modernity

1. Arnold, *Colonizing,* 203.
2. Klein, "Plague, Policy and Popular Unrest in British India".
3. Catanach, "Poona Politicians and the Plague" & Catanach, "Plague and the Tensions of Empire, 1896–1918".
4. Chandravarkar, "Plague Panic and Epidemic Politics in India, 1896–1914", 205.

5 Kidambi, "An Infection of Locality".
6. Sheel, "Bubonic Plague in South Bihar: Gaya and Shahabad Districts, 1900–1924".
7. Das, "Calcutta Plague: Epidemic, Colonial Intervention and Indigenous Society, 1898–1900".
8. Echenberg, *Plague Ports*, 71.
9. McNeill, *Plagues and Peoples.*
10. Echenberg, *Plague Ports*, 62. Echenberg later also offers ecological reasons for the absence of plague in Calcutta in terms of the specific species of flies and rats that were found there.
11. Attewell, 'Contesting Knowledges: Plague and Dynamics of the Unani Profession".
12. Having said this, it must be remembered that since Attewell's work engages the unani oeuvre, which itself operationalized a tradition that went beyond South Asia, Attewell's *al Taun*, ought not to be called a 'local' category either.
13. Once again this is not to suggest that European doctors working in India were immune to 'local' circumstances. It is merely to accent the fact that *daktars* were more closely integrated into the affective networks of the region.
14. Quoted in Arnold, *Colonizing:* 216.
15. Harrison, *Public Health,* 202–26; Arnold, *Colonizing,* 200–39.
16. Dipesh Chakrabarty has noticed similar 'contradictions' between the 'modernist aspirations and the search for a premodern identity in the plague discourse of middle-class nationalists like B. G. Tilak. Chakrabarty, however, designates these 'contradictory' moments as 'hesitance' (*didha*) rather than as moments of creative elaboration. Chakrabarty, *Shareer, Samaj O Rashtra: Oupanibeshik Bharatey Mahamari O Janasanskriti*": 173.
17. See Laden, "Recuperating the Archive: Anecdotal Evidence and the Questions of 'Historical Realism'".
18. Ray, "*Biubonik Plague Ba Mahamari*".
19. Bagchi, "*Achangamik Brodhno*".
20. Nandi, "*Chikisita Rogir Vivaran*", 256. Dr Nandi, however, describes himself as a 'homoeopathic phsycian'. Yet, it ought to be remembered that such designations, especially amongst the dispensary practitioners, were not always watertight, and in any case he would have still been within the ambit of the Plague Regulations which required anybody with knowledge of a plague case to report it immediately.
21. Ray, "*Biubonik Plague Ba Mahamari*", 326.

22. For a discussion of the British medical officer's zeal to diagnose plague, see Catanach, "Plague and the Indian Village", 241.
23. Basu, *Plague Tattwa*, 88.
24. Gupta, "*Sambad I*", 48.
25. File 2P/6-105, No. 148–49, Bengal Proceedings (Municipal Department, Medical Branch) Jan–Apr, 1897, A&AC Call No. P/5171.
26. In fact, evidence from the Surat plague of the 1990s suggests that the contentious and political nature of plague diagnosis remained true even after the immense diagnostic and techno-scientific advances of the nearly hundred years between the plague epidemics of the 1890s and the Surat plague. See Madan, "Editorial: Plague in India, 1994".
27. Good, "How Medicine Constructs Its Objects", 66.
28. Good, "How Medicine Constructs Its Objects", 68.
29. Gupta, "*Abar Plague*".
30. Ray "*Biubonik Plague*".
31. Gupta, "*Plague Nibaran Bishay Gobhernment-er Chesta*", 14.
32. Gupta, "*Plague-er Purbey Bombai*".
33. Rutherford, *Some Experiences of Plague.*
34. Rutherford, *Some Experiences of Plague,* 11.
35. Rutherford, *Some Experiences of Plague,* 9.
36. File 2-P/6-115, No. 160–61, Bengal (Municipal Department, Medical Branch) Proceedings, Jan–Apr, 1897, A&AC Call No. P/ 5171.
37. Having said this, it is still cogent to note that the classical ayurvedic texts such as the *Charak Samhita* did employ an explicitly spatial model to understand *Janapad-dhangshaniya Rogs* or Country-Destroying Diseases. See Sengupta et al, *Charak Samhita*, 328 .
38. Sarkar, *Swadeshi Movement in Bengal*, 47–62.
39. Gupta, "*Plague Nibaron*".
40. See Cullen, *Institutes of Medicine*, 8.
41. Sen, "*Swabhabik Rog-Badhok Shakti*", 137.
42. Arnold, " 'An Ancient Race Outworn' ".
43. Sen, "*Swabhabik Rog-Badhok Shakti*", 137.
44. Sen, "*Swabhabik Rog-Badhok Shakti*", 139.
45. Arnold's study of the Bengali writings on Malaria in the same period also locates the influence of this anxiety around 'effeminacy'. See Arnold, "'An Ancient Race Outworn'".
46. Chowdhury, *Frail Hero and Virile History*.
47. Gupta, "*Plague Sambandhey Amader Baktabya*".
48. Gupta, "*Plague Nibaron*".

49. Plague Notification No. 4, File No. 3–4/1–6, Bengal (Municipal Department, Medical Branch) Proceedings, Jan–Apr, 1897, A&AC Call No. P/ 5171.
50. Gupta, "*Plague Sambandhey Amader Baktabya*", 19.
51. Gupta, "*Plague O Sankirtan*".
52. Bandopadhyay, "*Daibya Shakti O Chikitsa Bigyan*".
53. Vivekananda, "The Plague Manifesto".
54. Basu, "Introduction", *Plague Tattwa.*
55. Chattopadhyay, *Grihadaha.*
56. The trope of the disease-ridden and unsanitary Bengali home had been developed by British writers since the beginning of the nineteenth century. See Chattopadhyay, *Representing Calcutta*, 66–67. Many of the seemingly novel inclusions in the Bengali description of *Galij* such as smoke, noise, darkness, etc., were already present in the writings of William Ward. The Bengali doctors, while having internalized these tropes, sought to inspire Bengalis themselves to address it.
57. Gupta, "*Plague Nibaron Upaye*", 279.
58. The typical Calcutta home often housed, other than the Bengali joint family, a number of sundry dependants in the form of servants, distant cousins or even people from the ancestral village who worked in the city but did not have sufficient means to run a household of their own. See Sastri, *Ramtonu.*
59. Gupta, "*Plague Sambandhey Amader Baktabya*", 19–20; Gupta., "*Plague Nibaron Upaye*", 279–83.
60. Gupta, "*Rogi Prithakikaran*".
61. Gupta, "*Plague Hoitey Shikhya*".
62. Nivedita, *The Master As I Saw Him*, 376.
63. Nivedita, "House on the Ganges".
64. Mark Nichter has observed that in lay medical frameworks of meaning, there is a correspondence between the *power* of pre-Brahmanic deities such as Kali and the *power* of 'western' medicine. Both are seen to be extremely powerful, but their powers are difficult to control and hence capable of causing both good and bad. This is in contrast to Brahmanic gods and ayurvedic medicines wherein powers are restrained and uniformly benevolent. See Nichter, "The Layperson's Perception of Medicine as Perspective into the Utilization of Multiple Therapy Systems in the Indian Context": 228 Vivekananda's reformulations of Hinduism and its relationship of epidemic disease and medicine added a new layer of complexity to these subtle contrasts and comparisons.
65. Nivedita, *The Master As I Saw Him,* 376.

66. Gupta, "*Plague*", 239.
67. Gupta, "*Plague Sambandhey Amader Baktabya*".
68. Gupta, "*Plague Chikitsa*".
69. Gupta, *Plague Nibaron Bishoy Gobhernment-er Chesta*", 15; Also see Gupta,. "*Swasthya Prasanga*".
70. Ahmed, *Tibb-e-Nobbi.*
71. Suyuti, *Jinn Jati-r Bismoykor Itihaash*, 134–35.
72. Kaviraj, "Filth and the 'Public Sphere'"; Chakrabarty, "Of Garbage, Modernity and the Citizen's Gaze".
73. Inden et al., *Kinship in Bengali Culture*, 21.
74. Das, *Munisipal- Darpan.*
75. This selective intellectual appropriation from British doctors and teachers clearly proves that the lower-level Bengali doctors were not passive agents of a seamless 'western' tradition. They were actively selecting what to adopt and what to ignore and framing it within their own medical rationality.
76. Bagchi, "Wealth and Work in Calcutta", Sinha, *Calcutta in Urban History.*
77. Chaturvedi, *Peasant Pasts*, 4.
78. With regard to these very different idioms in which the Gujarati and Bengali middle classes came to articulate their 'modernity' and hegemony, it is worth noting that while a full-blown Hindutva has in recent years dominated Gujarati politics, Bengali politics has long been dominated by a *bhodrolok*-dominated political bloc that, while being equally ready to use violence to enforce middle-class, neoliberal agendas of development, crucially remains invested in the altruistic rhetoric of Communism. For the middle-class affiliations of Bengali Communism see, Dasgupta, "Rhyming Revolution: Marxism and Culture in Colonial Bengal". For a more recent report on the violence inflicted in pursuit of neoliberal development, see Sarkar, "A Question Marked in Red" or Banerjee, "Peasant Hares and Capitalist Hounds of Singur".
79. Gupta, "*Plaguer Pradurbhabey Kolikatar Atith O Bartaman Obasthya*".
80. See Chattopadhyay, *Palli Mangal Granthavali.*
81. Anonymous, "*Plaguer Aushadh*".
82. Bhattacharya, *Sarbasiddhidata Pustak*, 454.
83. Tambiah, "The Magical Power of Words".
84. See Ray, "The Kahar Chronicles", 725.
85. Kiple et al., "Algae".
86. Sudarshan, "Slipada".
87. It is interesting to note in this respect that TC Rutherford had noted that villagers in northern India related some minor afflictions causing

glandular swellings with plague. See Rutherford, *Some Experiences of the Plague*, 3.

88. Karim, "Shamanism in Bangladesh", 294.
89. Spinage, *Cattle Plague: A History*, 477.

Chapter V. Endemic Commerce: Cholera and the Medical Market

1. Arnold, 'Cholera: Disease as Disorder".
2. Harrison "Cholera Theory and Sanitary Policy". Also see, Singh, "Cholera: Changing Perceptions of its Causality in the Last Two Centuries".
3. Singh, "'Clouds of Cholera' and Clouds around Cholera, 1817–70".
4. Klein, "Imperialism, Ecology and Disease: Cholera in India, 1850–1950".
5. The importance of these 'alternative' cures for cholera was comparatively more than that of other afflictions, since, in the case of cholera, authors like Seema Alavi have suggested with ample proof that Indian and Anglo-Indian management of the disease might have led rather than derived from 'western' practice. According to Alavi, many 'native' practices were adopted from 'native' physicians and then later exported to Britain. See Alavi, *Islam and Healing*: 109–121.
6. Breton, *Oauthar Vivaran*, 7–8.
7. Cited in Alavi, *Islam and Healing*: 114.
8. See Tables I & II .
9. Bengal Judicial (LP) Proceedings, dated, 27 Jun 1821, draft 245/1820–1, A&AC Call No. E/4/704, 201.
10. Breton, *Olauthar Vivaran*, 22–26.
11. Alavi: *Islam and Healing*: 118.
12. Prafullachandra Sen was one such appointee in 1913, working first at Jangipur and then at Bankipur. File 3A/2, Proceedings No. 136–37 B, Bengal Municipal (Medical Branch) Proceedings 1913, A&AC Call No. P/9145.
13. File 2A/15 Proceedings 27–28 B, Bengal Municipal (Medical Branch) Proceedings 1903, A&AC Call No P/6564.
14. For using 'petitions' to gauge people's expectations from the state, see Siddiqi, "The British Historical Context and Petitioning in Colonial India".
15. File 1P/7, Proceedings 341–42 B, Bengal Municipal (Medical Branch) Proceedings 1903, A&AC Call No P/ 9145.
16. Alavi, *Islam and Healing*: 129–47.

17. Lawrie, *Essay on Cholera*; Searle, *Cholera Its Nature, Cause, Treatment*; Thackrah, *Cholera in Character*.
18. Pinto, "Development Without Institutions: Ersatz Medicine and the Politics of Everyday Life in Rural North India".
19. Later in the century, however, the thriving market in cholera treatises may have been more important than any state instigation.
20. Ian Hacking has pointed out the centrality of centralised apparatuses of the state to the development of a statistical rationality in post-Napoleonic Europe. Hacking, *The Taming of Chance*, 27–34.
21. Das, "Medical Knowledge of the Body: Colonial Encounters", 119–20.
22. Hamilton, "Cholera: Its Endemic Area and Epidemic Progression", 142.
23. See Arnold, *Colonizing*, 160.
24. It may have been this singularly disturbing mode of death that prompted the popular belief that those dying of cholera became ghosts. The humorist Rajsekhar Basu used this belief as a plot for a comic sketch of the varieties of ghosts Bengalis believed in. See Basu, "*Bhusundir Math*".
25. Chattopadhyay, "*Kolera ba Olautha*".
26. The telegram bearing news of cholera was common at the time. The poet Rabindranath mentions receiving a telegram from Munger informing him of his son Samindranath's cholera in 1907. The anxious father rushed to Munger only to arrive in time to see his young son die. See "Letter to Maharajkumari Vidyavati Devi".
27. See for example, Uddin, "A Case of Cholera" or Hickman, "Treatment of Cholera with Sulphurous Acid".
28. Floyer, *Forty Two Histories*, v.
29. Millan, "Graeco-Roman Case Histories".
30. Wade, *Select Evidences*.
31. Khan, "On the Cure of Eliphantiasis".
32. Nowel-Smith, "Nineteenth Century Narrative Case Histories". I am grateful to Sarah Mitchell for pointing me to Nowel-Smith's work.
33. Jadunath Mukherji was a prolific writer and variously used both the anglicised form of his last name, i.e., 'Mukherji', as well as the more familiar 'Mukhopadhyay'. His books in the bibliography to this book follow his own usage and appear under both versions of the name depending upon his own choice in the respective cases.
34. In fact, the same story was repeated in the section on cholera in his later publication entitled *Chikitsa Darpan*, 81.
35. Mukhopadhyay, *Bishuchika Roger Chikitsa*, 11.

36. Though there have been some very interesting studies on the relationship between literature and medicine on the issue of cholera, most of it pertains to the influence of medicine on literature rather than the other way round. None of these studies, moreover, look at vernacular South Asian literatures at all. Seefor example, Otis, 'The Tigers of Wrath. Mann's Death in Venice as Myth and Medicine'. Otis points out that the vocabulary used to describe India as the source of cholera was strikingly similar in the writings of both Thomas Mann and Robert Koch. Though she does point out that the the politics and functions of this common vocabulary differed in the two authors, the words and images used remained the same and engaged with the ideologies of European imperialism. I am grateful to my friend and colleague Dr Thomas Rutten for this reference.
37. Tagore, *Gora.*
38. Tagore, *Galpaguchha III.*
39. Sen, *Brihat Banga Vol. I*, Introduction.
40. Das, *Murisipal-Darpan.*
41. Ganguly, '*Kolerar Pratishedhak*": 104.
42. In the previous decades, the few Bengali doctors who occupied important positions in the IMS usually chose to write in English than in Bengali. SCG Chuckerbutty and Gopaul Chunder Roy are good examples of this earlier era when medical status and Anglophony shared a much closer relationship.
43. Ganguly, '*Kolera Pratisedhak*': 104.
44. Basu, *Village Sanitation and a Manual of Hygiene*: 42–3.
45. *Alaler Gharer Dulal* is usually identified as the first Bengali novel and appeared in 1858. Bengali, until the nineteenth century, had lacked a well-developed prose form and the early novelists did much to develop a robust prose form. The connection between these developments and the Bengali medical writing is a tantalising story which will have to await another occasion for elaboration. See Bandopadhyay, *History of Modern Bengali Literature.*
46. Breton's list of names, however, seems to be limited in comparison with what later authors, like John Macpherson writing in 1872, mentioned. See Singh, 'Clouds of Cholera and Clouds around Cholera, 1817–1870': 145.
47. Breton, *Olauthar Vivaran*, 1.
48. Mukhopadhyay, *Natun Abhidhan*, 58, 283.
49. Morton, *Bengali Dictionary*: 81, 436.
50. Forster, *Vocabulary in Two Parts, Bongalee and English*: 70.

51. By the early 1830s, as cholera panic gripped Europe and metropolitan medical authors looked east in order to understand the disease, the equation of *Bishuchika* and cholera was internationalized. Writing in 1831, the very year when massive cholera epidemics broke out in northern England and Scotland, William MacMichael wrote that 'cholera spasmodica' was identical to the '*Sitanga*, a species of *Sannipata*' or '*Vishuchika*' of the 'ancient Hindoo' author 'Dhanwantari'. See MacMichael, *Is the Cholera Spasmodica of India A Contagious Disease?*: 32–3.
52. While in recent years there has been some investigation of the politics of place names and even personal names, little attention has been devoted to the 'politics of disease names'. One of the few exceptions to this rule is Levine, *Prostitution, Race and Politics* (especially Chapter 3). For places names see, Carter, *The Road to Botany Bay;* for personal names see Chaturvedi, "Vinayak and Me: Hindutva and the Politics of Naming".
53. Das, "*Bishuchi-Rakshan*".
54. Mukhopadhyay, *Bishuchika Roger Chikitsa*, 5–7.
55. Anonymous, "*Kolera Sambandhey Guti Kotok Katha*".
56. Chattopadhyay, "*Kolera ba Olautha*", 168.
57. Kar, *Bhisak Suhrid.*
58. Mukhopadhyay, "*Olautha*", *Biswakosh.*
59. Ramendrasundar Tribedi, "*Chikitsa Vaigyanik Paribhasha*". Tribedi was, significantly, also Secretary to the 'Scientific Vocabulary Association' [Vaiigyanik Paribhasha Samiti]. It is also interesting to note that the editors of the *Bhisak Darpan*, Drs Kalimohan Sen and Girishchandra Bagchi, added a note of dissent at the end of the essay, demonstrating with a few examples that using Vedic terminology might obscure contemporary connotations of particular words.
60. Incidentally, the copy that Tribedi used was loaned to him by Rabindranath Tagore and had originally belonged to the library of the *Tattwabodhini Sabha* before having stayed back with Tagore's father Debendranath when the *Sabha* became defunct.
61. Maitreya, "*Kaviraji Mothey Olautha Chikitsa*".
62. Maitreya, "*Bishuchika*".
63. For the 'new' cholera god of northern India in the nineteenth century, Hurdoul Lal, see Arnold, *Colonizing*, 171.
64. Nicholas, *Fruits of Worship*, 202–06.
65. This 'tinge' can be seen in the shift in the stance on popular Hinduism amongst *daktars* outlined in Chapter I.
66. Chakrabarty, "*Olabibir Gaan*", 31.
67. Rahim, *Dhakar Nawab Shaheber Punthi.*

68. Majumdar, *Kangal Fikirchand.*
69. Kipling, *Kim,* 246.
70. It is cogent to add here that such moralistic coding of cholera was not an uniquely colonial phenomenon. T. M. Greenhow, prolific medical author who had treated innumerable cholera cases in north eastern England since the first major outbreak in 1831, in a letter to James Hodgson, Mayor of Newcastle Upon Tyne, wrote in 1852, 'Sobriety, industry, honesty and religion maybe surely predicated as the inmates of the home characterised by order and cleanliness; but when, instead, dirt, slovenliness and disorder prevail, we may safely assume…that such a home is sure to be the resort of disease—fever, cholera or some other epidemic….'. See Greenhow, *Cholera From The East*: 7–8.
71. Chakrabarty, "*Shareer, Samaj O Rashtra: Oupanibeshik Bharatey Mahamari O Janasanskriti*": 169–78.
72. It is cogent to add Chakrabarty's own rider at this point, that to say that the premodern body is implicated in an imagination which trips up state power is not to romanticise the premodern. It must be remembered that premodern bodies, defined as they were often by caste, religion, ethnicity, gender, etc., were often implicative within their own networks of oppression. Chakrabarty, "*Shareer, Samaj O Rashtra: Oupanibeshik Bharatey Mahamari O Janasanskriti*": 177.
73. Basu Barman, *Karjoshadhok Oushodhgyan,* 88.
74. Datta, *Daktari Shikhya,* 62.
75. See first issue of *Gharer Katha.*
76. Ghosh, "*Kolera*".
77. Das, "*Bishuchi-Rakshan*".
78. Chattopadhyay, "*Kolera ba Olautha*", 133.
79. Sen, "*Udbhid Jeebanu*", 374.
80. Sircar, "*Olautha*".
81. Das, "*Bishuchi-Rakshan*".
82. Alavi has pointed out that cholera management in Britain had largely been shaped by the prior Indian experience. See Alavi, *Islam and Healing*: 109–21.
83. Greenhow, *Cholera As It Recently Appeared in the Towns of Newcastle & Gateshead*: 83.
84. Greenhow himself elsewhere mentions following the practice of these doctors and their greater expertise in cholera treatment owing to their Indian experience. See Greenhow, *Cholera: Its Non-Contagious Nature*: 9.
85. Letter to TM Greenhow, quoted in Greenhow, *Cholera as it Has Recently Appeared in Newcastle & Gateshead*: 85.

86. Lawrie, *Essay on Cholera*: 16.
87. Greenhow, *Hints on the Probable Approach of Cholera*, 8.
88. Ghosh, "*Kolera*", 53.
89. Ganguly, "*Kolera Pratisedhak*".
90. Latour, *Pandora's Hope.*
91. Basak, *Surapan;* Mukhopadhyay, *Tumi Je Sarbanese Gobardhan*; Mitra, *Madh Khawa Bara Daye*, etc.
92. The term *gurupak* appears regularly in nineteenth century Bengali adaptations of the older *dravya-guna* genre. See Sengupta, *Dravya Guna Shikhya.*
93. For a general survey of the ayurvedic position that relates digestion and health, see Pitman, "Food and Digesiton, Health and Disease".
94. Nichter, "*The Layperson's Perception of Medicine as Perspective into the Utilization of Multiple Therapy Systems in the Indian Context*": 299.
95. The negative effects of *gurupak* foods however are understood with reference to what Nichter has called *abhiyasa* (habituation). Thus, it is often said that those such as the English, who are more habituated to *gurupak* foods, can digest them. Unlike in Nichter's study, though, where *abhiyasa* is a matter of individual habit, in most of the nineteenth century texts *abhiyasa* is usually presented as a racial/national category, i.e., where the English and the Bengali have different *abhiyasa.*
96. Maitreya "*Ayurvediya Sadrisha Chikitsa*".
97. Sen, *Bhesaja Ratnavali*, 144–45.
98. The spatial proximity of the ideas within the space of the text, hence the material layout of the text, might also have reinforced such remappings.
99. Ghosh, "*Kolera*"; Chattopadhyay, "*Kolera ba Olautha II*"; Basu, "*Elopathy Mathey Olautharogey Udaradhman*"; Maitreya, "*Kaviraji Mathey Olautha Chikitsa*"; Mukharji, "*Bishuchika Darpan*".
100. Wujastyk, *The Roots of Ayurveda*, xviii–xix; Pitman, *The Nature of the Whole*, 83–140; Ecks, "Bodily Sovereignty as Political Sovereignty: 'Self-Care' in Kolkata, India".
101. Greenhow, *Hints on the Probable Approach of Cholera*: 8.
102. Prasad suggests that 'moderation' of diet was 'central to *bhodrolok's* discourses on food and gastronomy'. While this is unquestionably true, the prescriptions of British doctors like Greenhow show that as a *strategy* and *prescription* it was not unique to the *bhodrolok.* See Prasad, "Crisis, Identity, and Social Distinction", 258.
103. Greenhow, *Cholera As It Has Recently Appeared in the Towns of Newcastle & Gateshead*: 85.

104. Searle, *Cholera Its Nature, Cause, Treatment*: 27.
105. For ideas about the six 'non-naturals' which influenced calls for moderation in diet and exercise, see Emch-Deriaz, "The Non-Naturals Made Easy".
106. Michael Taussig calls this 'mimetic legitimation'. See Taussig, *Mimesis and Alterity*.
107. Das, "*Bishuchi-Rakshan*", 359.
108. Renbourn, "Flannel Binder and Cholera Belt".
109. Johnson, *The Influence of Tropical Climates*, 422.
110. Mitra, "*Amra O Amader Vyavsa*".
111. Chattopadhyay, "*Kolera ba Olautha*".
112. Chattopadhyay, "*Kolera ba Olautha*", 130 .
113. Advertisements of "Chlorodyne", *Gupta Press Dairektari Panjika 1322 BS;* Also see, Advertisement of "*Korpurarishto*" in the same publication.
114. Mukharji, "*Bishuchika Darpan II*".
115. See Mukherji, *Chikitsa Darpan*, 81.
116. Some scholars have recently turned their attention to the very different ways in which the body itself is imagined in different medical traditions and the different networks of power that such differential imaginations of power sustain. Unfortunately, these studies have remained, to varying extents, entrapped within a 'medical systems' framework. Developing these lines of enquiry without the constraining parameters of 'medical systems' promises to yield many new insights. See Chakrabarty, "*Shareer, Samaj O Rashtra: Oupanibeshik Bharatey Mahamari O Janasanskriti*"; Bhattacharya, "Anatomical Knowledge and East-West Exchange"; Das, "Medical Knowledge of the Body: Colonial Encounters".
117. Sanyal, *Chikitsa Kalpataru Vol I*, 207.
118. Mukherji, *Chikitsa Darpan*, 79.
119. Sanyal, *Chikitsa Kalpadruma Vol I*, 208–09.
120. Basu, "*Elopathy Mathey Olautharogey Udaradhman*", 96.
121. Sircar, "*Olautha*".
122. Anonymous, "*Kaolin Dwara Kolera Chikitsa*".
123. Chakrabarty, "*Olautha Nivaraner Upaya*", 95.
124. Anonymous, "*Prerita Patra*".
125. Anonymous, '*Olauthar Homiopathik Chikitsa*".
126. Das, "*Bishuchi-Rakshan II*", p. 408.
127. Chattopadhyay, "*Kolera ba Olautha*", 137; Basu, "*Elopathy Mathey Olautharogey Udaradhman*", 96; Sanyal, *Chikitsa Kalpadruma Vol I*, 209.
128. Anonymous, ' *Vaidya Mathey Chikitsita Rogir Vivaran*".
129. Anonymous, "*Olautha Chikitsa*".

130. Anonymous, "*Vaidik Vyavahar Sambandhey Prasna*".
131. Khan Choudhury, "*Paglami Kar?*".
132. Sanyal, *Chikitsa Kalpadruma Vol I*, 208.
133. Mukhopadhyay, *Bishuchika Roger Chikitsa*, 2–3.
134. Digby, *Making a Medical Living*.
135. Nichter, "*The Layperson's Perception of Medicine as Perspective into the Utilization of Multiple Therapy Systems in the Indian Context*": 226–27.
136. Mukherjee, *Calcutta: Myths and History*,10.
137. Pahari, *Unish Sataker Banglaye Sanatani Chikitsa Vyavasthyar Swarup*, 93–4.
138. Bajle Rahman Miah, "Cholerodyne" (Advertisement).
139. The advertisements for the specific appeared regularly in the *Grihasthya Mangal* throughout 1335 BS.
140. Shamsuddin J Sulemani, "*Olauthar Pratisedhak Aushadh*".
141. Das, "*Bishuchi-Rakshan*", 359.
142. File 146, dated march 1876 ('B' Proceeding 3 and 4), Bengal Medical Consultations 1876–77 A&AC Call No. P/873.
143. The notion of 'heteronomy' has been used by medical sociologists to designate a continuous scale stretching from complete subordination to the state on the one side, and complete autonomy on the other. Such a scale fluctuating between autonomy and subordination amply sums up the relationship of the state and market in medical matters. See Frankenberg, "Allopathic Medicine, Profession and Capitalist Ideology in India", 118.
144. Advertisement for "D Gupta & Company" in *Lord Ripon's Panjika* for 1290 BS.
145. Advertisement for "Indian Star Oil" in *Lord Ripon's Panjika* for 1290 BS.
146. Pol. Cons. 1858. National Archives of India, Delhi; Home Department, Political Consultations, 16 November 1858, Consultation No. 18.
147. Tarafdar, "*Kolera Roger Adhunik Chikitsa*", 357.
148. Das, "*Kolerar Prabal Hikkaye—Potash Iodide-er Upakarita*", 297.
149. Datta, *Prankrishanaushadhavali*, 102–3, 133.
150. Sengupta *Charitabhidhan*, 311. Also see Chapter II in this book.
151. Sobhan, *Elaj-e-Lokmani*, 3.
152. Referred to by Alavi, *Islam and Healing*, 127–29. Alavi also mentions that there was an older Mughal genre of encyclopaedic collections or recipe books such as the Nur-ul-Din Muhammad Shirazi's *Tibb-i-Darashikohi*. Unlike the later encyclopaedia's usually compiled by nonmedical men, however, these Persianate Mughal medical encyclopaedias were compiled by learned Persianate scholar-hakims. Alavi, *Islam and Healing*, 23, 35–43.

153. For collections 'sanitized' through rigorous scientific filters, see O'Shaughnessy, *Bengal Dispensatory*.
154. Basak, *Jalpan Bidhi & Prachin Aushadhavali.*
155. One of Biswas's remedies, for instance, involved the ingestion of a decoction made by crushing seven or nine jujubes, a clove and parched rice and then mixing it with water. However, it is said that the stems of the jujubes have to be set aflame before being crushed, and if they become brittle during the crushing rather than paste-like, then the patient will surely die. Datta, *Prankrishnaushadhavali*, 102–03, For other examples of cholera cures which straddle the herbal/magical divide, see Bhattacharya, *Sarba Siddhidata Pustak*, 366; Also quoted in Bhattacharya, *Brihat Indrajal*, 219.
156. Chattopadhyay, "*Kolera O Malaria Sambandhey Dui Khani Darkari Chithi*".
157. Chakrabarty, "*Shareer, Samaj O Rashtra: Oupanibeshik Bharatey Mahamari O Janasanskriti*", 169–71.
158. Buhnemann, "Selecting"; White, "Kamkala".
159. Acharya, *Brihat Indrajal*, 160.
160. Buhnemann, "Selecting", 172.
161. Maitreya, "*Homoeopathy O Elopathyr Darpa Churna*".
162. Perhaps somewhat strangely, Dr Ray's achievements are today almost totally forgotten. By the 1970s, Dr Ray was being referred to as the 'once-famous doctor'. See Basu, *Chhere Asha Gram*, 42.
163. Anonymous, *Daktar Dwarkanath Ray.*
164. Kaviratna, "*Sampadakiya Baktabya*".
165. Majumdar, *Kolera ba Olautha Chikitsa*; Nag, *Kolera Chikitsa*; Nag, *Sankhipta Kolera Chikitsa.*
166. Advertisement of "*Brihat Kolera Chikitsa*", *Gupta Press Dairektari Panjika* for 1322 BS.
167. File 3C/21 dated December 1897 ('B' Proceedings 148–49), Bengal Municipal (Medical Branch) Proceedings (November–December) 1897, A&AC Call No P/5173, 30.

Chapter VI. *Dhatu Dourbalya*: Diagnosing the Rhizoid Pathologies of Weakness

1. Deleuze et al., *A Thousand Plateaus.*
2. Wig, "Problems of Mental Health in India"; Yap, "Words and Things in Comparative Psychiatry".
3. Littlewood et al., "Culture Bound Syndromes": 105.
4. Hughes, "The Culture Bound Syndromes and Psychiatric Diagnosis".

5. Littlewood, "Cultural Comments on Culture Bound Syndromes".
6. Sumathipala et al., "Culture Bound Syndromes: The Story of *Dhat* Syndrome".
7. Jadhav, "Dhat Syndrome: A Re-Evaluation": 14.
8. How far post-independence India's 'quest for self-reliance' owed its origins to Gandhian ideals is suspicious. It is generally believed that the Nehruvian state's paradigms of development actually repudiated most of the Gandhian ideals in the name of achieving 'self-reliance'. For a good survey of the intellectual complexities of the Nehru–Gandhi dialogue on India's postcolonial future see, Zachariah, *Nehru.*
9. Jadhav, "*Dhat* Syndrome: A Re-Evaluation".
10. Bhugra et al., "Impotence in Ancient Indian Texts"; Chadha et al., "Dhat Syndrome: A Sex Neurosis of the Indian Subcontinent"; Sumathipala et al., "Culture Bound Syndromes: The Story of *Dhat* Syndrome".
11. Chattopadhyay, "*Dhatu-Dourbalya*", 22.
12. Interestingly, Siddha and Siddha influenced Bengali texts speak of 'mercury' as the sperm of the god Shiva. See Natarajan, "Divine Semen".
13. Mukhopadhyay, "*Dhatu*", *Biswakosh*, 251–52.
14. Sen, *Venereal Disease in Bengali*, 131–32.
15. Kar, *Bhisak Suhrid*, 414–16.
16. Bynum, "Spermatorrhoea".
17. Chattopadhyay, *"Dhatu Dourbalya I"*.
18. Sanyal et al., *"Prameha ba Dhater Pirha"*.
19. Maitreya, *"Jeeban Sahay"*.
20. Dr Gavin, "Spermatone".
21. *Amrita Bazar Patrika* [hereafter ABP], Calcutta, 23.08.06.
22. Home (Political) June, 1911, Part B, File No. 174-6. NAI. I have discussed this very interesting case in greater detail elsewhere. See Mukharji, "Sex, Medicine, Morality".
23. Bynum, *Medicine in the Nineteenth Century*, 49–50.
24. Foucault, *Order of Things,* 534.
25. Bynum, *Medicine in the Nineteenth Century*, 65; Foucault, "Body/Power".
26. Langford, *Fluent Bodies,* 21.
27. We are not putatively interested here in the ways in which certain diseases in themselves become metaphors for other social conditions, though undoubtedly *dhatu dourbalya* at one level was indeed an eloquent metaphor of the 'sapping debility' and 'impotence' of the colonized. These latter would to some extent be touched upon in the last section of the chapter. Here , however, we are interested in the way in which

the disease category itself is fashioned through a rational structure that functions through metaphors.

28. See Ricoeur, *The Conflict of Interpretations* and *The Rule of Metaphor;* For the role of metaphors in scientific theory See Livingstone et al., "Meaning Through Metaphor".
29. Lakoff et al., "Conceptual Metaphor in Everyday Language".
30. Merten et al., "Metaphor and Self: Symbolic Process in Everyday Life".
31. Sarkar, *Writing Social History,* 282–357.
32. Chattopadhyay, *"Dhatu Dourbalya I",* 222.
33. In this regard it is worth noting that stomach problems and digestive disorders have a singular importance in the middle-class urban Bengali mindscape that cannot wholly be reduced to causes acceptable to biomedical registers. See Ecks, "Bodily Sovereignity as Political Sovereignity: 'Self-Care' in Kolkata, India".
34. For the identification with Kaliyug see, Sarkar, *Writing Social History.*
35. Sanyal, *Banglar Samajik Itihas.*
36. Ayurvediya Bhesaj Ashram, *"Swarna-ghatita Makaranda Rasayan".*
37. Bynum, "Spermatorrhoea".
38. Gupta, *"Daihik Jama-Kharach".*
39. Charu Gupta's fascinating study of lowbrow Hindi print literature has highlighted how erotic advertisements negotiated questions of delicacy by recourse to the trope of Kaliyuga and appealing to the nationalist project. Though the Bengali physicians do not use the Kaliyuga trope in the same way, the nationalist project itself often justifies the violations of the norms of delicate prose, with *daktars* arguing that it is for the sake of the nation's future that they have had to throw delicacy to the wind. Another novel way by which Bengali doctors circumvent issues of delicacy is by refusing to write the more offensive words or phrases in Bengali. Dr Chattopadhyay thus confessed that the reason he was forced to use so much English in his 'description of the testes' was that they were too delicate to appear in Bengali. It was as if it was the language itself and not the reader whose sanctity was to be retained. See Gutpa, *Sexuality, Obscenity and Community.*
40. Gupta, *Bhaeprakash,* 54.
41. Sen, *Bhesaja Ratnavali,* 353.
42. Chakrabarty, *Bangla Dehatattwer Gaan,* 237.
43. For a detailed discussion of Baul rituals see, Bhattacharya, *Banglar Baul,* 369–437.
44. Sharif, *Madhyayuger,* 323.

45. Urban, *Songs of Ecstasy.*
46. Sen, *Bhesaj Ratnavali,* 353.
47. It is worth noting that this section will necessarily appear somewhat fragmentary to the reader. However, to render it seamless would defeat the very purpose behind it.
48. Kar, *Bhisak Suhrid,* 414–15.
49. Kar, *Bhisak Suhrid,* 415.
50. Sen, *Bhesaj Ratnavali,* 355.
51. Kar, *Bhisak Suhrid,* 414–16.
52. Sen, *Bhesaj Ratnavali,* 356.
53. Obeysekere, "The Impact of Ayurvedic Ideas on the Culture and the Individual in Sri Lanka".
54. Sarkar, *Susruta Samhita,* 178–79; Sengupta et al., *Charak Samhita,* 285–90.
55. Chakrabarti, *Religious Processes.*
56. According to these legends, King Ballal Sena had been enamoured by a woman who wished to bring the royal court into disrepute by encouraging the King to accept the Tantric heterodox practices frowned upon by the orthodoxy. See Sanyal, *Samajik Itihas,* 37–40.
57. Majumdar, *Bangiya Kulashashtra,* 25.
58. Natarajan, "Divine Semen".
59. Sharif, *Madhyayug,* 35.
60. Hatley, "Islamic Yoga of Bengal".
61. Sengupta, *Sharangadhar,* 61.
62. Gupta, *Bhabprakash,* 57–58.
63. Bhattacharya, *Banglar Baul,* 256–57.
64. Gupta, *Bhabprakash,* 176.
65. Advertisement for *Sibshakti Batika* in *Gupta Press Dairektari Panjika* for 1322 BS; Also see Advertisement of *Swopnoshanti* in *Gupta Press Dairektari Panjika* for 1322 BS.
66. O'Flaherty, *Dreams,* 17.
67. O'Flaherty, *Dreams,* 65.
68. Green, "Roles of Dreams".
69. Khater, *Khwabnama Pahela Balam;* Khater, *Khwabnama Dusra Balam;* Khater, *Talenama.*
70. The well-known *Chandshi* medical tradition, for instance, refers to its origins in a dream from the goddess Monosha. Bijoygupta's fifteenth-century text, the *Padmapuran,* refers to the author having received divine inspiration through a dream, and the massive Kali temple of Dakshineshwar near Calcutta owes its origins to a Rani Rashmoni being

commanded in a dream. These examples however are merely some of the best known. Nearly every village in Bengal has its own dream legends.

71. Das, *"Bukchapa* (Nightmare)".
72. Chattopadhyay, *"Dhatu Dourbalya"*, 22–23.
73. Chattopadhyay, *"Dhatu Dourbalya* I", 222–23.
74. Wigglesworth (Edmund Sears Morgan ed.), *The Diary*, 5, 79, 93; Also see, Cherniavsky, "Night Pollution and the Floods of Confession in Michael Wigglesworth's Dairy".
75. Murray, "Men's Bodies, Men's Minds".
76. It is interesting to note that the 1710 tract was published as an advertising text to promote the sale of the 'Strengthening Tincture' and the 'Prolifick Powder'. Though scholars tend to look at Tissot as the father of the medical anxieties over semen loss—especially through masturbation—this anonymous tract was in no way of marginal importance, as it had gone into nineteen editions by 1750. See Bennet et al., *Solitary Pleasures.*
77. Quoted from the 1764 edition of *Onanisme* in Stengers et al., *Masturbation.*
78. Donoghue, "Imagined More than Women".
79. Acton, *The Functions and Disorders,* 138.
80. Acton, *The Functions and Disorders,* 138–44.
81. Chattopadhyay, *"Dhatu Dourbalya I"*, 223.
82. Balfour, *Sexual Science.*
83. Chattopadhyay, *"Dhatu Dourbalya"*, 23.
84. Kar, *Bhisak Suhrid,* 416.
85. For references to recent use of this category See Gautham et al., "Genital Symptoms Experienced by Men in Rural India", 387.
86. See Advertisement for *Someshwar Modok, BMP,* 12.
87. Reddy, *With Respect to Sex.*
88. Ibid, 245.
89. Sweet, "The First Medicalization".
90. Sen, *Bhesaj Ratnavali,* 358.
91. Misra, *Bhavaprakash,* 27.
92. Vanita, "Born of Two Vaginas". Interestingly, Vanita's work has shown that in the Bengal region in particular—perhaps, she suggests, under the impact of Tantrism—such ideas gained a firmer hold and not only remained in circulation, but were also expanded upon in the medieval period.
93. Gupta, *"Dourbalya"*, 78.
94. Gupta, *"Dourbalya I"*.
95. Gupta, "Dourbolyo".

96. Though it does not directly speak of the world of the *keranis*, Rajnarayan Basu's influential critique of the urban modernity had given a detailed account of the way quotidian personal rhythms of work and relaxation had been drastically altered under colonialism. Basu, *Se Kal Ar Ekal*, 38–52; For a more vivid account of the urban drudgery of the *keranis*, see Ray, *Deb Ganer Marte Agaman*, 424–27; Also see Tagore, *"Banshi"*.
97. Basu, *"Rajbhog"*, 80–81.
98. Even in the 1930s, advertisements for reinvigorating medicines apparently made from electricity were still to be seen. See Advertisements of Elektro-Ayurvedic Farmesi in the *Grihasthya Mangal*.
99. It is important to note that this discourse is distinct from, and should not be equated with, the discourse on male hysteria. Other 'associated terms' not discussed here in greater detail, such as *snayubik durbalata* or 'nervous weakness', do suggest a proximity to the discourse on male hysteria. Yet, that proximity—established through other associated terms—should not be equated with the extension of hysteria into male hysteria. For male hysteria, see Link-Heer et al., "Male Hysteria".
100. Trollope-Kumar, "Cultural and Biomedical Meanings of the Complaint of Leukorrhea in South Asian Women".
101. Advertisement for *Mahashakti Rasayan* in *Brihat Mohammadiya Panjika* for 1318 BS.
102. Advertisement for *Amritashakti Rasayan* in *Brihat Mohammadiya Panjika* for 1318 BS.
103. Mukhopadhyay, *Biswakosh*, 251–52.
104. Chakrabarti, *Andare Antare.*
105. See Attewell, "Treating Women".
106. Much of the framework for conceptualizing hysteria as a disease of the 'wandering womb' derived from Thomas Sydenham's revival of the writings of Hypocrates on the topic in the middle of the seventeenth century. See Wright, "Hysteria and the Mechanical Man".
107. Advertisement of *"Prameha Kalyan Bori"*; Also see, Advertisement of *"Prameha Shanti Batika"*, both in in *Gupta Press Dairektari Panjika* for 1322 BS.
108. Advertisement of *"Mahashakti Rasayan"*, in *Gupta Press Dairektari Panjika* for 1322 BS.
109. Sinha, *Colonial Masculinity;* Chowdhury, *Frail Hero and Virile History.*
110. Sontag, *Illness as Metaphor*, 29.
111. Scheper-Hughes and Lock argue that there are three distinct levels at which the body is articulated. First, the level at which the self experiences it; second, the level at which others perceive it and finally, the level at which it is enumerated, manipulated and controlled at the level of distant

objects coded as anonymous 'populations'. Scheper-Hughes et al., "The Mindful Body". Kirmayer suggests that there is a fourth level—the 'indexical'—where the self itself perceives a certain state of the body through the interpretation of certain indexes, such as the reading of a thermometer. Kirmayer, "The Body's Insistence on Meaning".

112. Gupta, "*Shikhya O Swasthya*"; McCay, *Standards of the Constituents of the Urine and the Blood of the Bengalis.*
113. The works of Sinha and Choudhury have done much to enlighten us about a good many of these political rivalries/aspirations, social anxieties literary tropes, etc. Sinha, *Colonial Masculinity,* Choudhury, *Frail Hero and Virile History.*
114. Maitreya "*Jeeban Sahay*"; Advertisement of *Nabashakti (Sarbaprakar Dhatu Dourbalya Roger Jom)* in the *Gupta Press Dairekttari Panjika* for 1322 BS.
115. Advertisement for "Amrita Sindhu Salsa" in *Gupta Press Dairektari Panjika* for 1322 BS.
116. Rack, *Race, Culture,* 101–05.
117. Jadhav et al., "Cultural Experience of Depression among White Britons in London".
118. Advertisement by G. K. Nag & Co. in the *Gupta Press Dairektari Panjika* for 1322 BS.
119. Advertisement by D. Gupta & Co. in *Lord Ripon's Panjika* for 1290 BS.
120. Advertisement by Navashakti Aushadhalaya in the *Gupta Press Dairektari Panjika* for 1322 BS.
121. Advertisement by Navashakti Aushadhalaya in the *Gupta Press Dairektari Panjika* for 1322 BS.
122. Parascandola, "Patent Medicines and the Public's Health".
123. Austin, "A Review on Indian Sarsaparilla".
124. Smith, "The Contagious Diseases Acts Reconsidered": 214.
125. See Advertisement by GK Nag & Co in the *Gupta Press Dairektari Panjika* for 1322 BS.
126. See, for instance, advertisements for *Amrita Sagar Salsa or Sarsa Vito;* both appeared in *Gupta Press Dairektari Panjika* for 1322 BS.
127. Alter, *Yoga in Modern India:* 40–41.
128. The fear of mercury poisoning can be seen in the innumerable advertisements which protested that their drugs—unlike those of others—did not use any mercury. Mohamed Abdul Rab of Jalpaiguri, for example, commenced his advertisement by 'swearing in the name of Allah' *(Allah kasam)* that his medicines did not contain mercury. Advertisements of Mohamed Abdul Rab in the *Brihat Mohammadiya Panjika* for 1318 BS.

129. Advertisement of *London Medical Hall in the Chikitsa Prakash* throughout 1920.
130. Advertisement of *Parke Davis & Co in the Chikitsa Prakash* throughout 1920.
131. Ecks, "Pharmaceutical Citizenship: Antidepressant Marketing and the Promise of Demarginalization in India".
132. Ecks particularly draws attention to the notion of *mon kharap* ('bad-mind'), which, under the influence of late nineteenth and early twentieth century neo-Hindu ideologies, has actually remained strong and resisted the easy insertion of 'depressive' mental states into a medical market. See Ecks, "Pharmaceutical Citizenship: Antidepressant Marketing and the Promise of Demarginalization in India".

Conclusion

1. Latour, *Pandora's Hope:* 266–92.
2. For a detailed discussion of 'double articulation', see Deleuze et al., *Thousand Plateaus:* 44–83.
3. Ghosh, *E Myanual oph Injekshan Chikitsa.*
4. Shamsuddin, "Influnza Heart".
5. Basu, "*Chikitsa Sankat*".
6. Das, "*Gil-Dhil-Pill-Bill-Kill*".

Bibliography

1. Durga Das Gupta, better-known as D. D. Gupta, was the editor of the journal called *Swasthya.* The journal did not explicitly mention whether all the published pieces were indeed written by the editor or not. In view of this, we have attributed authorship of all the pieces from the *Swasthya* to Gupta. It is cogent to add that other Bengali medical periodicals are known to have existed in the period, where the 'editor' is explicitly known to have authored all the pieces appearing in it. Jadunath Mukherji's *Chikitsa Darpan* and Pulinchandra Sanyal's *Chikitsa Kalpataru* are examples of such individually authored medical periodicals.

BIBLIOGRAPHY

English Works

Acton, William. *The Functions and Disorders of the Reproductive Organs in Childhood, Youth, Adult Age and Advanced Life*. (London: John Churchill 1867)

Agamben, Giorgio. *Homo Sacer: Sovereign Power and Bare Life*. Daniel Heller-Roazen, trans. (Stanford: Stanford University Press 1998)

Alam, Muzaffar and Sanjay Subrahmanyam. "The Making of a Munshi." *Comparative Studies of South Asia, Africa and the Middle East* 24, no. 2 (2004): 61–72

Alavi, Seema. *Islam and Healing: Loss and Recovery of an Indo-Muslim Medical Tradition, 1600–1900*. (Basingstoke: Palgrave Macmillan, 2008)

________. "Unani Medicine in the Nineteenth Century Public Sphere." *Indian Economic and Social History Review* 42, no. 1 (2005): 101–29

Alter, Jospeh S. "Gandhi's Body, Gandhi's Truth: Nonviolence and the Biomoral Imperative of Public Health." *Journal of Asian Studies* 55, no. 2 (1996): 301–22

________. *Yoga in Modern India: The Body between Science and Philosophy*. (Princeton: Princeton University Press 2004)

Amin, Shahid. *Event, Metaphor, Memory: Chauri-Chaura 192292*. (Berkeley: University of California Press 1995)

Amin, Sonia. *The World of Muslim Women in Colonial Bengal 1876–1939*. (Leiden: Brill 1996)

Anderson, Warwick. "Excremental Colonialism: Public Health and the Poetics of Pollution." *Critical Inquiry* 21, no. 3 (1995): 640–69

________. "Introduction: Postcolonial Technoscience." *Social Studies of Science* 32, no. 5–6 (2002): 643–58

________. "The Possession of Kuru: Medical Science and Biocolonial Exchange." *Comparative Studies in Society and History* 42, no. 4 (2000): 713–44

Anonymous. "Bengal Water Hyacinth Bill." *Indian Annual Register*. (Calcutta: The Annual Register Office 1936): 177

________. "Committee." *The Modern Review* (Allahabad: Prabasi Press Pvt Ltd. 1923): 100

________. "Obituary: Khan Tamiz Khan Bahadur." *Indian Medical Gazette*, XXXVII (1882): 187

________. "Prize Essay on Plague Prevention." *Indian Medical Gazette*, XLII (1907): 303–4

Appadurai, Arjun. ed., *The Social Life of Things: Commodities in Cultural Perspective*. (Cambridge: Cambridge University Press 1986)

Apple, Rima. *Vitamania: Vitamins in American Culture*. (New Brunswick: Rutgers University Press 1996)

Arnold, David and Sumit Sarkar. "In Search of Rational Remedies: Homeopathy in Nineteenth Century Bengal." In Waltraud Ernst, ed., *Plural Medicine, Tradition and Modernity, 1800–2000* (London: Routledge 2002): 40–57

Arnold, David. "'An Ancient Race Outworn': Malaria and Race in Colonial India, 1860–1930." In Bernard Harris and Waltraud Ernst, ed., *Race, Science and Medicine, 1700–1960* (London: Routledge 1999)

________. "Cholera: Disease as Disorder." *Colonizing the Body: State Medicine and Epidemic Disease in Nineteenth Century India.* (Berkeley: University of California Press 1993): 159–99

________. *Colonizing the Body: State Medicine and Epidemic Disease in Nineteenth Century India.* (Berkeley: University of California Press 1993)

________. "Plurality and Transition: Knowledge Systems in Nineteenth-Century India." Unpublished Paper presented at The Princeton History of Science Seminar, October 2003. available at http://www.princeton.edu/~hos/WorkshopIpapers/Arnold History ofSciencepaper.htm (accessed 21 October 2008)

________. *The New Cambridge History of India III. 5: Science, Technology and Medicine in Colonial India* (Cambridge: Cambridge University Press 2002)

Arnold, David. ed., *Warm Climates and Western Medicine.* (Amsterdam: Rodopi 1996)

Attewell, Guy Nicolas Anthony. "Contesting Knowledges: Plague and Dynamics of the Unani Profession." In unpublished PhD Thesis "Authority, Knowledge and Practice in Unani Tibb, c. 1890–1930." London: School of Oriental and African Studies: 49–92

________. "Crossing the Faultlines of Historiography: *Tiryaq*, Transregional Trade and Therapeutic Transformation." Unpublished paper, presented at the "Crossing Colonial Historiographies of Medicine." Conference at Oxford, September 2008

________. *Refiguring Unani Tibb: Plural Healing in Late Colonial India.* (Hyderabad: Orient Longman 2007)

________. "Treating Women: Women's Engagement with Unani Tibb and its Engagement with Women in Early Twentieth Century India." In Unpublished PhD Thesis, "Authority, Knowledge and Practice in Unani Tibb in India, c. 1890–1930. (London: School of Oriental and African Studies 2004): 184–227

Austin, Anoop. "A Review on Indian Sarsaparilla, *Hemidesmus indicus* (L.) R. Br." *Journal of Biological Sciences* 8, no. 1 (2008): 1–12

Bagchi, Amiya Kumar. "Wealth and Work in Calcutta: 1860–1921." In Sukanta Chaudhuri, ed., *Calcutta: The Living City, Volume I.* (Calcutta: Oxford University Press 1990): 212–23

Bala, Poonam. *Imperialism and Medicine in Bengal: A Socio-Historical Perspective.* (New Delhi: Sage Publications 1992)

Balfour, John. A *Sexual Science: A Guidebook for Married and Single Men.* (Bombay: Century Publishing Co. 1894)

Bandyopadhyay, Asitakumar. *History of Modern Bengali Literature: Nineteenth and Twentieth Centuries.* (Calcutta: Modern Book Agency 1986)

Banerjee, Madhulika. "The Long Road to Khari Baoli: Environmental Discourse and the Market for Medicinal Plants." Unpublished paper presented at the Seventh Annual Conference of the International Association for the Study of Common Property at Vancouver, June 1998. Available at http://www.indiana.edu/~iascp/Final/banerjee.pdf (accessed 21 October 2008)

Banerjee, Sumanta. "Peasant Hares and Capitalist Hounds of Singur." *Economic and Political Weekly* 41, no. 52 (2006): 5296–99

Banerji, Nripendra Chandra. *At the Cross-roads, 1885–1946: The Autobiography of Nripendra Chandra Banerji.* (Calcutta: Jignasa, 1974)

Barrett, Ron. *Aghor Medicine: Pollution, Death, and Healing in Northern India.* (Berkeley: University of California Press 2008)

Basalla, George. "The Spread of Western Science." *Science* 156, no. 3775 (1967): 611–22

Bashford, Alison and Claire Hooker. *Contagion: Historical and Cultural Studies.* (London: Routledge 2001)

Basu, Chunilal. *Village Sanitation and a Manual of Hygiene.* (Calcutta: np, 1931)

Basu Raychaudhury, Anasua. "Nostalgia of 'Desh', Memories of Partition." *Economic and Political Weekly* 39, no. 52 (2004)

Bayly, C. A. *Empire and Information: Intelligence Gathering and Social Communication in India, 1780–1870.* (Cambridge: Cambridge University Press 1995)

Bennet, Paula and Vernon Rosario II. eds., *Solitary Pleasures: The Historical, Literary, and Artistic Discourses of Autoeroticism.* (New York: Routledge 1995)

Berger, Rachel. *Ayurveda, State and Society in Colonial North India, 1895–1947.* Unpublished PhD Thesis. University of Cambridge, 2008

Bernutz, Gustave and Goupil Ernest. *Clinical Memoirs of the Diseases of Women Vol. II.* (London: New Sydenham Society, 1867)

Bewell, Alan J. *Romanticism and Colonial Disease.* (Baltimore: Johns Hopkins University Press 1999)

Bhattacharya, Jayanta. "Anatomical Knowledge and East-West Exchange." Unpublished Paper presented at the Third Conference of the Asian Society for History of Medicine at Jawaharlal Nehru University, November 2006

Bhattacharya, Nandini, Caroline Procter and Sarah Hodges. "Medical Garbage and the Limits of Global Governance in Contemporary Tamil Nadu, India." Garnet Working Paper no. 43/08, May 2008. Available at http://www.garnet-eu.org/fileadmin/documents/working_papers/4308.pdf (accessed 21 October 2008)

Bhattacharya, Sanjoy. *Expunging Variola: The Control and Eradication of Small Pox in India, 1947–77.* (New Delhi: Orient Longman 2006)

Bhattacharya, Tithi. *The Sentinels of Culture: Class, Education and the Colonial Intellectual in Bengal.* (New Delhi, Oxford University Press 2005)

Bhugra, D. and A. Buchanan. "Impotence in Ancient Indian Texts." *Sexual and Marital Therapy* 4, no. 1 (1989): 87–92

Blair, Harry W. "Mrs Gandhi's Emergency, the Indian Elections of 1977, Pluralism and Marxism: Problems with Paradigms." *Modern Asian Studies* 14, no. 2 (1980): 237–71

Bloch, Marc. *Feudal Society.* L. A. Manyon, trans. (Chicago: University of Chicago Press 1964)

Bode, Maarten. "Taking Traditional Knowledge to the Market: The Commoditization of Indian Medicine." *Anthropology & Medicine* 13, no. 3 (2006): 225–36

Bruchhausen, Walter. "Medicine by Non-Doctors? 'Tribal Dressers' in Tanganyika between Health Care and Politics, 1926–1951." Unpublished Paper presented at "Imagining and Practising Imperial and Colonial Medicine, 1870–1960." Conference at St Anthony's College, Oxford, January 2008

Buckingham, Jane. *Leprosy in Colonial South India: Medicine and Confinement.* (New York: Palgrave Macmillan 2002)

________. "Patient Welfare Vs. the Health of the Nation: Governmentality and Sterilisation of Leprosy Sufferers in Early Post-Colonial India." *Social History of Medicine* 19, no. 3 (2006): 483–99

Buhnemann, Gudrun. "Selecting and Perfecting Mantras in Hindu Tantrism." *Bulletin of the School of Oriental and African Studies* 54 no. 2 (1991): 292–306

Burdett, Henry C. *Hospitals and Asylums of the World: Their Origin, History, Construction, Administration, Management and Legislation.* (London: J & A Churchill 1893)

Burnham, John C. *How the Idea of Profession Changed the Writing of Medical History. Medical History,* Supplement no. 18. (London: Wellcome Institute for the History of Medicine 1998)

Bynum, Bill. "Spermatorrhoea." *The Lancet* 357 (2001): 726

Bynum W. F. and Janice Wilson. "Periodical Knowledge: Medical Journals and their Editors in Nineteenth Century Britain." In W. F. Bynum, Stephen Lock and Roy Porter, eds., *Medical Journals and Medical Knowledge.* (London: Routledge 1992): 29–48

________. *Science and the Practice of Medicine in the Nineteenth Century.* (Cambridge: Cambridge University Press 1994)

Calcutta University. *Minutes 1873–74.* (Calcutta: Calcutta University 1874)

Carter, Paul. *The Road to Botany Bay: An Essay in Spatial History.* (London: Faber & Faber 1987)

Catanach, I. J. "Plague and the Indian Village." In Peter Robb, ed., *Rural India: Land, Power, Society Under British Rule.* (Richmond: Curzon Press 1983): 216–43

________. "Plague and the Tensions of Empire, 1896–1918." In David Arnold, ed., *Imperial Medicine and Indigenous Society.* (Manchester: Manchester University Press 1998): 149–71

________. "Poona Politicians and the Plague." *South Asia* 7, no. 2 (1984): 1–18

Chadha C. and N. Ahuja. "Dhat Syndrome: A Sex Neurosis of the Indian Subcontinent." *British Journal of Psychiatry* 159 (1991): 577–79

Chakrabarti, Kunal. *Religious Processes: The Puranas and the Making of a Regional Tradition.* (Delhi: Oxford University Press 2004)

Chakrabarti, Pratik. "Medical Marketplace beyond the West: Bazaar Medicine, Trade and the English Establishment in Eighteenth Century India." In Patrick Wallis and Mark Jenner, eds., *Medicine and the Market in Early Modern England and its Colonies.* (Basingstoke: Palgrave Macmillan 2007): 196–215

________. "Science Nationalism and Colonial Contestations: PC Ray and his Hindu Chemistry." *Indien Economic and Social History Review* 37, no. 2 (2000): 185–213

________. *Western Science in Modern India: Metropolitan Methods, Colonial Practices.* (Delhi: Permanent Black 2004)

Chakrabarty, Dipesh. *Habitations of Modernity: Essays in the Wake of Subaltern Studies.* (Chicago: University of Chicago Press 2002)

________. "Modernity and the Past: A Critical Tribute to Ashis Nandy." *Habitations of Modernity: Essays in the Wake of Subaltern Studies.* (Chicago: University of Chicago Press 2002): 28–50

________. "Of Garbage, Modernity and the Citizen's Gaze." *Habitations of Modernity: Essays in the Wake of Subaltern* Studies. (Chicago: University of Chicago Press 2002): 65–79

________. "Remembered Villages: Representations of Hindu-Bengali Memories in the Aftermath of the Partition." In D. A. Low and Howard Brasted, eds., *Freedom, Trauma, Communities: North India and Independence.* (New Delhi: Sage 1998): 318–37

________. "Romantic Archives: Literature and the Politics of Identity in Bengal." *Critical Inquiry* 30 no. 3 (2004): 654–83

________. "The Difference-Deferral of (A) Colonial Modernity: Public Debates on Domesticity in British Bengal." *History Workshop* 36, no. 1 (1993): 1–34

Chandravarkar, Rajnarayan. "Plague Panic and Epidemic Politics in India, 1896–1914." In Terence O. Ranger and Paul Slack, eds., *Epidemics and Ideas: Essays on the Historical Perception of Pestilence.* (Cambridge: Cambridge University Press 1999): 203–40

Charles, Cathcart. "Pelvic Floor, Peritonium, Dermatitis." *Edinburgh Medical Journal* 34, pt. 2 (1889): 716–1101

Chatterjee, Kumkum. "History as Self-Representation: The Recasting of a Political Tradition in Late Eighteenth Century Eastern India." *Modern Asian Studies* 32, no. 4 (1998): 913–48

Chatterjee, Partha. "Modernity, Democracy and a Political Negotiation of Death." *South Asia Research* 19 no. 1 (1999): 103–19

________. *Nation and Its Fragments: Colonial and Postcolonial Histories.* (Princeton: Princeton University Press 1993)

________. *Our Modernity.* (Rotterdam: SEPHIS 1997)

Chattopadhyay, Debiprasad. *Science and Society in Ancient India.* (Amsterdam: BR Gruner 1977)

Chattopadhyay, Swati. *Representing Calcutta: Modernity Nationalism and the Colonial Uncanny.* (London: Routledge 2006)

Chaturvedi, Vinayak. *Peasant Pasts: History and Memory in Western India.* (Berkeley: University of California Press 2007)

________. "Vinayak and Me: Hindutva and the Politics of Naming." *Social History* 28, no. 2 (2003): 155–73

Cherniavsky, Eva. "Night Pollution and the Floods of Confession in Michael Wigglesworth's Dairy." *Arizona Quarterly* 45 no. 2 (1989): 15–33

Chowdhury, Indira. *Frail Hero and Virile History: Gender and the Politics of Culture in Colonial Bengal.* (Delhi: Oxford University Press 1998)

Ciccetti, Jane. *Dreams, Symbols & Homoeopathy: Achetypal Dimensions of Healing.* (Berkeley: North Atlantic Books 2003)

Cifuentes, Lluis. "Vernacularization as an Intellectual and Social Bridge. The Catalan Translations of Teodorico's *Chirurgia* and of Arnau De Villanova's *Regimen Sanitatis.*" *Early Science and Medicine* 4, no. 2 (1999): 127–48

Cobb, Richard. *The Sense of Place.* (London: Duckworth 1976)

Cohen, Lawrence. "The Other Kidney: Biopolitics Beyond Recognition." *Body & Society* 7, no. 2/3 (2001): 9–29

Conrad, Lawrence and Dominic Wujastyk. *Contagion: Perspectives from Pre-Modern Societies.* (Aldershot: Ashgate 2000)

Cook, Harold J. "Good Advice and Little Medicine: The Professional Authority of Early Modern English Physicians." *Journal of British Studies* 33, no. 1 (1994): 1–31

Cooper, Frederick. "Conflict and Connection: Re-thinking Colonial African History." *The American Historical Review* 99, no. 5 (1994): 1516–45

Crawford, D. G. *A History of the Indian Medical Service 1600–1913 Vol. II.* (London: W Thacker & Co 1914)

Crossgrove, William. "The Vernacularization of Science, Medicine and Technology in Late Medieval Europe: Broadening Our Perspectives." *Early Science and Medicine* 5, no. 1 (2000): 47–63

Cullen, William. *Institutes of Medicine: Part I Physiology.* (Edinburgh: Charles Elliot 1772)

Daeschel, Markus. *The Politics of Self Expression: The Urdu Middle Class Milieu in Mid Twentieth Century India and Pakistan.* (London: Routledge 2006)

Darnton, Robert. *The Great Cat Massacre and Other Essays*. (Colchester: Vintage Books 1998)

Das, Amal. "Calcutta Plague: Epidemic, Colonial Intervention and Indigenous Society, 1898–1900." In Chittabrata Palit and Achintya Kumar Dutta, eds., *History of Medicine in India: The Medical Encounter*. (Delhi: Kalpaz Publications 2005): 87–110

Das, Anirban. "Medical Knowledge of the Body: Colonial Encounters." *Re-thinking Marxism* 13, no. 2 (2001): 109–31

Das, Sisir Kumar. *Sahibs and Munshis: An Account of the College at Fort William*. (New Delhi: Orion Publications 1978)

Dasgupta, Rajarshi. "Rhyming Revolution: Marxism and Culture in Colonial Bengal." *Studies in History* 21, no. 1 (2005): 79–98

Datta, Pradip Kumar. "'Dying Hindus': Production of Hindu Communal Common Sense in Early 20th Century Bengal." *Economic and Political Weekly* 28, no. 25 (1993): 1305–19

De Landa, Manuel. *Intensive Science and Virtual Philosophy*. (London: Continuum 2003)

Deleuze, Gilles and Felix Guattari. "10,000 BC: The Geology of Morals. (Who does the Earth think it is?)." In Giles Deleuze and Felix Guattari eds., *A Thousand Plateaus: Capitalism and Schizophrenia*. Brian Massumi, trans. (London: Continuum 2004): 44–82

________. *A Thousand Plateaus: Capitalism and Schizophrenia*. Brian Massumi, trans. (London: Continuum 2004)

________. "Instincts and Institutions." *Desert Islands and Other Texts (1953–74)*. (Los Angeles: Semiotext(e) 2004): 19–21

Derrida, Jacques. *Archive Fever: A Freudian Impression*. Eric Prenowitz, trans. (Chicago: University of Chicago Press 1996)

Digby, Anne. *Making a Medical Living: Doctors and Patients in the English Market*. (Cambridge: Cambridge University Press 1994)

Donoghue, Emma "Imagined More than Women: Lesbians as Hermaphrodites, 1671–1766." *Women's History Review* 2, no. 2 (1993): 199–216

Dutta, Achintya Kumar. "Upendranath Brahmachari in Pursuit of *Kala-Azar*." In Chittabrata Palit and Achintya Kumar Dutta, eds., *History of Medicine in India: The Medical Encounter*. (Delhi: Kalpaz Publications 2005): 139–58

Echenberg, Myron. *Plague Ports: The Global Urban Impact of Bubonic Plague, 1894–1901*. (London: New York University Press 2007)

Ecks, Stefan. "Bodily Sovereignty as Political Sovereignty: 'Self-Care' in Kolkata, India." *Anthropology and Medicine* 11, no. 1 (2004): 75–89

________. "Pharmaceutical Citizenship: Antidepressant Marketing and the Promise of Demarginalization in India." *Anthropology and Medicine* 12, no. 3 (2005): 239–54

Eisenstadt, Shmuel. 'Multiple Modernities." *Daedalus* 129, no. 1 (2000): 1–29

Emch-Deriaz, Antoinette. "The Non-Naturals Made Easy." In Roy Porter, ed., *The Popularization of Medicine, 1650–1850*. (London: Routledge 1992), 134–59

Ernst, Waltraud. "Beyond East and West. From the History of Colonial Medicine to a Social History of Medicine(s) in South Asia." *Social History of Medicine*. Advance Access Publication, November 13, 2007.

________. "Colonial Psychiatry, Magic and Religion: The Case of Mesmerism in British India." *History of Psychiatry* 15, no. 1 (2004): 57–71

________. *Mad Tales from the Raj: European Insane in British India*. (London: Routledge 1991)

Ernst, Waltraud, ed., *Plural Medicine, Tradition and Modernity, 1800–2000*. (London: Routledge 2002)

Feierman, Steven. "History of Pluralistis Medical Systems. Change in African Therapeutic Systems." *Social Science & Medicine* 13b, no. 4 (1979): 277–84

Floyer, John. *A Comment on Forty Two Histories.* (London: J. Isted 1726)

Foot, John. "Micro-history of a House: Memory and Place in a Milanese Neighbourhood, 1890–2000." *Urban History* 34, (2007): 431–52

Foucault, Michel. "Body/Power." *Power/Knowledge.* Colin Gordon, trans. (New York: Random House 1977): 55–62

________. "Governmentality." In Graham Burchell, Colin Gordon and Peter Miller, eds., *The Foucault Effect: Studies in Governmentality.* Rosi Braidotti, trans. (Chicago: University of Chicago Press 1991): 87–104

________. *History of Sexuality Volume I: An Introduction.* (London: Penguin Books 1990)

________. "The Ethic of Care for the Self as a Practice of Freedom." In James Bernauer and David Rasmussen, eds., *The Final Foucault.* (Boston: MIT Press 1988): 1–20

________. *The Order of Things: An Archaeology of the Human Sciences.* (London: Tavistock Publications 1970)

Frankenberg, Ronald. "Allopathic Medicine, Profession and Capitalist Ideology in India." *Social Science and Medicine* 15a, no. 2 (1981): 115–25

Furdell, Elizabeth Lane. *Publishing and Medicine in Early Modern England.* (Rochester: University of Rochester Press 2002)

Gait, E. A. *Census of India, 1901: The Lower Provinces of Bengal and their Feudatories Volume IV, Part I.* (Calcutta: Bengal Secretariat Press 1902)

Gaudilliere, Jean-Paul and Ilana Lowy. *Heredity and Infection: The History of Disease Transmission.* (London: Routledge 2001)

Gautham Meenakshi, Rajesh Singh, Helen Weiss, Ruairi Brugha, Vikram Patel, Nimesh G. Desai, Deoki Nandan, Karina Kielmann and Heiner Grosskurth. "Socio-cultural, Psycho-sexual and Bio-medical Factors Associated with Genital Symptoms Experienced by Men in Rural India." *Tropical Medicine and International Health* 13, no. 3 (2008): 384–95

Ghosh, Anindita. *Power in Print: Popular Publishing and the Politics of Language and Culture in a Colonial Society.* (Delhi: Oxford University Press 2006)

________. "Revisiting the 'Bengal Renaissance': Literary Bengali and Low-Life Print in Colonial Calcutta." *Economic and Political Weekly* 37, no. 42 (2002): 19–25

Ginzburg, Carlo, John Tedeschi and Anne C. Tedeschi. "Microhistory: Two or Three Things I Know About It." *Critical Inquiry* 20, no. 1 (1993): 10–35

Gole, Nilufer. "Snapshots of Islamic Modernities." *Daedalus* 129, no. 1 (2000): 91–117

Good, Byron. "How Medicine Constructs its Objects." *Medicine, Rationality and Experience: An Anthropological Perspective.* (Cambridge: Cambridge University Press 1994): 65–87

Goswami, Manu. *Producing India: From Colonial Economy to National Space.* (New Delhi: Permanent Black 2004)

Government of Bengal. *Provincial Autonomy in Bengal: Being a Report of the Work Done by the Government of Bengal.* (Calcutta: Directorate of Public Instruction 1937)

Green, Nile. "The Religious and Cultural Roles of Dreams and Visions in Islam." *Journal of the Royal Asiatic Society Series 3* 13, no. 3 (2003): 287–313

Greenblatt, Stephen. *Learning to Curse: Essays in Early Modern Culture.* (New York: Routledge 1992)

Greenhow, T. M. *Cholera as it has Recently Appeared in the Towns of Newcastle and Gateshead including cases illustrative of its Physiology and Pathology.* (London: S Highley 1832)

________. *Cholera from the East. A Letter addressed to James Hodgson, Mayor of Newcastle.* (Newcastle Upon Tyne: E Charnley 1852)

________. *Cholera: Its Non-Contagious Nature. A Letter addressed to the Mayor of Newcastle.* (Newcastle Upon Tyne: Emerson Charnley 1831)

———. *Hints on the Probable Approach of Cholera. A Letter addressed to Stephen Lowrey, Mayor of Newcastle.* (Newcastle Upon Tyne: Emerson Charnley 1848)

Guha, Ranajit. *Dominance without Hegemony: History and Power in Colonial India.* (Cambridge, MA: Harvard University Press 1997)

———. "The Prose of Counter-Insurgency." in *Selected Subaltern Studies.* Ranajit Guha and Gayatri Chakravorty Spivak, eds., (New York: Oxford University Press 1988): 45–88

Gupta, Brahmananda. "Indigenous Medicine in Nineteenth and Twentieth Century Bengal." In *Asian Medical Systems: A Comparative Study I.* Charles Leslie ed., (Berkeley: University of California Press 1976): 368–78

Gupta, Charu. *Sexuality, Obscenity and Community: Women, Muslims and the Hindu Public in Colonial India.* (New Delhi: Permanent Black 2000)

Gupta, Swarupa. 'Samaj, Jati and Desh: Reflections on Nationhood in Late Colonial Bengal." *Studies in History* 27, no. 2 (2007): 177–203

Habib, S Irfan and Dhruv Raina. *Domesticating Modern Science: A Social History of Science and Culture in Colonial India.* (New Delhi: Tulika Books 2004)

Hacking, Ian. *The Taming of Chance.* (Cambridge: Cambridge University Press 1990)

Hall, Donald Eugene. ed., *Muscular Christianity: Embodying the Victorian Age.* (Cambridge: Cambridge University Press 1994)

Hamilton, Surgeon Major. "Cholera: Its Endemic Areas and Epidemic Progression." *Indian Medical Gazette* XX (1885): 142–47

Hamlin, Christopher. "Predisposing Causes and Public Health in Early Nineteenth Century Medical Thought." *Social History of Medicine* 5, no. 1 (1992): 43–70

Hardiman, David, ed., *Healing Bodies, Saving Souls: Medical Missions in Asia and Africa.* (Amsterdam: Rodopi 2006)

Harrison, Mark. "Book Reviews: Anil Kumar, Medicine and the Raj." *Science, Technology & Society* 4, no. 2 (1999): 360–65

———. "Cholera Theory and Sanitary Policy." *Public Health in British India: Anglo-Indian Preventive Medicine 1859–1914.* (Cambridge: Cambridge University Press 1994): 99–116

———. *Climates and Constitutions: Health, Race and Environment in British Imperialism in India, 1600–1850.* (Delhi: Oxford University Press 2002)

———. *Public Health in British India: Anglo-Indian Preventive Medicine 1859–1914.* (Cambridge: Cambridge University Press 1994)

Hatley, Shaman. "Mapping the Esoteric Body in the Islamic Yoga of Bengal." *History of Religions* 46, no. 4 (2007): 351–68

Hickman, A. "Treatment of Cholera with Sulphurous Acid." *Indian Medical Gazette.* December (1882): 321

Hodges, Sarah. "Chennai's Biotrash Chronicles: Chasing the Neo-Liberal Syringe." Garnet Working Paper no. 44/08, May 2008. Available at http://www.garnet-eu.org/fileadmin/documents/working_papers/4408.pdf (accessed 21 October 2008)

———. "Governmentality, Population and the Reproductive Family in Modern India." *Economic and Political Weekly* 39, no. 11 (2004): 1157–63

———. "Indian Eugenics in an Age of Reform." In *Reproductive Health in India: History, Politics, Controversies.* Sarah Hodges, ed., (Delhi: Orient Longman 2006): 115–38

Hughes, C. C. "The Culture Bound Syndromes and Psychiatric Diagnosis." In *Culture and Psychiatric Diagnosis: A DSM—IV Perspective.* J. Mezzich, A. Kleinman, H. Fabrega, eds., (Washington: APA, 1996): 298–308

Hume, Joseph Chandler Jr. "Rival Traditions, Western Medicine and Unan-i-Tibb in the Punjab, 1849–1889" *Bulletin of the History of Medicine* 51, no. 2 (1977): 214–31

Iliffe, John. *East African Doctors: A History of the Medical Profession*. (Cambridge: Cambridge University Press 1998)

Inden, Ronald B. and Ralph W. Nicholas. *Kinship in Bengali Culture*. (New Delhi: Chronicle Books 2005)

Iqbal, Iftekhar. "Towards an Environmental History of Colonial East Bengal: Paradigms and Praxis." *Journal of the Asiatic Society of Bangladesh: Golden Jubilee Volume* (online edition). Available at http://www.asiaticsociety.org.bd/journals/Golden_jubilee_vol/ index.html

Jadhav, Sushrut. "*Dhat* Syndrome: A Re-Evaluation." http://www.indianpsychiatry.com/dhat.pdf (accessed 23 April 2008)

Jadhav, Sushrut, M. G. Weiss and R. Littlewood. "Cultural Experience of Depression among White-Britons in London." *Anthropology & Medicine* 8, no. 1 (2001): 47–69

Janzen, John M. *The Quest for Therapy in Lower Zaire*. In collaboration with William Arkinstall. (Berkeley: University of California Press 1978)

Johnson, James. *The Influence of Tropical Climates*. (London: J Callow 1826)

Johnson, T. "Imperialism and the Professions. Notes on the Development of Professional Occupations in Britain's Colonies and the New States." In *Professionalisation and Social Change*. Paul Halmos, ed., (Keele: University of Keele 1973): 281–309

Karim, Anwarul. "Shamanism in Bangladesh." *Asian Folklore Studies* 47, (1988): 277–309

Kaviraj, Sudipta. "An Outline of a Revisionist Theory of Modernity." *European Journal of Sociology* 46, no. 3 (2005): 497–526

________. "Filth and the 'Public Sphere.'" *Public Culture* 10, no. 1 (1997): 83–113

________. "Introduction: Ideas of Civil Society." In *Civil Society: History and Possibilities*. Sudipta Kaviraj and Sunil Khilnani, eds., (Cambridge: Cambridge University Press 2001): 1–8

Kaviraj, Sudipta and Khilnani, Sunil eds., *Civil Society: History and Possibilities*. (Cambridge: Cambridge University Press 2001)

Khan, At'har Ali'. "On the Cure of Elephantiasis." *Asiatic Researches*, II (1800): 149–58

Khare, R. S. "*Dava*, Daktar and *Dua*: Anthropology of Practised Medicine in India." *Social Science & Medicine* 43, no. 5 (1996): 837–48

Kidambi, Prashant. "'An Infection of Locality': Plague, Pythogenesis and the Poor in Bombay, c. 1896–1905." *Urban History* 31, no. 2 (2004): 249–67

Kiple, Kenneth F. and Kriemhild Conee Ornelas. "Algae." *The Cambridge World History of Food*. (Cambridge: Cambridge University Press 2000): 231–32

Kipling, Rudyard. *Kim*. (Suffolk: The Chaucer Press 1978)

Kirmayer, Laurence J. "The Body's Insistence on Meaning: Metaphor as Presentation and Representation in Illness Experience." *Medical Anthropology Quarterly* 6, no. 4 (1992): 323–46

Klein, Ira. "Imperialism, Ecology and Disease: Cholera in India, 1850–1950." *Indian Economic and Social History Review* 31, no. 4 (1994): 491–518

________. "Plague, Policy and Popular Unrest in British India," *Modern Asian Studies* 22, no. 4 (1988): 728–53

Kopf, David. *British Orientalism and the Bengal Renaissance: The Dynamics of Indian Modernization, 1773–1835*. (Berkeley: University of California Press 1969)

Kothari, Manu L. and Lopa A. Mehta. "Violence and Modern Medicine." In *Science, Hegemony and Violence: A Requiem for Modernity*. Ashis Nandy, ed., (Delhi: Oxford University Press 1988): 167–210

Kumar, Anil. "Emergence of Western Medical Institutions in India 1822–1911." In *History of Medicine in India: The Medical Encounter*. Chittabrata Palit and Achintya Kumar Dutta, eds., (Delhi: Kalpaz Publications, 2005): 159–76

________. *Medicine and the Raj: British Medical Policy in India, 1835–1911.* (New Delhi: Sage 1998)

Kumar, Deepak. 'Medical Encounters in British India, 1820–1920." *Economic and Political Weekly* 32, no. 4 (1997): 166–70

________. *Science and Empire: Essays in Indian Context (1700–1947).* (Delhi: Anamika Prakashan 1991)

________. *Science and the Raj: 1857–1905.* (New York: Oxford University Press 1995)

Kumar, Deepak, ed., *Disease and Medicine: A Historical Overview.* (New Delhi: Tulika Books 2001)

Laden, Sonja. "Recuperating the Archive: Anecdotal Evidence and the Questions of 'Historical Realism.'" *Poetics Today* 25, no. 1 (2004): 1–28

Lakoff, George and Mark Johnson. "Conceptual Metaphor in Everyday Language." *The Journal of Philosophy* 77, no. 8 (1980): 453–86

Langford, Jean M. *Fluent Bodies: Ayurvedic Remedies for Post-colonial Imbalance.* (Durham NC: Duke University Press 2003)

Laport, Dominique. *History of Shit.* Nadia Benabid and Rodolphe El-Khoury, trans. (Cambridge MA: MIT Press 2002)

Latour, Bruno. *Pandora's Hope: Essays on the Reality of Science Studies.* (Cambridge, Mass: Harvard University Press 1999)

Lawrie, James Adair. *Essay in Cholera Founded on Observations of the Disease in Various Parts of India and in Sunderland, Newcastle and Gateshead.* (Glasgow: John Smith & Sons 1832)

Le Goff, Jacque. *The Medieval Imagination.* Arthur Goldhammer, trans. (Chicago: University of Chicago Press 1988)

Lepore, Jill. "Historians Who Love Too Much: Reflections on Microhistory and Biography." *The Journal of American History* 88, no. 1 (2001): 129–44

Leslie, Charles. ed., *Asian Medical Systems: A Comparative Study.* (Berkeley: University of California Press 1976)

Lethbridge, Roper. *The Golden Book of India.* (New York: Elbiron 2005 (1893)).

Link-Heer, Ursula and Jamie Owen Daniel. "Male Hysteria: A Discourse Analysis."*Cultural Critique* 15, (1990): 191–220

Littlewood, R. "Cultural Comments on Culture Bound Syndromes." In *Culture and Psychiatric Diagnosis: A DSM—IV Perspective.* J. Mezzich, A. Kleinman, H Fabrega, eds., (Washington: APA 1996): 309–12

Littlewood, R. and M. Lipsedge. "Culture Bound Sundromes." In *Recent Advances in Clinical Psychiatry.* K. Granville-Grosman. ed., (Edinburgh: Churchill Livingstone 1985): 105–42

Livingstone, David N. and Richard T. Harrison. "Meaning Through Metaphor: Analogy as Epistemology.' *Annals of the Association of American Geographers* 71, no. 1 (1981): 95–107

Livingstone, Julie. *Debility and the Moral Imagination in Botswana.* (Bloomington: Indiana University Press 2005)

Long, Rev. James. *Descriptive Catalogue of Bengali Books.* (Calcutta: Sanders, Cones and Co. 1855)

Lourdusamy, J. *Science and National Consciousness in Bengal: 1870–1930.* (New Delhi: Orient Longman 2004)

MacMichael, William. *Is the Cholera Spasmodica of India a Contagious Disease? Question Considered in a Letter addressed to Sir Henry Halford.* (London: John Murray 1831)

Madan, T. N. "Editorial: The Plague in India, 1994." *Social Science and Medicine* 40, no. 9 (1995): 1167–68

Marriott, McKim. "Hindu Transactions: Diversity Without Dualism." In *Transactions and Meaning: Directions in Anthropology of Exchange and Symbolic Behaviour.* Bruce Kapferer, ed., (Philadelphia: Institute for the Study of Human Issues 1976): 109–42

McCandless, Peter. "Dangerous to Themselves and Others: The Victorian Debate Over the Prevention of Wrongful Confinement." *Journal of British Studies* 23, no. 1 (1983): 84–104

McCay, D. *Standards of the Constituents of the Urine and Blood and the Bearing of the Metabolism of Bengalis on the Problems of Nutrition.* (Calcutta: Superintendent Government Printing 1908)

McNeill, William H. *Plagues and Peoples.* (New York: Anchor Books 1998)

Merten, Don and Gary Schwartz. "Metaphor and Self: Symbolic Process in Everyday Life." *American Anthropologist* 84, no. 4 (1982): 796–810

Meulenbeld, Gerrit-Jan. "Reflections on the Basic Concepts of Indian Pharmacology." In *Studies on Indian Medical History, Papers presented at the International Workshop on the Study of Indian Medicine held at the Wellcome Institute for the History of Medicine, 2–4 September 1985.* G. Jan Meulenbeld and Dominik Wujastyk, eds., (Groningen: Egbert Forsten 1987): 1–17

Millan, Christina Alvarez. "Greaco-Roman Case Histories and their Influence on Medieval Clinical Accounts." *Social History of Medicine* 12, no. 9 (1993): 19–43

Mills, Jim. *Cannabis Britannica: A Social and Political History of Cannabis and the British Government, 1800–1928.* (Oxford: Oxford University Press, 2005)

Morgan, L. M. "'Properly Disposed of': A History of Embryo Disposal and the Changing Claims on Fetal Remains." *Medical Anthropology* 21, no. 3–4 (2002): 247–74

Mouat, F. J. "Hindu Medicine." *Calcutta Review* Vol. VIII (1847): 379–433

Mukharji, Projit Bihari. "Bangali Ayurbed: Frames, Texts and Practices." *The Calcutta Historical Journal* 25, no. 2 (2005)

________. "Going Beyond Elite Medical Traditions: The Case of Chandshi." *Asian Medicine* 2, no. 2 (2006): 277–91

________. "Sex, Medicine, Morality: The Modernization of Sexed Bodies." Forthcoming

________. "Structuring Plurality: Locality, Caste, Class and Ethnicity in Nineteenth Century Bengali Dispensaries." *Health and History* 9, no. 1 (2007): 80–105

Mukherjee, S. N. *Calcutta: Myths and History.* (Calcutta: Subarnarekha 1977)

Mukherjee, Sushilkumar. *The Story of the Calcutta Theatres, 1753–1980.* (Calcutta: K.P. Bagchi and Company 1982)

Murray, Jacqueline. "Men's Bodies, Men's Minds: Seminal Emissions and Sexual Anxiety in the Middle Ages." *Annual Review of Sex Research* 8, (1997): 1–26

Nanda, Meera. "Hindu Nationalism and Vedic Science." *Prophets Facing Backwards: Postmodern Critiques of Science and Hindu Nationalism in India.* (Piscataway: Rutgers University Press 2003): 37–124

Nandy, Ashis. *Alternative Sciences: Creativity and Authenticity in Two Indian Scientists.* (Delhi: Oxford University Press 1995)

________. "Defiance and Conformity in Science: The Identity of Jagadis Chandra Bose." *Science Studies* 2, no. 1 (1972): 31–85

________. "Introduction: Science as a Reason of State." In *Science, Hegemony and Violence: A Requiem for Modernity.* Ashis Nandy, ed., (Delhi: Oxford University Press 1988)

________. *The Intimate Enemy: Loss and Recovery of the Self under Colonialism.* (Delhi: Oxford University Press 1983)

Nandy, Ashis. ed., *Science, Hegemony and Violence: A Requiem for Modernity.* (Delhi: Oxford University Press 1988)

Nappi, Carla. "Winter Worm, Summer Grass: Historicizing Identity in Colonial Chinese Medicine." Unpublished paper, presented at the "Crossing Colonial Historiographies of Medicine" conference at Oxford, September 2008

Natarajan, Kanchana. "'Divine Semen' and the Alchemical Conversion of Iramatevar." *The Medieval History Journal* 7, no. 2 (2004): 255–78

Nicholas, Ralph W. *Fruits of Worship: Practical Religion in Bengal.* (New Delhi: Orient Longman 2003)

Nichter, Mark. "The Layperson's Perception of Medicine as Perspective into the *Utilization* of Multiple Therapy Systems in the Indian Context." *Social Science & Medicine* 14b, no. 4 (1980): 225–33

Nivedita, Sister. "House on the Ganges." In Swami Vivekananda's Collected Works, Volume IX, dated 3 May 1898. http://www.ramakrishnavivekananda.info/vivekananda/complete_works.htm (accessed 21 March 2008)

________. *The Master As I Saw Him.* (London: Longmans, Green & Co. 1910)

Nowel-Smith, Harriet. "Nineteenth Century Narrative Case Histories: An Enquiry into Stylistics and History." *Bulletin Canadien d'Histoire de la Medecine* 12, (1995): 47–67

O'Donnell, C. J. *Census of India, 1891: The Lower Provinces of Bengal and their Feudatories Volume III.* (Calcutta: Bengal Secretariat Press 1893)

O'Flaherty, Wendy Doniger. *Dreams, Illusions and Other Realities.* (Chicago: University of Chicago Press 1984)

Obeysekere, Gananath. "The Impact of Ayurvedic Ideas on the Culture and the Individual in Sri Lanka." In *Asian Medical Systems: A Comparative Study.* Charles Leslie, ed., (New Delhi: Motilal Banarsidass 1998): 211–12

Ogborn, Miles. *Indian Ink: Script and Printing in the Making of English East India Company.* (Chicago: Chicago University Press 2007)

Oldham, C. F. *What Is Malaria And Why Is It Most Intense In Hot Climate?* (Calcutta and London: HK Lewis 1871)

Orwell, George. *Burmese Days.* (Harmondsworth: Penguin Books 1969)

Osseo-Asare, Abena Dove. "Bioprospecting and Resistance: Transforming Poisoned Arrows into Strophantin Pills in Colonial Gold Coast, 1885–1922." *Social History of Medicine* 21, no. 2 (2008): 269–90

Otis, Laura. "The Tigers of Wrath. Mann's Death in Venice as Myth and Medicine." In *Teaching Literature and Medicine.* A. Hunsaker Hawkins and M. Chandler McEntyre, eds., (New York: The Modern Language Association, 2000): 243–51

Palit, Chittabrata *Science and Nationalism in Bengal 1876–1947.* (Kolkata: Institute of Historical Studies 2004)

Palit, Chittabrata and Achintya Kumar Dutta, eds., *History of Medicine in India: The Medical Encounter.* (Delhi: Kalpaz Publications 2005)

Pande, Ishita. "Excrement, Class and Citizenship in a Late Nineteenth Century Calcutta." Unpublished paper, presented at the "Crossing Colonial Historiographies of Medicine" conference at Oxford, September 2008

Parascandola, J. "Patent Medicines and the Public's Health." *Public Health Reports*, 114, no. 4 (1999): 318–21

Patton, Adell. *Physicians, Colonial Racism and Diaspora in West Africa.* (Gainesville: University Press of Florida 1996)

Pati, Biswamoy and Mark Harrison. *Health, Medicine and Empire: Perspectives on Colonial India.* (Delhi: Sangam Books 2001)

Pelling, Margaret. *Cholera, Fever and English Medicine, 1825–65I.* (Oxford: Oxford University Press 1978)

Pickstone, John. "Dearth, Dirt and Fever Epidemics: Re-writing the History of British 'Public Health', 1780–1850." In *Epidemics and Ideas: Essays on the Historical Perception of*

Pestilence. Terence Ranger and Paul Slacks, eds., (Cambridge: Cambridge University Press 1999): 125–48

Pinto, Sarah. "Development without Institutions: Ersatz Medicine and the Everyday Life in Rural North India." *Cultural Anthropology* 19, no. 3 (2004): 337–64

Pitman, Vicki. "Food and Digestion, Health and Disease." In *The Nature of the World: Holism in Ancient Greek and Indian Medicine.* (Delhi, Motilal Banarsidass 2006): 83–140

Pollock, Sheldon. "Cosmopolitan and Vernacular in History." *Public Culture* 12, no. 3 (2000): 591–625

Prakash, Gyan. "A Different Modernity." In *Another Reason: Science and the Imagination of Modern India.* (Princeton, Princeton University Press 1999): 201–26

________. *Another Reason: Science and the Imagination of Modern India.* (Princeton, Princeton University Press 1999)

Prasad, Srirupa. "Crisis, Identity, and Social Distinction: Cultural Politics of Food, Taste, and Consumption in Late Colonial Bengal." *Journal of Historical Sociology* 19, no. 3 (2006): 245–65

Prins, Gwyn. "'But what was the Disease?' The Present State of Health and Healing in African Studies." *Past and Present* 124, no. 1 (1989): 159–79

Quaiser, Neshat. "Politics, Culture and Colonialism: *Unani's* Debate with *Doctory*," In *Health, Medicine and Empire: Perspectives on Colonial India.* Biswamoy Pati and Mark Harrison, eds., (Hyderabad: Orient Longman 2001): 317–55

Rack, Philip. *Race, Culture and Mental Disorder.* (London: Tavistock Publications 1982)

Raj, Kapil. *Relocating Modern Science: Circulation and the Constitution of Scientific Knowledge in South Asia and Europe, 1650–1900.* (Basingstoke: Palgrave Macmillan 2007)

Ramanna, Mridula. "Ranchordlal Chotalal: Pioneer of Public Health in Ahmedabad." In *History of Medicine in India: The Medical Encounter.* Chittabrata Palit and Achintya Kumar Dutta, eds., (Delhi: Kalpaz Publications 2005): 311–26

________. *Western Medicine and Public Health in Colonial Bengal, 1845–1895.* (New Delhi: Orient Longman 2002)

Ramasubban, Radhika. "Imperial Health in British India, 1857–1900." In *Disease, Medicine and Empire: Perspectives on Western Medicine and the Experience of European Expansion.* Roy MacLeod and Milton Lewis, eds., (London: Routledge 1988): 38–60

Ray, Kabita. *Food for Thought: Food Adulteration in Bengal 1836–1947.* (Calcutta: Papyrus 2003)

________. "Voluntary Associations and Public Health in Bengal 1900–1947." In *History of Medicine in India: The Medical Encounter.* Chittabrata Palit and Achintya Kumar Dutta, eds., (Delhi: Kalpaz Publications 2005): 327–40

Ray, Rajat Kanta. *Felt Community: Commonality and Mentality Before the Emergence of Indian Nationalism.* (New Delhi: Oxford University Press 2003)

________. "The Kahar Chronicles." *Modern Asian Studies* 21, no. 4 (1987): 711–49

Raychaudhuri, Tapan. "Translator's Note." In *The Memoirs of Dr Haimabati Sen: From Child Widow to Lady Daktar.* Geraldine Forbes and Tapan Raychaudhuri, eds., (New Delhi: Roli Books 2000): 9

Reddy, Gayatri. *With Respect to Sex: Negotiating Hijra Identity in South Asia.* (Chicago: University of Chicago Press 2005)

Renbourn, E. T. "The History of the Flannel Binder and Cholera Belt." *Medical History* 1, no. 3 (1957): 211–25

Ricoeur, Paul. *The Conflict of Interpretations.* (Evanston, Ill: Northwestern University Press 1974)

________. *The Rule of Metaphor.* (Toronto: University of Toronto Press 1979)

Risley, H. H. *The Tribes and Castes of Bengal. Vol. I.* (Calcutta: 1892)

Robinson, Francis. "Islamic Reform and Modernities in South Asia." *Modern Asian Studies* 42, no. 2/3 (2008): 259–81

Rose, Nicolas. *Inventing Our Selves.* (Cambridge: Cambridge University Press 1996)

Ross, Fiona Georgina Elisabeth. *The Evolution of the Bengali Character from 1778 to 1978.* Unpublished PhD Thesis. London: School of Oriental and African Studies (1988)

Ross, J. T. C. *General Report on the Lunatic Asylums, Vaccinations and Dispensaries in the Bengal Presidency, 1868.* (Unpublished Report, V/24/664)

Roy, Porter. *Quacks: Fakers & Charlatans in English Medicine.* (Gloucester: Tempus Publishing 2000)

Roy, Srirupa. *Beyond Belief: India and the Politics of Postcolonial Nationalism.* (Durham, NC: Duke University Press 2007)

Roy, Tapti. "Disciplining the Printed Text: Colonial and Nationalist Surveillance of Nationalist Literature." In *Texts of Power: Emerging Disciplines in Colonial Bengal.* Partha Chatterjee, ed., (Minneapolis: University of Minnesota Press 1995): 30–62

Royle, J. F. *An Essay on the Antiquity of Hindoo Medicine.* (London: William H. Allen 1837)

Ruth Vanita. "Born of Two Vaginas: Love and Reproduction Between Co-Wives in Some Medieval Indian Texts." *GLQ* 11, no. 4 (2005): 547–77

Rutherford, Thomas Corrie. *Some Experiences of Plague in India and Burma. December 1903 to June 1906.* Unpublished Dissertation. Newcastle University, Newcastle Upon Tyne: 1906

Sangvai, Sanjay. "Narmada Displacement: Continuing Outrage." *Economic and Political Weekly* 37, no. 22 (June 2002): 2132–33

Sangwan, Satpal. *Science, Technology and Colonization: An Indian Experience 1757–1857.* (Delhi: Anamika Prakashan 1991)

Sardar, Ziauddin. *The Revenge of Athena: Science, Exploitation and the Third World.* (London: Mansell 1989)

Sarkar, Sumit. "A Question Marked in Red." *Indian Express*, 9 January 2007

________. *Swadeshi Movement in Bengal, 1903–1908.* (Delhi: People's Publishing House 1973)

________. *Writing Social History.* (Delhi: Oxford University Press 1997)

Scheper-Hughes, Nancy. "Ishi's Brain, Ishi's Ashes: Anthropology and Genocide." *Anthropology Today* 17, no. 1 (2001): 12–18

Scheper-Hughes, Nancy. "The Globalization of Organ Stealing Rumours." *Anthropology Today* 12, no. 3 (1996): 3–11

Scheper-Hughes, Nancy and Margaret Lock. "The Mindful Body: A Prolegomenon to Future Work in Medical Anthropology." *Medical Anthropology Quarterly* 1, no.1 (1987): 6–41

Searle, Charles. *Cholera Its Nature, Cause, Treatment.* (London: S. Highley 1831)

Sen Gupta, P. C. "Soorjo Coomar Goodeve Chuckerbutty: The First Indian Contributor to Modern Science." *Medical History* 14, no. 2 (1970): 183–91

Shankar, Darshan and Ram Manohar. "Ayurveda Today—Ayurveda at the Crossroads." In *An Illustrated Guide to the Asian Arts of Healing.* Mark De Fraeye, ed., *Oriental Medicine:* (London: Serindia Publications 1995): 99–105

Shapin, Steven. "'Nibbling at the Teats of Science': Edinburgh and the Diffusion of Science in the 1830s." In *Metropolis and Province: Science in British Culture, 1780–1850.* Ian Inkster and Jack Morrell, eds., (London: Hutchinson 1983): 151–78

Sharma, Madhuri. "Creating a Medical Consumer: An Analytical Study of Advertisements." In *Society, Medicine and Politics: Colonial India, 1850–1940.* Biswamoy Pati and Mark Harrison, eds., (London: Routledge, Forthcoming, Expected 2008)

Sheel, Alok. "Bubonic Plague in South Bihar: Gaya and Shahabad Districts, 1900–1924." *Indian Economic and Social History Review* 35, no. 4 (1998): 421–42

Siddiqi, Majid. *The British Historical Context and Petitioning in Colonial India.* (XXIInd Dr M. A. Ansari Memorial Lecture) (Delhi: Aakar Books 2005)

Singh, Dhrub Kumar. "Cholera: Changing Perceptions of its Causality in the Last Two Centuries—A Cursory Appraisal." In *History of Medicine in India: The Medical Encounter.* Chittabrata Palit and Achintya Kumar Dutta, eds. (Delhi: Kalpaz Publications 2005): 67–86

________. "'Clouds of Cholera' and Clouds around Cholera, 1817–70." In *Disease and Medicine in India: A Historical Overview.* Deepak Kumar, ed., (New Delhi: Tulika Books 2001): 144–165

Sinha, Mrinalini. *Colonial Masculinity: The "Manly Englishman" and the "Effeminate Bengali" in the Late Nineteenth Century.* (New York: Manchester University Press 1995)

Sinha, Pradip. *Calcutta in Urban History.* (Calcutta: Firma KLM 1978)

Sinha, Sandeep. *Public Health Policy and the Indian Public: Bengal 1850–1920.* (Calcutta: Vision Publications 1998)

Sivaramakrishnan, Kavita. *Old Potions, New Bottles: Recasting Indigenous Medicine in Colonial Punjab, (1850–1945).* (Hyderabad: Orient Longman 2006)

Skinner, Quentin. "Meaning and Understanding in the History of Ideas." In *Meaning and Context: Quentin Skinner and his Critics.* J. Tully, ed., (Cambridge: Polity Press 1988): 29–67

Smith, F. B. "The Contagious Diseases Acts Reconsidered." *Social History of Medicine* 3, no. 2 (1990): 197–215

Smoult, W. H. "*The Neilgherries….*" *Calcutta Review*, XVIII (1857): xiii–xvii

Sontag, Susan. *Illness as Metaphor and AIDS and Its Metaphors.* (New York: Picador 2001)

Spinage, Clive A. *Cattle Plague: A History.* (New York: Plenum Publishers 2003)

Stengers, Jean and Anne van Neck. *Masturbation: The History of a Great Terror.* Kathryn Hoffman, trans. (New York: Palgrave 2001)

Stewart, George R. *Pickett's Charge: A Microhistory of the Final Attack at Gettysburg, July 3, 1863.* (Boston: Mariner Books 1959)

Stone, Lawrence. "Prosopography." *Daedalus* 100, no. 1 (1971): 46–71

Sudarshan, S. R., ed., "Slipada." *Encyclopaedia of Indian Medicine.* (Delhi: Popular Prakashan 2005): 228–30

Sumathipala, A, S. H. Siribaddana and D. Bhugra. "Culture Bound Syndromes: The Story of *Dhat* Syndrome." *British Journal of Psychiatry* 184 (2004): 200–9

Swami Vivekananda. "The Plague Manifesto." http://www.ramakrishnavivekananda.info/vivekananda/complete_works.htm (accessed 20 March 2008)

Sweet, Michael J. and Leonard Zwilling. "The First Medicalization: The Taxonomy and Etiology of Queerness in Classical Indian Medicine." *Journal of the History of Sexuality* 3, no. 4 (1993): 590–607

Taavitsainen, Irma and Paivi Pahta. "Vernacularisation of Medical Writing in English: A Corpus-Based Study of Scholasticism." *Early Science and Medicine* 3, no. 2 (1998): 157–85

Tagore, Rabindranath. "Letter to Maharajkumari Vidyavati Devi." Letter dated 27 December 1935. In *Selected Letters of Rabindranath Tagore.* Krishna Dutta and Andrew Robinson, eds., (Cambridge: Cambridge University Press 2005): 462–63

Tambiah, Stanley. "The Magical Power of Words." *Man* 3, no. 2 (1968): 175–208

Tarkunde, V. M. "Nuclear Tests and the 'Nation.'" *Economic and Political Weekly* 33, no. 27 (1998): 1696–7

Taussig, Michael. *Mimesis and Alterity: A Particular History of the Senses.* (New York: Routledge 1993)

Thackrah, C. T. *Cholera Its Character and Treatment with Remarks on the Identity of the Indian and English and a Particular Reference to the Disease now existent at New Castle and its Neighbourhood.* (Leeds: J. Baines 1832)

Thompson, John. *An Account of the Life, Lectures and Writings of William Cullen MD Vol. II.* (Edinburgh: William Blackwood and Sons 1832)

Trollope-Kumar, Karen. "Cultural and Biomedical Meanings of the Complaint of Leukorrhea in South Asian Women." *Tropical Medicine and International Health* 6, no. 4 (2001): 260–66

Uddin, Iktidar. "A Case of Cholera." *Indian Medical Gazette* XVII (December 1882): 320

Urban, Hugh B. *Songs of Ecstasy: Tantric and Devotional Songs from Colonial Bengal.* (New York: Oxford University Press 2001)

Vaughan, Megan. *Curing their Ills: Colonial Power and African Illness.* (Stanford: Stanford University Press 1991)

Wade, John Peter. *Select Evidences of a Successful Method of Treating Fever and Dysentery in Bengal.* (London: J. Murray 1761)

Ward, William. *A View of the History, Literature, Mythology of the Hindoos Vol. I.* (Serampore: The Mission Press 1818)

Waring, Edward J. "Notice of Aegle Marmelos." *The Medical Times and Gazette* 1, (1864): 198–99

Watson, Thomas. *Lectures on the Principles and Practice of Physic Delivered at the King's College.* 3rd American Edition. (Philadelphia: Blanchard and Lea, 1855)

Wear, Andrew. "Popularization of Medicine in Early Modern England." In *The Popularization of Medicine, 1650–1850.* Roy Porter, ed., (London: Routledge 2001): 17–41

White, David Gordon. "Transformations in the Art of Love: Kamkala Practices in Hindu Tantric and Kaula Traditions." *History of Religions* 38 no. 2 (1998): 172–98

Whorton, James C. *Inner Hygiene: Constipation and the Pursuit of Health in Modern Society.* (Oxford: Oxford University Press 2000)

Wig, N. N. "Problems of Mental Health in India." *Journal of Clinical and Social Psychiatry* 17, no. 2 (1960): 48–53

Wigglesworth, Michael. *The Diary of Michael Wigglesworth, 1653–1657: The Conscience of a Puritan* Edmund Sears Morgan, ed., (New York: Harper's & Co. 1965)

Wilson, H. H. "*Kushta*, Or Leprosy as Known to the Hindus." *Transactions of the Medical and Physical Society of Calcutta* 1 (1825)

Wise, Thomas Alexander. *Commentary on the Hindu System of Medicine.* (Calcutta: Thacker Spink & Co. 1845)

———. *Review of the History of Medicine* (London: J Churchhill 1867)

Worboys, Michael. "Germs, Malaria and the Invention of Mansonian Tropical Medicine: From 'Diseases in the Tropics' to 'Tropical Diseases.'" In *Warm Climates and Western Medicine.* David Arnold, ed., (Amsterdam: Rodopi 1996)

———. *Spreading Germs: Disease Theories and Medical Practice in Britain, 1865–1900.* (Cambridge: Cambridge University Press 2000)

Wright, John P. "Hysteria and the Mechanical Man." *Journal of the History of Ideas* 41, no. 2 (1980): 233–47

Wujastyk, Dominik. *The Roots of Ayurveda.* (London: Penguin Books 2003)

Yap, P. M. "Words and Things in Comparative Psychiatry with Special Reference to Exotic Psychosis." *Acta Psychatria Scandinavia* 38 (1962): 157–82

Zachariah, Benjamin. *Developing India: An Intellectual and Social History, c.1930–50*. (Delhi: Oxford University Press 2005)
________. *Nehru*. (London: Routledge 2004)

Bengali Works

Ahmed, Hafez Nazar. *Tibb-e Nobbi*. Maulana Mohammed Nuruj Jaman, trans. (Dhaka: Madrasa Darul Ulum 1997)
Ahmed, Mohammed Reyajuddin. *Brihat Mohammadiya Panjika for 1318 BS*. (Calcutta: Kaji Osman Ali 1911)
Ali, Lakshmikanta. "*Epidemik Dropsi ba Samkramak Shoth*." *Bhisak Darpan* 19, no. 9 (1909): 328–35
Anonymous. *Daktar Dwarkanath Ray Mohashoyer Shongkhipta Jeebori*. (Calcutta: Art Press 1926)
________. "*Deshiya Swasthya Vigyan*." *Chikitsa Sammilani* 2, no. ? (1888): 101–02
________. "*Gabsthrailokya—Matarah*." *Swasthya Samachar* 16, no.1 (1927): 19–20
________. "*Gata Varsha*." *Chikitsa Sammilani* 4, no. 1 (1887): 1–7
________. "*Kaolin Dwara Kolera Chikitsa*." *Swasthya Samachar* 17, no. 3 (1928): 87–8
________. "*Khadya-Dravya Pariksha*." *Gharer Katha* 2, no. 1 (1929): 21–31
________. "*Kolera Sambandhey Guti Kotok Katha*." *Chikitsa Sammilani* 5, no. ? (1888): 335–44
________. "*Mulyaprapti*." *Chikitsa Sammilani* 3, no. 1 (1887): Two initial unnumbered pages and pages 2–4.
________. "*Mulyaprapti I*." *Chikitsa Sammilani* 4, no. 1 (1888): i–iv
________. "Nucleo-Poroteid Compound." *Chikitsa Prakash* 13, no. 1 (1920): 4–5
________. "Nuctarlin." *Chikitsa Prakash* 13, no. 6/7 (1920): 245–47
________. "*Olautha Chikitsa*." *Chikitsak O Samalochak* 1, nos. 5 & 6 (1895): 152–53
________. "*Olauthar Homiopathik Chikitsa*." *Chikitsa Sammilani* 3, no. ? (1887): 27–9
________. "*Plaguer Aushadh*." *Chikitsak* 3, no. 4 (1899): 74–5
________. "*Prerita Patra*." *Chikitsa Prakash* 13, no. 1 (1920): 341
________. *Shokavijay*. (Calcutta: np 1881)
________. "*Vaidik Vyavahar Sambandhey Prasna*." *Bhishak Darpan* 10, no. 8 (1900): 351–2
________. "*Vaidya Mathey Chikitsita Rogir Vivaran*." *Chikitsa Sammilani* 2, no. ? (1888): 191–2
________. "Zahiruddin Ahmed." *Bhisak Darpan* 6, no. 1 (1898): 1
Ayurvediya Bhesaj Ashram. "*Swarna-ghatita Makaranda Rasayan*." (Advertisement) in Kaviraj, Sukhdeb *Kaviraji Mushtiyog*, fifth edition. (Calcutta: Gupta Press (nd))
Bagchi, Girishchandra. "*Ashangamik Brodhno*." *Bhisak Darpan* 5, no. 5 (1896): 194–201
________. "*Pet Bedana—Shul*." *Bhisak Darpan* 23, no. 3 (1913): 83–98
________. "*Sampadak Parivartan*." *Bhisak Darpan* 10, no. 1 (1900): Inside front cover
Bagchi, Gyanendranarayan. *Bagher Baccha*. (Calcutta: Bijoykumar Mitra 1920)
Bandopadhyay, Kalipada. *Prakritik Chikitsa*. (Calcutta: ? 1894)
Bandopadhyay, Surendranath. "*Daibya Shakti o Chikitsa Bigyan*." *Chikitsak O Samalochak* 2, no. 3 (1896): 41–55
Bandopadhyay, Tarashankar. *Arogya Niketan*. (Calcutta: Prakash Bhavan 2007)
Basak, Bhubanchandra. *Jalpan Bidhi*. (Calcutta: Gyan Ratnakar Yantra 1884)
________. *Prachin Aushadhavali*. (*Lolimbaraj Mathey*). (Calcutta, nd)
Basak, Gyanchandra. *Surapan*. (Calcutta, 1888)
Basak, Harimohan. *Grihamushtiyoga*. (Dhaka: Nababpur Narayan Yantra 1900)
Basu, Amritakrishna. *Plague Tattwa*. (Calcutta: Taruni Press 1899)

Basu, Anjali, ed. *Samsad Bangali Charitabhidhan*. Second edition. (Calcutta: Sishu Sahitya Samsad 2002)

Basu, Charuchandra. "Acetonuria." *Bhisak Darpan* 20, no. 7 (1910): 241–5

________. "Indicanuria." *Bhisak Darpan* 19, no. 8 (1909): 293–6

Basu, Chunilal. *Palli Vasir Prati Nivedan*. Second edition. (Calcutta: np, 1919)

Basu, Dakshinaranjan. *Chhere Asha Gram*. (Calcutta: Jignasa 1975)

Basu, Jagadbandhu. "*Elopathy Mathey Olautharogey Udaradhman*." *Chikitsa Sammilani* 2, no. ? (1888): 95–9

Basu, Panchanan. "*Bhaitameen Kichhu*." *Swasthya Samachar* 16, no. 4 (1927): 120–2

Basu, Pradeep Kumar. *Samoyiki: Bijnan O SomajI*. (Calcutta: Ananda Publishers 1998)

Basu, Rajnarayan. *Se Kal Ar Ekal*. (Calcutta: Bangiya Sahitya Parishad 1956)

Basu, Rajsekhar. '*Bhusundir Math*' in *Parasuram Granthavali*. (Calcutta: MC Sarkar & Sons Pvt Ltd 1987): 52–62

________. "*Chikitsa Sankat*." In *Parasuram Granthavali*. (Calcutta: Print-O-Graph 1987): 19–30

________. "*Daktari O Kaviraji*." In *Parasuram Granthavali*. (Calcutta: Print-O-Graph 1987): 228–35

________. "*Jodu Daktarer Patient*." *Parasuram Granthavali*. (Calcutta: Print-O-Graph 1987): 183–90

________. "*Rajbhog*." in *Parasuram Granthavali*. (Calcutta: Print-O-Graph 1987): 78–81

Basu Barman, Fakirchandra. *Karyasadhak Aushadhgyan*. (Calcutta: Nutan Bangla Yantra 1876)

Bhadra, Gautam. *Jal Rajar Golpo: Bardhamaner Protapchand*. (Calcutta: Ananda Publishers 2002)

________. "*Nera Bot-tolaye Jaye Kobar?*" In *Abaabhash*. Rushati Sen, ed., (Calcutta 2006)

________. "*Unish Satake Bangla Boi-er Bigyapan*." (Calcutta: Susobhan Sarkar Memorial Lecture 2000)

Bhattacharya, Charuchandra. *Bangalir Khadya*. (Calcutta: Gurudas Chattopadhyay & Sons., nd)

Bhattacharya, Nrisingha, ed., *Brihat Indrajal*. (Calcutta: Rajendra Library, nd)

Bhattacharya, Sukhdeb, comp. *Sarba Siddhidata Pustak*. (Calcutta: Rajendra Library, nd)

Bhattacharya, Sukhdeb. *Sarbasiddhidata Pustak*. (Calcutta: Rajendra Library, nd)

Bhattacharya, Surendramohan. *Dakini Vidya*. (Calcutta: Bengal Medical Library 1911)

Bhattacharya, Upendranath. *Banglar Baul O Baul Gaan*. (Calcutta: Orient Book Company 2001)

Bhuttacharya, Amritalal. *A Practical Treatise on Malarious Fevers with Their Complications and Sequelae*. (Calcutta: Elm Press 1897)

Bidyanidhi, Srichandra. *Lord Ripon's Panjika for 1290 BS*. (Calcutta: Bidyaratna Yantra 1883)

Biswas, Sailendra. *Samsad Bengali-English Dictionary*. (Calcutta: Sahitya Samsad 2000)

Breton, Peter. *Olauthar Vivaran*. (Calcutta: Calcutta School Book Society 1826)

Buchanan, W. J. "*Sankramak Rogl*." *Bhisak Darpan* 15, no. 7 (1905): 241–59

Chakrabarti, Sambuddha. *Andarey Antarey: Unish Satake Bangali Bhadramahila*. (Calcutta: Stree 1995)

Chakrabarty, Amarkrishna. "*Olabibir Gaan*." *Shahitya Parishad Patrika* 3, no. 4 (1983): 30–41

Chakrabarty, Amulyaratan. *Captain Narendranather Jeebonkotha*. (Calcutta: Nava Shakti Press 1952)

Chakrabarty, Dipesh. '*Shareer, Samaj o Rashtra: Oupanibeshik Bharatey Mahamari o Janasanskriti*." In *Nimnabarger Itihaas*. Gautam Bhadra and Partha Chattopadhyay, eds., (Kolkata: Ananda Publishers 2001): 161–180

Chakrabarty, Haridas. "*Oluatha Nivaraner Upaya.*" *Chikitsa Sammilani* 8, no. ? (1891): 92–95
Chakrabarty, Hariprasad. *Daktari Abhidhan.* (Dhaka: 1889)
Chakrabarty, Hariprasad. *Homiopathic Bhaisajyatattwa o Chikitsa Pradarsika.* (Dhaka: 1880)
Chakrabarty, Ramakanta. "*Haridaser Guptakatha.*" *Bangalir Dharma, Samaj O Sanskriti.* (Calcutta: Subarnarekha 2002): 190–203
________. "*Hindu Punarutthyaner Tattwavali.*" *Bangalir Dharma, Samaj O Sanskriti.* (Calcutta: Subarnarekha 2002): 252–67
Chakrabarty, Sachindranath. *Saral Totka Chikitsa.* (Calcutta: Akshay Press, nd)
Chakrabarty, Saradaprasad. *Bishuchika Chikitsa Sar.* (Calcutta: Berini & Co. 1892)
________. *Saral Chikitsa Tattwa.* (Calcutta: The Author 1914)
Chakrabarty, Satyasaran. "*Rog: Todutpotti O Kromobikash.*" *Bhisak Darpan* 19, no. 6 (1909): 212–23
Chakrabarty, Sudheer. *Bangla Dehatattwer Gaan.* (Calcutta: Pustak Bipani 1990)
Chattopadhyay, Aswinikumar. "*Kolera o Malaria Sambandhey Dui Khani Darkari Chithi.*" *Grihasthya Mangal* 1, no. 9 (1927): 352–3
Chattopadhyay, D. N. "*Kolera ba Olautha.*" *Bhisak Darpan* 23, no. 4 (1913): 126–37
________. "*Kolera ba Olautha II.*" *Bhisak Darpan* 23, no. 5 (1913): 168–73
Chattopadhyay, Lalitmohan. "*Dhatu Dourbalya.*" *Bhisak Darpan* 6, no. 1 (1896): 20–23
________. "*Dhatu Dourbalya I.*" *Bhisak Darpan* 10, no. 6 (1900): 221–24
________. "*Paras-Bai.*" *Bhisak Darpan* 6, no. 5 (1896): 188–89
Chattopadhyay, Saratchandra. "*Grihadaha.*" *Sarat Rachanavali.* (Calcutta: Sarat Samiti 1976): 231–400
Chaudhuri, Sarachchandra. *Garhasthyavigyan.* (Mymensingh: 1880)
Chottopadhyay, Ashwinikumar. *Palli Mangal Granthavali.* (Calcutta: Palli Mangal Office 1938–40)
Choudhury, Abdul Ajed Khan. "*Chikitshokgoner Sochehoritro O Neeti Shikhya.*" *Bhisak Darpan* 6, no. 4 (1896): 133–38
________. "*Paglami Kar?*" *Bhisak Darpan* 10, no. 9 (1900): 360–73
Das, Kunjabihari. "*Bishuchi-Rakshan.*" *Bhisak Darpan* 10, no. 9 (1900): 353–60
________. "*Bishuchi-Rakshan II.*" *Bhisak Darpan* 10, no. 10 (1900): 404–13
________. "*Bukchapa* (Nightmare)." *Bhisak Darpan* 6, no. 11 (1897): 441–47
Das, Mukunda. *Palliseva.* (Barisal: np, 1931)
Das, Satyaranjan. "*Kolerar Prabal Hikkaye—Potash Iodide-er Upakarita.*" *Chikitsa Prakash* 13, no. 8 (1920): 294–8
Das, Sundarimohan. "*Gil-Dhil-Pill-Bill-Kill.*" *Swasthya Samachar* 16, no. 6 (1927): 186–90
________. "*Gramer Sekal o Ekal.*" *Grihasthya Mangal* 4, no. 12 (1930): 310–11
________. *Munisipal Darpan.* (Calcutta: Prabhakar Yantra 1892)
Dasgupta, Kaliprasanna. *Ledi Daktar.* (Calcutta: Emerald Friting Works 1921)
________. *Pallir Pran.* (Calcutta: np, 1919)
Datta, Manindrabhushan. "Rai Nabinchandra Datta Bahadur." *Navyabharat* 38, no. 3 (1920): 129–38
Datta, Nafarchandra. *Sachitra Sahaj Daktari Shikhya.* (Calcutta: Sudharnab Press 1905)
________. *Sahaj Daktari Sikhya.* (Calcutta: Amritalal Datta 1905 [5th Edn.])
De, Umacharan. *Garhasthya Chikitsabhidhan. Second edition.* (Calcutta: The Author 1880)
Deb, Kunjabihari. *Thengapathic Bhnuiphod Daktar.* (Calcutta: Manimohan Rakshit 1887) The text was published under the authorship of 'Ami' (Me). However, the Blumhardt catalogue of the British Library's collection identifies the author as Kunjabihari Deb.

Dutta, Jadunath. *Prankrishnaushadhavali.* Fifth reprint (Calcutta: Sudharnav Yantra 1877)
Elektro-Ayurvedic Farmesi. "Elektro-Ayurvedic Aushadhavali." *Grihasthya Mangal* 4, no. 1 (1930): front cover
Forster, H. P. *Vocabulary in Two Parts, Bongalee and English and Vice Versa Part II.* (Calcutta: Post Press 1802)
Gangopadhyay, Jadunath. "*Banglar Chikitsak Samaj.*" *Chikitsa Sammilani* 6, nos. 5, 6 & 7 (1889): 178–92
Ganguly, Brajendranath. "*Kolerar Pratisedhak.*" *Grihasthya Mangal* 1, no. 3 (1927): 103–4
Gavin, Dr "Spermatone." (Advertisement). *Grihasthya Mangal* 4, no. 1 (1930): 1
Ghosh, Biharilal. *Bangiya Garhasthya Chikitsa.* (Calcutta: 1878–9)
Ghosh, Doyal Krissen. *Malaria.* (Calcutta: np, 1878)
Ghosh, Gopinath. *Tattwayoga ba Varnachikitsa.* (Calcutta: 1921)
Ghosh, Harinath. "*Kolera.*" *Bhisak Darpan* 22, no. 2 (1912): 49–56
Ghosh, Kiran Chandra. *E Myanual oph Injekshan Chikitsa.* Second edition, 1923. Third edition, 1926. (Calcutta: 1921)
Ghosh, Mahendranath. "*Bhakkhya Dravya ba Khadya.*" *Bhisak Darpan* 19, no. 7 (1909): 266–73
Ghosh, Pramathanath. *Sarpaghater Chikitsa.* (Calcutta: 1868)
Ghoshal, Lalmohan. "*Banglar Jwar Sambandhe Mantabya.*" *Bhisak Darpan* 16, no. 7 (1906): 245–47
Goswami, Jayanta. *Samaj Chitre Unabingsha Satabdir Bangla Prahasan.* (Calcutta: 1974)
Guha, Kulachandra. "*Ekti Rogir Vivaran.*" *Bhisak Darpan* 22, no. 11 (1912): 423–28
________. "*Pratirodh Shakti.*" *Bhisak Darpan* 22, no. 12 (1912): 441–51
________. "*Pratirodh Shakti I.*" *Bhisak Darpan* 22, no. 11 (1912): 428–40
________. "*Shishuder Tiubarkel.*" *Bhisak Darpan* 19, no. 8 (1909): 296–309
________. "*Shustha Shareere Vyamer Prayajaniyata o Karjya.*" *Bhisak Darpan* 20, no. 1 (1910): 29–2
Guha Thakurta, Manoranjan. *Ashapradeep.* (Barisal: Manomohan Chakravarty 1887)
Gupta, Anandamohan. "*Koshtabaddhata.*" *Grihasthya Mangal* 5, no. 1(1931): 14
Gupta, Bipinbihari. *Mushtiyoga Sarsamgraha.* (Calcutta: Kamalakanta Press 1902)
Gupta D. D.[1] "Abar Plague." Swasthya 5, no. 11 (1901): 321–22
________. "Aharer Pariman." Swasthya 4, no. 2 (1900): 46–50
________. "Anahar o Durbhikkya." Swasthya 4, no. 2 (1900): 55–57
________. "Bajarer Khabar." Swasthya 4, no. 6 (1900): 175–7
________. "Bangali Saheb Nahe." Swasthya 5, no. 2 (1901): 36–37
________. "Bari Bhada." Swasthya 4, no. 8 (1900): 230–32
________. "Basagriha." Swasthya 2, no. 1 (1898): 5–7
________. "Beg Rodher Apakarita." Swasthya 2, no. 8 (1898): 193
________. "Daihik Jama-Kharach." Swasthya 3, no. 8 (1899): 232–36
________. "Dokaner Mithai." Swasthya 3, no. 8 (1899): 231–32
________. "Dourbalya I." Swasthya 3, no. 7 (1899): 207–09
________. "Dourbalya." Swasthya 4, no. 3 (1900): 78–81
________. "Grihasthya o Janjal." Swasthya 4, no. 11 (1900): 321–22
________. "Grishmakale Pallir Gram." Swasthya 2, no. 11 (1898): 265–66
________. "Jalasaucha." Swasthya 2, no. 8 (1898): 169–70
________. "Koshtabaddhata", Swasthya 5, no. 10 (1901): 314–19
________. "Naitrojen Khadya." Swasthya 5, no. 3 (1901): 81–82
________. "Palligramer Paniya Jal." Swasthya 2, no. 11 (1898): 244–46
________. "Pathya Nirdharan." Swasthya 4, no. 6 (1900): 171–75

________. "Plague Chikitsa." In *Basu, Pradeep Kumar Samoyiki: Bijnan O Somaj* (Calcutta: Ananda Publishers 1998): 245–47

________. "Plague-er Purbey Bombai." Swasthya 3, no. 1 (1899): 22–24

________. "Plague Hoitey Shikhya." In *Samoyiki: Bijnan O Somaj*. Pradip Kumar Basu, ed., (Calcutta: Ananda Publishers 1998): 248–50

———. "Plague Nibaran Bishay Gobhernment-er Chesta." Swasthya 4, no. 1 (1900): 13–16

________. "Plague Nibaron." In *Samoyiki: Bijnan O Somaj*. Pradip Kumar Basu, ed., (Calcutta: Ananda Publishers 1998): 256–57

________. "Plague Nibaron Upaye" In *Samoyiki: Bijnan O Somaj*. Pradip Kumar Basu, ed., (Calcutta: Ananda Publishers 1998): 279–83

________. "Plague O Sankirtan." Swasthya 3, no. 12 (1899): 351–54

________. "Plaguer Pradurbhabey Kolikatar Atith O Bartaman Obasthya." Swasthya 2, no. 4 (1898): 80–83

________. "Plague Sambandhey Amader Baktabya." Swasthya 4, no. 1 (1900): 16–20

________. "Pratarutthan." Swasthya 2, no. 1 (1898): 2–3

________. "Rogi Prithakikaran." Swasthya 2, no.1 (1898): 16–17

________. "Saharer Dudh." Swasthya 2, no. 7 (1898): 146–47

________. "Sambad I." Swasthya 2, no. 2 (1898): 46–48

________. "Sambad." Swasthya 2, no. 5 (1898): 119–20

________. "Samkramak Rog o Deshiya Pratha." Swasthya 2, no. 2 (1898): 27–28

________. "Shikhya O Swasthya." Swasthya 5, no. 7 (1901): 195–203

________. "Shishuder Khadyer Pariman." Swasthya 2, no. 7 (1898): 153–55

________. "Streediger Swasthya." Swasthya 4, no. 7 (1900): 218–24

________. "Swasthya Prasanga." in Pradeep Kumar Basu ed., Samoyiki: Bijnan O Somaj (Calcutta: Ananda Publishers, 1998): 288–89

________. "Ucchhistha Dosh." Swasthya 4, no. 6(1900): 163–64

________. "Vividha I." Swasthya 2, no. 11 (1898): 259–61

________. "Vividha II." Swasthya 2, no. 8 (1898): 190–91

________. "Vividha III." Swasthya 2, no. 10 (1898): 237–38

________. "Vividha Vishaya O Sambad." Swasthya 4, no. 3 (1900): 11–14

________. "Vyam Charcha." Swasthya 4, no. 3 (1900): 81–84

Gupta, Haralal. *Ayurved Bhasabhidhan.* (Calcutta: Kalika Yantra 1888)

Gupta, Rasiklal. *Bhabprakash.* (Title page missing. Possibly Calcutta: 1883)

Haldar, Dheerendranath. "*Change ba Hawa Paribartan.*" *Chikitsa Prakash* 14, no. 1 (1921)

Jyotirbhushan, Kunjabihari. "*Shuddhachar.*" *Bhisak Darpan* 20, no. 9 (1910): 348–53

Kar, Durgadas. *Bhaisajya Ratnavali.* (Calcutta: np, 1868)

________. *Bhisak Bandhu.* Radhagobinda Kar, comp. Second edition. (Calcutta: 1879)

Kar, Radha Gobinda. *Bhisak Suhrid or the Physicians' Vade Mecum Designed for the Use of Students Preparing for Examination & Practitioners.* (Calcutta: The Author 1880)

Kaviratna, Avinashchandra. "*Amader Katha.*" *Chikitsa Sammilani* 9, no. 1 (1893): 35–38

________. "Daktar Annadacharan Khastagir." *Chikitsha Sammilani* 4, no. 4 (1887): unnumbered pages inserted between pp. 36 and 37.

________. "*Sampadakiya Baktabya.*" *Chikitsa Sammilani* 9, no. ? (1893): 230–31

Khater, Mohammed. *Asrar al-Khwabnama: Dusra Balam.* (Calcutta: Harihar Yantra 1877)

________. *Asrar al-Khwabnama: Pahela Balam.* (Calcutta: Harihar Yantra,1877)

________. *Solemani Talenama.* (Calcutta: Sudharnav Press, 1880)

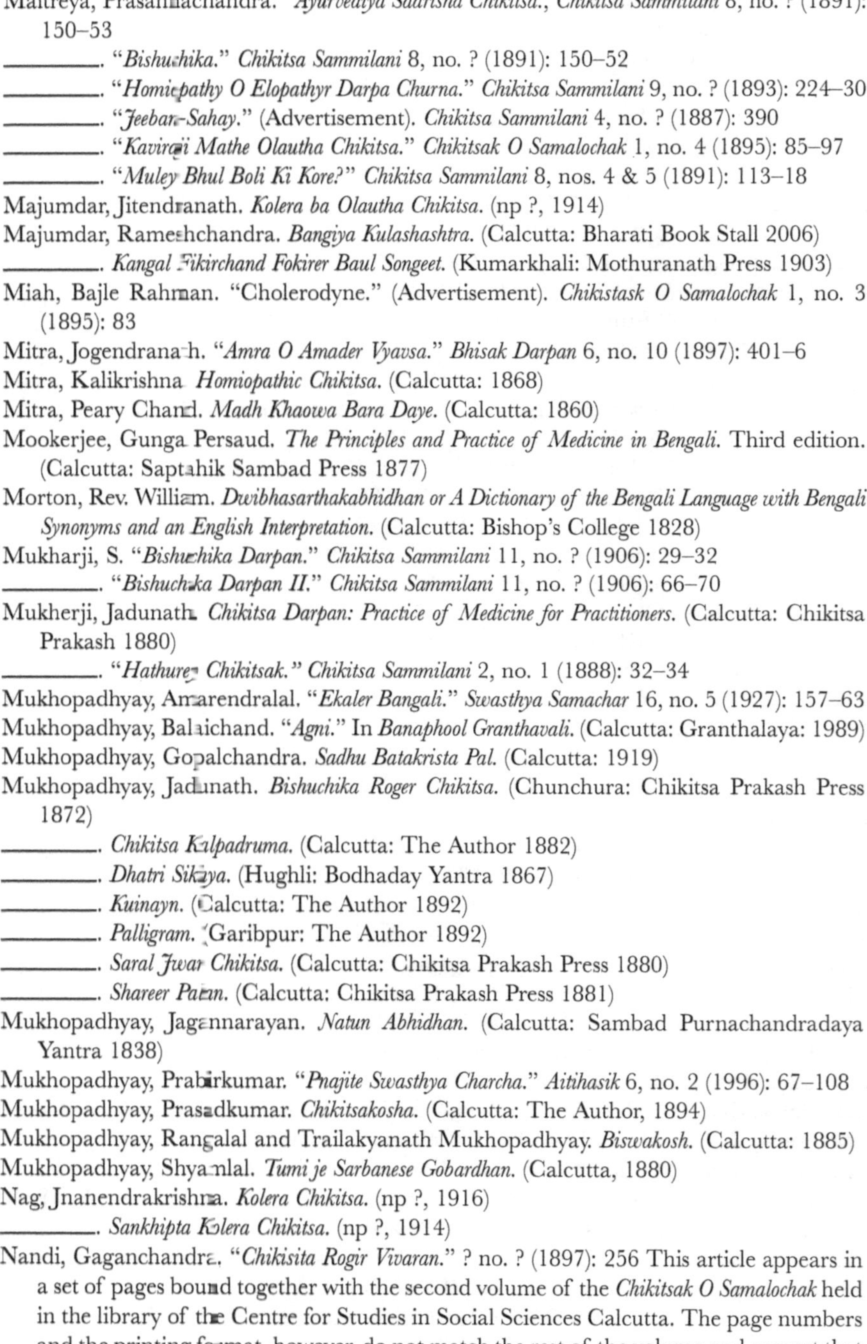

Maitreya, Prasannachandra. "*Ayurvediya Sadrisha Chikitsa.*, *Chikitsa Sammilani* 8, no. ? (1891): 150–53

________. "*Bishuchika.*" *Chikitsa Sammilani* 8, no. ? (1891): 150–52

________. "*Homiopathy O Elopathyr Darpa Churna.*" *Chikitsa Sammilani* 9, no. ? (1893): 224–30

________. "*Jeeban-Sahay.*" (Advertisement). *Chikitsa Sammilani* 4, no. ? (1887): 390

________. "*Kaviraji Mathe Olautha Chikitsa.*" *Chikitsak O Samalochak* 1, no. 4 (1895): 85–97

________. "*Muley Bhul Boli Ki Kore?*" *Chikitsa Sammilani* 8, nos. 4 & 5 (1891): 113–18

Majumdar, Jitendranath. *Kolera ba Olautha Chikitsa.* (np ?, 1914)

Majumdar, Rameshchandra. *Bangiya Kulashashtra.* (Calcutta: Bharati Book Stall 2006)

________. *Kangal Fikirchand Fokirer Baul Songeet.* (Kumarkhali: Mothuranath Press 1903)

Miah, Bajle Rahman. "Cholerodyne." (Advertisement). *Chikistask O Samalochak* 1, no. 3 (1895): 83

Mitra, Jogendranath. "*Amra O Amader Vyavsa.*" *Bhisak Darpan* 6, no. 10 (1897): 401–6

Mitra, Kalikrishna *Homiopathic Chikitsa.* (Calcutta: 1868)

Mitra, Peary Chand. *Madh Khaowa Bara Daye.* (Calcutta: 1860)

Mookerjee, Gunga Persaud. *The Principles and Practice of Medicine in Bengali.* Third edition. (Calcutta: Saptahik Sambad Press 1877)

Morton, Rev. William. *Dwibhasarthakabhidhan or A Dictionary of the Bengali Language with Bengali Synonyms and an English Interpretation.* (Calcutta: Bishop's College 1828)

Mukharji, S. "*Bishuchika Darpan.*" *Chikitsa Sammilani* 11, no. ? (1906): 29–32

________. "*Bishuchika Darpan II.*" *Chikitsa Sammilani* 11, no. ? (1906): 66–70

Mukherji, Jadunath. *Chikitsa Darpan: Practice of Medicine for Practitioners.* (Calcutta: Chikitsa Prakash 1880)

________. "*Hathurer Chikitsak.*" *Chikitsa Sammilani* 2, no. 1 (1888): 32–34

Mukhopadhyay, Amarendralal. "*Ekaler Bangali.*" *Swasthya Samachar* 16, no. 5 (1927): 157–63

Mukhopadhyay, Balaichand. "*Agni.*" In *Banaphool Granthavali.* (Calcutta: Granthalaya: 1989)

Mukhopadhyay, Gopalchandra. *Sadhu Batakrista Pal.* (Calcutta: 1919)

Mukhopadhyay, Jadunath. *Bishuchika Roger Chikitsa.* (Chunchura: Chikitsa Prakash Press 1872)

________. *Chikitsa Kalpadruma.* (Calcutta: The Author 1882)

________. *Dhatri Sikhya.* (Hughli: Bodhaday Yantra 1867)

________. *Kuinayn.* (Calcutta: The Author 1892)

________. *Palligram.* (Garibpur: The Author 1892)

________. *Saral Jwar Chikitsa.* (Calcutta: Chikitsa Prakash Press 1880)

________. *Shareer Palan.* (Calcutta: Chikitsa Prakash Press 1881)

Mukhopadhyay, Jagannarayan. *Natun Abhidhan.* (Calcutta: Sambad Purnachandradaya Yantra 1838)

Mukhopadhyay, Prabirkumar. "*Pnajite Swasthya Charcha.*" *Aitihasik* 6, no. 2 (1996): 67–108

Mukhopadhyay, Prasadkumar. *Chikitsakosha.* (Calcutta: The Author, 1894)

Mukhopadhyay, Rangalal and Trailakyanath Mukhopadhyay. *Biswakosh.* (Calcutta: 1885)

Mukhopadhyay, Shyamlal. *Tumi je Sarbanese Gobardhan.* (Calcutta, 1880)

Nag, Jnanendrakrishna. *Kolera Chikitsa.* (np ?, 1916)

________. *Sankhipta Kolera Chikitsa.* (np ?, 1914)

Nandi, Gaganchandra. "*Chikisita Rogir Vivaran.*" ? no. ? (1897): 256 This article appears in a set of pages bound together with the second volume of the *Chikitsak O Samalochak* held in the library of the Centre for Studies in Social Sciences Calcutta. The page numbers and the printing format, however, do not match the rest of the volume and suggest that it was an issue from some other publication—perhaps the *Chikitsa Sammilani*—which were bound together by mistake at some point.

Pahari, Subrata. *Unish Sataker Banglaye Sanatani Chikitsa Vyavasthyar Swarup*. (Calcutta: Progressive Publishers 2001)

Porter, William Henry. "*Antrik Ajirna Rog, Tahar Juktijukta Chikitsa o Pathya Vyavasthya*." *Bhisak Darpan* 6, no. 1 (1896): 2–7

Rafdhar, R. E. "*Madhu Makkhika, Bolta ebam Bhimrul Dangshan*." *Bhisak Darpan* 6, no. 1 (1896): 9–16

Rahim, Abdur. *Dhakar Nawab Saheber Punthi*. (Calcutta: Reyajul Islam Press 1906)

Ray, Binodbihari. "*Bayu, Pittwa, Kaph*." *Chikitsak* 1, no. 3 (1889): 52–56

Ray, Devendranath. "*Bangalir Shareer Poshan*." *Bhisak Darpan* 20, no. 2 (1910):58–61

________. *Bhaisajya Sutra O Vyavahara: Principles and Practice of Medicine*. (Calcutta: 1895)

________. "*Biubonik Plague*." *Bhisak Darpan* 6, no. 5 (1896): 185–87

________. "*Samkramak Shoth*." *Bhisak Darpan* 19, no. 2 (1909): 51–55

________. "*Shareer Poshane Chittenden*." *Bhisak Darpan* 19, no. 6 (1909): 223–27

Ray, Durgacharan. *Deb Ganer Marte Agaman*. (Calcutta: Ranjan Press 1911)

Ray, Satyacharan. "*Biubonik Plague Ba Mahamari*." *Chikitsak O Samalochak* 2, no. 12 (1896): 319–28

Raychaudhury, Rajkrishna. *Naradeha Nirnaya*. (Calcutta: 1869)

Roy, Benoybhusan. *Unish Satake Banglar Chikitsa Vyavasthya, Deshiya Bhesaj o Sarkar*. (Delhi: International Centre for Bengal Studies 1998)

Roy, Binodbihari. "*Nivedan*." *Chikitsak* 1, no. 5 (1889): inside front cover

Roy, Kamakhyaprasad. *Mayapuri*. (Calcutta: Surathkumar Sarkar 1937)

Roy, Nibaranchandra. "*Vaigyanik Iswar*." *Bhisak Darpan* 23, no. 1 (1913): 1–13

Roy, Rajkrishna. *Daktarbabu*. (Calcutta: Beena Yantra 1889)

Roy, Satyakrishna. "*Bhumika*." *Chikitsak O Samalochak* 1, no. 1 (1896): 1–11

Roy, Taraknath. "*Jeevanishakti* (Vital Force)." *Bhisak Darpan* 14, no.12 (1904): 441–47

Sambuddha (Amulyakumar Dasgupta). "*Kaviraj*." In *Sambuddha Rachanavali Vol. 1*. Prabir Mukhopadhyay, ed., (Calcutta: Ababhaas 2007): 339–45

Sanyal, Durgacharan. *Banglar Samajik Itihas*. (Kolkata: Model Publishing House 1997)

Sanyal, Pulinchandra. *Chikitsa Kalpataru Vol. III*. (Calcutta: Bengal Medical Library, 1904)

________. *Chikitsa Kalpataru Vol. IV*. (Calcutta: Bengal Medical Library 1916)

________. "*Muley Bhul*." *Chikitsa Sammilani* 8, nos. 2 and 3 (1890): 41–47

Sanyal Pulinchandra and Avinashchandra Kaviratna. "*Prameha ba Dhater Pirha*." *Chikitsa Sammilani* 5, no. ? (1888): 193–94

Sarkar, Jashodanandan. *Susruta Samhita (Mul O Banganuvad)*. (Calcutta: Bangabasi Steam Meshin Press 1894)

Sedgewick, William. "*Roganukrome Sambandhe Abhijattyer Adhipattya*." *Bhisak Darpan* 6, no. 1 (1896): 16–19

Sen, Binodlal. *Ayurvediya Dravyabhidhan*. (Calcutta: Ayurved Yantra 1876)

________. *Bhesaja Ratnavali*. (Calcutta: Ayurved Yantra 1884)

Sen, Dineshchandra. *Brihat Banga Vol. I*. (Calcutta: De's Publishing 1992)

Sen, Harimohan. "*Banga Desher Swasthya*." *Bhisak Darpan* 20, no. 8 (1910): 281–98

________. "*Smashan Kalkata*." *Bhisak Darpan* 22, no. 7 (1912): 249–52

________. "*Swasthya Rakshya O Swasthya Unnatir Upaya*." *Bhisak Darpan* 21, no. 11 and 12 (1911): 401–28

________. "*Udbhid Jeebanu*." *Bhisak Darpan* 21, no. 10 (1911): 361–82

Sen, Hemchandra. "*Swabhabik Rog-Badhok Shakti.*" *Chikitsa Sammilani* 12 no. ? (1900): 137–43

Sen, Hur Chunder. *Venereal Disease in Bengali.* (Calcutta: Gupta Press 1882)

Sen, Pearymohan. "*Shesh Nivedan., Chikitsa Sammilani* 4, no. ? (1887): Unnumbered page preceding p. 133

Sengupta, Debendranath and Upendranath Sengupta. *Charak Samhita (Banganuvad).* (Calcutta: Dhanwantari Steam Meshin Yantra 1909)

Sengupta, Nagendranath. *Dravya Guna Shikhya.* (Calcutta: 1902)

Sengupta, Pearymohan. *Sharangadhar Samgraha.* (Calcutta: Benimadhab De & Co. 1889)

Sengupta, Sachindranath. *Narsin Hom.* (Calcutta: Gurudas Chattopadhyay & Sons 1940)

Sengupta, Subodhchandra and Anjali Ghosh. *Samsad Bangali Charitabhidhan.* (Calcutta: Sahitya Samsad 1976)

Shamsuddin, M. "*Influenjar Notun Murti. Influnza Heart.*" *Chikitsa Prakash* 13, no. 2 (1920): 58–62

Sharif, Ahmed. *Medhyayuger Sahitye Samaj O Sanskritir Rup.* (Dhaka: Shomoy 2000)

Shastri, Shibnath. "*Brahmo Dharmer Prabhaber Hrash O Hindu Dharmer Punarutthyaner Suchana.*" In *Ramtonu Lahiri O Tatkalin Banga Samaj.* Baridbaran Ghosh, ed., (Calcutta: New Age Publishers 2007): 200–9

________. "*Daktar Mahendralal Sircar.*" In *Ramtonu Lahiri O Tatkalin Banga Samaj.* Baridbaran Ghosh, ed., (Calcutta: New Age Publishers 2007): 193–99

________. "*Navya Banger Trithiya Yuger Netribrinda.*" In *Ramtonu Lahiri O Tatkalin Banga Samaj.* Baridbaran Ghosh, ed., (Calcutta: New Age Publishers 2007): 210–32

________. *Ramtonu Lahiri o Tatkalin Banga Samaj.* Baridbaran Ghosh, ed., (Calcutta: New Age Publications 2007)

Singha, Kaliprasanna. *Satik Hutam Pnechar Naksha.* Arun Nag, ed., (Calcutta: Subarnarekha 1996)

Sircar, Mahendralal "*Olautha.*" *Chikista Sammilani* 3, no. ? (1887): 20–4

Sircar, Nilratan. "*Chikitsa Vyavsaya.*" *Chikitsa Sammilani* 8, nos. 10, 11, 12 (1891): 373–80

Sobhan, Abdus. *Sahi Elaj-e-Lokmani* (Dhaka: Azimi Press 1921) Name of the real author appears only on the last page; the title page attributes authorship to the author's spiritual perceptor Hakim Hafeez Muazzem Ali.

Sripantha (Nikhil Sarkar). *Bot-tola.* (Calcutta: Ananda Publishers 1996)

________. *Jokhon Chhapa Khana Elo.* (Calcutta: Paschim Banga Sahitya Akademi 1996)

Sulemani, Shamsuddin J. "*Olauthar Pratisedhak Aushadh.*" Letter to the Editor, *Bhisak Darpan* 10, no. 8 (1900): 346–47

Suyuti, Allama Jalaluddin *Jinn Jati-r Bismoykor Itihaash.* Mohammed Hadiujjaman, trans. and ed. (Dhaka: Modina Publications 2001)

Tagore, Rabindranath. "*Banshi.*" In *Rabindro Rachanavali.* (Calcutta: Vishwa Bharati 1961): 63–5

________. *Galpaguchha III.* (Calcutta: Vishwa Bharati 1927)

________. *Gora.* (Calcutta: Vishwa Bharati 1924)

________. "*Nation Ki?*" *Rabindra Rachanavali Vol. II.* (Calcutta: Vishwa Bharati Prakashan 1986): 620–67

Tarafdar, Bidhubhusan. "*Kolera Roger Adhunik Chikitsa.*" *Chikitsa Prakash* 13, no. 10 (1920): 354–64

Tribedi, Ramendrasundar. "*Chikitsa Vaigyanik Paribhasha.*" *Bhisak Darpan* 10, no. 2 (1900): 62–75

Vadley, Palmer. "*Chikitsa Shastra Itihas.*" *Bhisak Darpan* 6, no. 2 (1896): 45–56

Hindi, Urdu and Persian Works

Anonymous. *Kitab-i-Daktari.* Unpublished Manuscript. Dhaka University Manuscript Collection, No. DU/189

________. *Nizamat-tibb.* Unpublished Manuscript: Dhaka University Manuscript Collection, No. DU/73

________. *Nushkhajat.* Unpublished Manuscript: Dhaka University Manuscript Collection, No. DU/437

________. *Nushkhajat.* Unpublished Manuscript: Dhaka University Manuscript Collection, No. AK/1

Misra, Brahmshankar. *Bhavprakash.* (Benares: Chowkhamba Sanskrit Office 1938)

India Office Records

(*Individual Files cited are mentioned in Footnotes*)

Board of Control Records, 1784–1858

Bengal Proceedings, 1860–1920

Various Dispensary Reports, 1840–1912

INDEX

A

24 Pergunnahs 62
abhijattya 117 [see also Heredity, *kulaja*, *kaulik*]
acetonuria 122
Acharya, Adwaitya 136
Acting Native Doctor' 62
Acton, William 218, 235, 236, 306
Adhya, Udaychandra 81
adulteration 105, 125, 129–32, 203, 286, 287 (see also Bengal Municipal Act, Bengal Food Adulteration Act, *Gharer Katha*, *Moira*)
Age of Consent Bill 39
Agnivesa 215
Agra 4–5
Ahmed, Moulvi Zahiruddin 40, 94, 99, 269, 293
Ahuja, N. 215
ajirna 127, 138, 224, 278
Alavi, Seema 4, 15, 30–1, 76–8, 113, 181, 261, 262, 264, 268, 270, 273–4, 281, 294, 298, 301
Ali, Lakshmikanta 115, 116, 282
Ali, Mir Ashraf 96
Ali, Najaf 60
Allahabad 4–5
Almora 50, 51
Alter, Joseph 24, 266
American anisette 45
Amin, Shahid 36, 268, 270
Amrita Bazar Patrika 154, 221, 272, 303
Amritashakti Rasayan 239–40, 307
Anatomical and Pathological Museums 39
Anderson, Warwick 10–12, 128, 263, 266, 286
Anglo-Sikh War 38
Annual Dispensary Reports 84
Anwara 48
Apothecary 3
Aquinas, Thomas 234
Aristotle 115, 215
Arnold, David 9, 14 (see n. 64), 17–19, 26, 83, 147, 150, 179, 183, 190, 262, 264–5, 267, 272, 274–5, 285, 289–91, 294–5, 297
Arrah 62, 209, 269
Arsenevalle 159
Aryan/s 135, 144, 162
Assistant Surgeon 5, 6, 40, 68, 84, 283
atmashakti 158–9, 163
Attewell, Guy 9, 26, 76, 148–9, 263, 267, 273, 275–7, 284, 290, 307
Australia 104, 111; Medical Journal, 39, 268
Awadh 76
Awasthi, Rameshwar 4–5, 80–1
aye-byaye [Income-Expenditure] 126, 226
Ayodhya District 50
Ayurveda 10, 26–7, 44, 67, 79, 80, 82–3, 85, 89–91, 93, 96, 109, 142, 144, 172, 203, 216, 267, 279, 281, 284–5, 299

B

baghi 151–2, 175
Baksh, Mohammed 60
Baksh, Sheikh Jahangir 60
Bala, Poonam 9
Balfour, John 235, 306
Balloo 2
Bandopadhyay, Tarashankar 63, 68, 78, 174, 271, 272, 274
Banerjee, Harinarayan 61
Banerjee, Hemchandra 204
Banerjee (also Bandopadhyay), Surendranath 158, 161, 292
Bangiya Sahitya Parishad 190
Bareilly 4–5
Baruipur 62
Basak, Gobindachandra 205, 302
Basalla, George 17, 265
Bashford, Alison 111, 112, 281
Basu Barman, Fakirchandra 92, 276, 298
Basu, Amritakrishna *Plague Tattwa*, 153, 162, 170, 291, 292
Basu, Bholanath 96
Basu, Charu Chandra 57, 283
Basu, Chunilal (also Rai Chunilal Basu Bahadur) 126, 128, 139, 186, 285, 288–9, 296
Basu, Jagadbandhu 200, 299, 300
Basu, Kailash Chandra 57
Basu, Kartikchandra 53, 143, 144, 145
Basu, Rajnarayan 21, 44, 307
Basu, Rajsekhar (Parashuram) 64, 104–5, 106, 223, 239, 272, 280, 281, 295, 307, 309
Bathgate & Co 66
Baudrillard, Jean 101, 279
Baul 176, 226–7, 304
Bayaaz (unani prescription collections) 63, 271
bayu 88, 152; (as air), 137, 143; *jal-bayu*, 145; *mol-dushito bayu*, 193
Beard 215
Beatson, JF 61–2
Benares 5; City Hospital 4
Bengal Food Adulteration Act 129
Bengal Immunity Company 57
Bengal Medical Library 90
Bengal Municipal Act 129
Bengal Renaissance 43, 75–6, 149, 270, 275
Bengalee 158
Bentley, CA 141, 288
Berger, Rachel 26, 100, 104, 113, 267, 279, 281
Beriberi 114
Bernier, Francois 1
Bethune College 46, 47
Misra, Bhab 226, 232, 306
Bhabanipur 5
Bhabprakash 226, 232, 237, 304, 305
Bhadra, Gautam 36, 101, 268, 273, 275, 279
Bhaitameen/s 124, 284
Bharat Samskar Sabha 136, 196
Bharatborsho 164
Bhatt, Adhar 2, 3
Bhattacharya, Charuchandra 122, 283, 285
Bhattacharya, Iswarchandra 81
Bhattacharya, Sanjoy 19, 265
Bhattacharya, Surendramohan 90, 276
Bhisak Darpan (BD) 15, 68, 92–5, 97, 99, 100, 117, 156, 268–9, 278, 297
Bhisak Suhrid 77, 90, 189, 218, 268, 273, 297, 303, 305, 306
bhodrolok 48, 76, 114, 121–2, 125, 129, 130, 150–1, 158–9, 161, 166, 168, 171–2, 174–6, 191, 205, 224, 242, 254, 258, 293, 299

Bhose, Dharmadas 5
Bhugra, D. 215, 303
bhut 45
Bidyabinod, Khirodeprosad 204
Bihar 147, 231
billiards 120
Binodini 47
Biomedicine 10, 32, 259
biomorality 24–5; biomoral, 117, 123, 213, 281
biopolitics 24
bio-power 9, 24–5
bishuchika 187–92, 196–7, 297 [see also *olautha*, *naamutha*]
Biswakosh 218, 240, 297, 303, 307
Biswas, Prankrishna 78–9, 89, 205, 302
Black Doctor 3, 79, 249
Black Hospital Assistant 2
Bloc, Marc 36, 268
Boerhaave 115
Bogra 61
boidyo 40, 47, 60, 81, 191
Bojrojogini (village) 141
Bombay 2, 64, 209, 235; Plague, 147–9, 156
Bongiyo Mohila Mohabidyaloy 46
'Bordeaux & London' 63
Bot-tola 33, 75, 89, 91, 250, 273
bradhna 152, 175
Brahmachari, Upendranath (U.N.) 135, 263
Brahmo 43–5, 47–8, 52–3, 136, 143, 164, 208, 209; Samaj, 44, 270
Breton, Peter 77, 79, 87, 88, 187–8, 190, 255, 274, 294, 296
Bruchhausen, Walter 11, 263
Bubonic Plague 153, 161
Buchanan Major 53
Buchanan, W. J. 117, 282
Buckingham, Jane 19, 262
Burdett, Sir Henry 80, 274
Burma 31, 42, 57, 156, 269
Butter 85
Butto Kristo Paul & Co. 103, 280
Bynum, William. F. 93, 218, 222, 223, 225, 277, 303, 304

C

Calcutta Review 82
Calcutta 3, 38, 39, 42–4, 46, 48–9, 55, 64, 66, 68, 71, 78–9, 89, 97, 101, 103, 105, 107, 114, 128–30, 132, 136, 138, 149, 151, 169, 171, 173, 183, 201, 203–4, 208–9, 224, 233, 247, 261, 277, 281, 286, 287, 292–93, 301, 305; College, 7; High Court, 97; Madrasa, 3, 80; Medical and Physical Society, 79; Medical Board, 2, 49–50, 53, 154, 180; Medical Club, 114; Medical College (CMC), 3–5, 8, 16, 38, 42, 48, 55–6, 60, 80–1, 122, 136, 149, 202, 208, 268, 274–5; Medical College Hospital, 39; Medical School, 68, 121, 169; Medical Society, 37, 39, 47; Municipal Corporation, 131–2; Native Medical Institution (NMI), 3–4, 79–80, 83, 261, 274; Plague, 22, 147, 148, 152–56, 161–3, 168, 290; Physi-Surgic Club, 65; University, 5, 268
Campbell Medical School 39–40, 43, 94
Cassian, John 234
Cassirer, Ernest 155
Catanach, Ian 147, 289, 291
Celsus 215
Chadha, C. 215, 303
Chakrabarti, Kunal 231, 305
Chakrabarti, Pratik 14, 21, 125, 264, 266, 285

Chakrabarty, Amarkrishna 191, 297
Chakrabarty, Amulyaratan 56–7, 270
Chakrabarty, Dipesh 20, 29, 168, 170, 192, 206, 266, 267, 287, 288, 290, 293, 298, 300, 302
Chakrabarty, Hariprasad 87, 88, 275, 276
Chakrabarty, Prasannakumar 55
Chakrabarty, Ramakanta 75, 266, 270, 273
Chakrabarty, Satyasaran 114, 282
Chandavarkar, Rajnarayan 147, 148, 289
Changayani Sudha 239
Charak 89, 215–16, 217, 218, 257, 258, 282; *Samhita*, 190, 215, 230, 291, 305
charitable dispensary (CD) 39, 80, 88, 152, 271
chakras/mokams Chari Mokam Bhed, 231; *tattwa*, 231
Chatterjee, Partha 21, 24, 171, 266, 269
Chatterjee, Rajkrishna 60–1
Chatterjee, Rajkrista 4
Chattopadhyay, Bankimchandra 21
Chattopadhyay, D. N. 183, 189, 193, 195, 198–9, 201, 295, 297, 298, 299, 300
Chattopadhyay, Lalibhamohan 88
Chattopadhyay, Lalitmohan 217, 219–22, 225 234, 236, 275, 303, 304, 306
Chattopadhyay, Purnananda 66
Chattopadhyay, Saratchandra (also Chatterjee) 31, 90, 164, 292
Chaturvedi, Vinayak 171, 293, 297
Chaudry, Premchand 89–90
Medical Officer Chief, 50, 204; Executive, 60; in-Charge, 88, 152, 218
Chikitsa Darshan 102
Chikitsa Kalpadruma 99, 276, 278, 300, 301
Chikitsa Prakash 123, 200, 309
Chikitsa Sammilani (CS) 92– 99, 161, 200, 201, 277, 278
Chikitsak O Samalochak 98
Chikitsak 93, 96, 97, 98, 172, 277
Chill Theory 116, 282
Chittagong 4–5, 40–1, 46–9, 53–4, 59–60, 271; district court, 41; Government Collegiate School, 48, 54; Jail Hospital, 50
Chodok (festival) 25, 53, 143, 267
Chopra Committee 31
Choudhury, Abdul Ajed Khan 52, 94, 202, 270, 301
Choudhury, Badanchandra 5
Choudhury, Deen 72, 108
Chowdhury, Indira 159, 291
Chromopathy 89, 91, 276
Chuckerbutty, Soorjo Coomar Goodeve 6, 37–8, 40, 55
Civil Society 24, 169, 254
Civil Sub-Medical Department 3
Civil Surgeon 43, 61, 66, 74
Hooker, Claire 111–2
Cobb 153–4, 157, 268 (see also Simpson, W. J.)
Cohen, Lawrence 12, 24, 263, 266–7
Col Banerjee 72, 74
'College Boys' 45
colonial science 17, 18, 19
Comilla 54–5; District school, 54; Victoria College, 55
Commissioner of Bardhaman 63
Composite Individuals' 36
Compounder 2, 3, 4, 6, 7, 27, 38, 62, 68, 72, 249, 277 [see also *Hospital Assistant*]
Conrad, Lawrence 112, 281
constipation [*kosthokatthinyo*] 105, 109, 126–9, 187, 220, 285, 286
'constructive Swadeshi' 135, 140

Cook, Harold 14–15, 264
coolie ship 49
Cooper, Fredrick 12, 263
Copland, James 115
Crawford, J. R. 107, 261–2
Cricket 120
Crossgrove, William 30, 268
Cuddalore 2
Cullen, William 115, 119, 158, 291
'Culture Bound Syndrome' (CBS) 213–15, 247, 257
Cunningham, D. D. 154
Cuttack 63, 277

D

D. Gupta & Co 103, 204, 243, 308
Daeschel, Markus 105, 280
Dak Munshi 60
daishik 134 [see also *desh-dharmak*, Endemic Diseases]
Darpan (as genre) 105, 280
Das, Amal 147–8, 290
Das, Anirban 182, 262, 265, 295, 300
Das, Bharatcharan 63
Das, Chintamoni 62
Das, Durgamohon 44
Das, Gobinda 89, 90, 196, 226, 227, 229, 230, 237
Das, Kunjabihari 188–9, 193–5, 198, 201, 204, 234, 297, 298, 300, 301, 306
Das, Mukunda 139, 288
Das, Ramlal 151, 154
Das, Ramnarayan 4–5
Das, Sundarimohan 105, 121, 130, 132, 169, 170, 259, 280, 283, 286, 287, 293, 296, 309
Dasgupta, Kaliprasanna 108–9, 139, 281, 288
Dasgupta, Neemchand 60
Datta, Jadunath 89, 276
Datta, Nabinchandra 48–53, 270
Datta, Nafarchandra 67, 91–2, 102, 192, 272, 276, 298
Datta, Narendranath 54–8, 65, 70–1, 72, 270
Datta, Neelmani 4–5
Datta, Shyamacharan 4–5
Davies 85
De Souza, L. 5
Deb, Kunjabihari 66, 68, 105, 272, 281
debility 115, 118–9, 135, 219, 221, 224, 228, 239, 242, 243, 245, 303 [see also *durbalata*, weakness]
dehatattwa 232
DeLanda, Manual 21
Deleuze, Giles 213, 284, 302, 309
Delhi 4–5, 50, 97, 148, 149, 301
Derrida, Jacques 27, 267
desh 93, 108, 134, 136–7, 142; *-dharmak*, 134 [see also *daishik*, Endemic Diseases]; *-samskar*, 47, 137
Dey Bahadur, Rai Kanailal
Dey, Kalachand 5
Dey, Pulinchandra 84–5
Dey, Rajkrista 4
Dey, Rev. Lal Behari 174
Dhaka 4–5, 42, 88, 97, 140–41, 191, 204–5, 208; College, 208; dispensary, 60; University, 62; lunatic asylum, 73
Dhara, Jadabchandra 5
Dhat 213–20, 222, 230, 239, 247, 256, 303
Dherkanal 50
Dhwajabhanga 220–1, 228, 237, 241
Digby, Anne 203, 301
Djinns 63, 167
d'Orta, Garcia 1
Dr Fraser 2
Dr Gavin 221, 303
Dr Khastagir Girl's High School 46
Dresser 3, 4

DSM-IV 215
Duncan, J. 61
Durbalata 115, 119, 237–9, 240, 307 [see also weakness, debility]
Dutt, Bepin Behari 154–5, 157
Dutt, Udaychandra 96
Dutta, Achintya Kumar 11
Dutta, Akshoykumar 44

E

Echenberg, Myron 148, 290
Ecks, Stefan 101 197, 247, 279, 299, 304, 309
Education Gazette 206
Edward's Moondie-Essence 68
Eisenstadt, S. N. 29, 267
Embezzlement 74
Endemic 33, 62, 133–5, 137, 179, 209–10, 25-, 270, 289, 295
Endemic Diseases 134, 289 [see also *Daishik, Desh-Dharmak*]
Epidemic Dropsy 114 [see also *sankramak shoth*]
Epidemic 6, 33, 62, 74, 79, 111, 114, 125, 133–4, 147–51, 153, 155–6, 160, 162, 176, 181, 192, 194, 206, 207, 249, 253–5, 289, 290–2, 295, 297–8
Epidemiological Society of London 39, 268
Ernst, Waltraud 17, 18, 262, 265
ersatz doctors' 67–8, 181
Esquirol 215
Essence of Jamaica Sarsaparilla 243
Exciting Causes 114 [see also *uddipok*]

F

Factish 251–5
Fakir 68, 175–6, 191, 226–7
Farrukhabad 5
fever 47, 89, 91, 135, 151, 222, 230, 298; Bengal (*banglar jwor*), 115; Burdwan, 47; malarious/ Malarial, 85, 88, 116, 136; Enteric, 133; epidemic, 125; remittent, 199; scarlet, 208; 'slow fever', 39; tri-humoural, 153
Floyer, John 184, 295
Folk 172, 176–7, 205, 286
Football 120
Forth, Christopher E. 119
Foucault, Michel 9, 11–12, 17, 24, 28, 118, 218, 222–3, 266, 282, 285, 303
Fragment [also fragmentary, fragmented] 35–6, 59, 76, 97, 167, 173, 205–6, 249, 305
Freeship 55
Freud 215

G

Gafoor, Abdul 62
Galen 115, 184
Galij 164, 167, 292
Gandhi, Mohandas Karamchand [Gandhian] 21, 36, 143–4, 171, 215, 266, 286–7, 303
Gangopadhyay, Jadunath 96, 97, 278
Ganguly, Dwarkanath 44
Ganguly, Iswarchandra 4–5, 80–4
garhasthya chikitsa 89, 276
Gaudilliere, Jean-Paul 113, 281
Gaya 5
Germ Theory 114, 133, 144, 282
Gharer Katha 129–30, 298
Ghosh, Anindita 75–6, 273
Ghosh, Aurobindo 158
Ghosh, Doyalkrishna 133
Ghosh, Harinath 193, 195
Ghosh, Kiranchandra 258

Ghosh, Mahendranath 122
Ghosh, Pramathanath 89, 276
Ghosh, Surjyonarayon 221
Ghoshal, Lalmohan 115–6, 282
Ginzburg, Carlo 151, 268
Bagchi, Girishchandra 94, 97, 152, 195, 278, 290, 297
GK Nag & Co. 209, 243, 280, 308
Gobind, Seo 60
Golden Age 73, 142
Gole, Nilufer 29, 267
Good, Byron 155, 291
Gorgori, Jodunondon 64
Goswami, Mahatma Bijoykrishna 52, 136
Goswami, Manu 21, 266
Government Medical Stores 38
governmentality 9, 118, 262, 282
Greeks 117, 204
Greenblatt, Stephen 28, 267
Greenhow, Thomas Michael 194, 197, 298, 299
Guattari, Felix 213
Guha, Kulachandra 69–70, 114, 119–20, 126, 130–1, 134–5, 137, 141, 272, 282, 283, 285, 286, 287, 289
Gupta Press Dairektari Panjika 102, 103, 219, 244, 246, 276, 279, 280, 282, 285, 300, 302, 305, 307, 308
Gupta, Annadamohan 126, 285
Gupta, Biharilal 47
Gupta, Brahmanand 9
Gupta, Charu 101, 280
Gupta, Durga Das (D. D.) 122–3, 142, 153–4, 156, 160, 167, 225–6, 237–8, 274, 281, 283–86, 288, 289, 291, 292, 293, 304, 306, 308, 309
Gupta, Dwarkanath 4
Gupta, Haralal 89, 276
Gupta, Madhusudan 35, 37, 39, 81–2, 90, 96
Gupta, Swarupa 134, 287
gurupak 130, 196–7, 299
Gyan Prakash 20–1, 266
Bagchi, Gyanendranarayan 53, 70–2, 74, 108, 143, 267, 270, 272, 281

H

Habib, Irfan 11, 263
Hakim 99, 106, 279
Haldar, Dheerendranath 145, 289
Hamilton Bell, Geoffrey 194, 255
Hamlin, Christopher 112, 133, 281, 282
Hardiman, David 18, 265
Hardinge, Sir Henry 38
Harrison, Mark 9, 13, 17–19, 179, 262, 265, 290, 294
Hemming, R. 4
herbaria 39
Heredity 113, 114, 117, 146, 281 [see also *abhijattya*, *kulaja* and *kaulik*]
Hijras 236
Hindu Satkar Samiti 163
Hippocrates 115, 184, 215
Hodges, Sarah 14, 18, 262, 264, 265, 266
Homoeopathy 43–4, 46, 67, 86–7, 91, 95, 102, 202, 207–10, 269
Hospital Assistant 2, 6, 8, 27, 35, 37, 52, 259
Hospital Mate 2, 3
Hossain, Syed Abul 104, 280
Hossein (also Hussain), Syed Enayat 4–5
Hossein, Syed Luteef 62
Howrah 66
Hughes, C. C. 214, 302
Hughli 1, 5, 48, 63–4; Factory, 2
Hybridization 9, 30
Hydropathy 89, 90, 205
Hysteria 228, 239–41, 307

I

ICD-10 215
Ichhabhedi Batika 127
Iliffe, John 1, 7, 11, 261, 263, 264
Inden, Ronald 169, 293
Indian Aryanism 135
Indian Medical Gazette 6, 37, 262
Indian Medical Service (IMS) 16, 19, 32, 81, 84, 95, 108, 148, 193, 275, 284, 296
Indian Mutiny 68
indicanuria 122
Iran 56, 57
Iraq 56, 57
Izal 16

J

Jabbalpur 5
jalsaucha 129
Jamalkhana 49
Jamoakandi 61
Jeevanishakti 114, 117, 137, 143, 282 [see also vital force]
Jewish Native Doctor 4, 60, 261
Jog Kalandar 231
Johnson, James 79, 125, 180, 194, 198, 285, 300
Johnson, Mark 223, 304
Jorasanko 48
Jyotirbhushan K, Kunjabihari 145, 289

K

kaaph 88, 152, 229–30
Kabiratna, Abinashchandra 201, 220
Kaliyug 224, 304
Kandy 230
Kanpur 4–5, 50; dispensary, 60
Kar Samhita 77, 273
Kar, Durgadas 39, 68, 86, 87, 90, 91, 92, 96, 99, 272, 275, 276
Kar, Radhagobinda (R. G.) 39, 68, 77, 86, 189, 218, 219, 220, 228–9, 232, 236, 268, 273, 297, 303, 305, 306
Karim, Anwarul 175–6, 294
Karmakar, Shib Charan 39
Karpurashab 127
kaulik 113 [see also *abhijattya*, *kulaja*, heredity]
Kaviraj, Sudipta 24, 29, 168, 266, 267, 293
Keranis 104, 224–5, 228, 238–9, 280, 307
Khan Bahadur, Khan Moulvi Tamiz 37–40, 58, 268
Khan, Gohur 5, 58–65, 66
Khan, Jaumat Ali 204
Khastagir, Annadacharan 40–8, 49, 50, 58, 88, 95, 96, 97, 201, 269, 270, 276
Khater, Mohammed 233, 305
Kherupara 140
Khilnani, Sunil 24
Kidambi, Prashant 147, 148, 290
Kidderpore Dock Yards 55
Kinu Goala-r Goli 132
Kipling, Rudyard 46, 192, 270, 298
Kishanganj 2
Kishenprasad 60
Klaibya 237
Klein, Ira 147, 179, 289, 294
Knowledge 11, 14, 80, 218, 252; Local 189, 205–6; Traditional 264; Medical 30–1, 65, 78–80, 84, 95, 151, 172, 262, 265, 295, 300
Kokhyastha Granthisphithi Rog 152
Kothari, Manu 20, 266
Krishnokumar 54
kulaja 113 [see also *abhijattya*, *kaulik*, heredity]
Kumaon 38, 156
Kumar, Anil 7, 18, 261–2, 265

Kumar, Deepak 1, 11, 13, 18, 261–5, 267
Kumar, P. 86
Kumudini 47

L

Lahore 31, 38–9, 50, 99
Lakoff, George 223, 304
Lal, Chiman 5
Lalan Fakir 191, 226–7
Langford, Jean 222, 303
Latour, Bruno 21, 195, 251–3, 266, 284, 299, 309
Lawrie, James Adair 181, 194, 255, 295, 299
Lazarus, Edward John 5, 60, 80, 261
Lepore, Jill 37, 268
LGBT 237
Liebermeister 116
Lipsedge, M. 214
Littlewood, R. 214, 302–3
local native doctor' 59, 61–3, 270 (see also, 'locally entertained native doctor')
locally entertained native doctor' 32, 59, 181, 249 (see also, 'local native doctor')
lokayata 204–5
Lona-laga 138
Long, Rev James 82, 86, 274, 275, 276
Lord Northbrook 46
Lourdusamy, J. 19, 266
Lower Primary School 54
Lowy, Ilana 113
Lausanne 235
Lucknow 4, 5, 50, 156

M

Macaulay, T. B. 159
Madhab Kar 82, 89
Madhuri Sharma 100, 264, 279
Madhusudan Gupta 35, 37, 39, 81–2, 90, 96, 274–5
Madras 3
Marfati 226, 233
magical' cures 180, 207
Mahashakti Rasayan 239, 241, 246, 307
Maitreya, Prasannachandra 96, 190–1, 196, 200, 207–8, 220, 278, 297, 299, 302, 303, 308
Major Buchanan 53
Majumdar, Harinath (Fikirchand) 191, 298
Malaria 47, 88, 115, 116, 119, 133–7, 139, 141, 143, 152, 159, 265, 282, 287, 291, 302
Malaria Commission of Egypt 47
Malaysia 57
Malboidyo 89
Malda 43, 50, 74, 272
Manucci, Niocolao 1
Marriott, McKim 25, 266
Marwari 114, 116
Masturbation [*Onania, L'Onanisme*] 228, 235, 306
Mathura 5, 42; dispensary, 60
Maudsley 215
Mauritius 31, 49
Mayurakshi 64
McCay, David 122–3, 308
McNeill, William 148, 290
Medical Market 14–6, 33, 68, 88, 92, 104, 109, 127, 179–80, 203–4, 206, 208–10, 213, 221–3, 238, 239, 246–7, 251, 253, 256–7, 264, 284, 294, 309
Medical Registration Act/s 7, 69, 70, 73, 93, 95
Medical Reporter 201
Medical Systems 7, 9–10, 13, 26, 82, 85, 92, 100, 106, 109, 262, 267, 300
Medinipur 62
Mehta, Lopa 20

Mercury 79, 200–1, 218, 231, 245, 303, 308
Mesmerism 89, 90, 161, 276
Mess In-Charge [Messes/'Messing' houses] 56 130, 224
'metaphorical rationality' 223, 225, 257
Microhistory 35, 268
Middle Vernacular School 54
Milk, adulteration of 131–2, 286–7
Millan, Christina Alvarez 184, 295
Mitra, Jogendranath 198–9, 332
Mitra, Kalikrishna 87, 275
Mitra, Nabinchandra 4
Mitra, Satyasaran 114, 116
Mitter, Prosonno Coomar 39
Modern Review 140
modern science 12, 20, 32, 221
Mohammadiya Panjika 104, 280, 307, 308
Mohammed, Jan 204
Mohammed, Shukur 227
Mohan Mela 49
Mohanto, Dinabandhu 62
Moira 130
Manamohini 47
Montague-Chelmsford 140
Mookerjee, Gunga Persaud 96, 113–16, 119–22, 127, 133–4, 137, 139, 281, 282, 283, 287, 288
Moradabad 4–5, 50
Morar Purvoe 2
Morton, Rev William 188, 296
Mouat, F. J. 38, 82, 275
Ms Newton, Chambers & Co 16
Mukharji, Rajkrishna 81
Mukherjee, Kishori Mohun 154–5
Mukherjee, N. 155
Mukhopadhyay (also Mukherji), Jadunath 65, 69, 70, 89, 92, 184–5, 188–9, 193, 198, 199, 202, 272, 276, 278, 295, 297, 300, 301, 309
Mukhopadhyay, Balaichand (Banaphool) 108, 281
Mukhopadhyay, Jagannarayan 187
Mukhopadhyay, Prasadkumar 88, 276
Mukhopadhyay, Rangalal 189
Mukhopadhyay, Trailakyanath 189
Mulford Company 246
Mullick, Indumadhab 58
Mullick, Sadhucharan 5
Mullick, Lakshminarayan 174–6
Munshi 38, 40–1, 268–9, 273
Munshi Ramchandra 41, 48
Murshidabad 4–5, 149
mushtiyoga 89, 91, 276

N

Naamutha 187–8 [see also *bishuchika*, olautha]
Nainital 50
naitrojen 122–4, 251–3, 283–4 [see also Nitrogen, acetonuria, indicanuria]
Na-mardangi 228, 236–7, 241
Nanda, Meera ['reactionary modernity'] 141, 189
Nandan Ayurvediya Aushadhalay 127
Nandy, Ashis 20, 23, 266, 282
Nathpanthi Tantric 226, 231
national diet' 124–32
National Indian Association for Social Progress 39
national science 19–21
national' businesses 58
nationalism 19, 20, 21, 22, 111, 130, 135, 142, 149, 171, 251, 253, 261, 266
Native Doctor 2, 6, 32, 58–63, 84, 181, 249, 270
Native Dresser 3
Native Hospital 3

Native Medical Institution 3–4, 59, 79–80, 83, 261, 274
Naun, Maheshchandra 5
Navashakti Aushadhalaya 243, 308
Nepal 68
Nervigor 243
Nervous affliction 219
New Dispensation 44, 46
New Historicism 28, 30
New Sydenham Society 39
Nicholas, Ralph 169, 190, 297
Nichter, Mark 16, 196, 203, 265, 292, 299, 301
Nicola 3
Nilkanth/Nilchand 2
Nitrogen 252, 283–4, 122–3 [see also *naitrojen,* acetonuria, indicanuria]
Nobo Bidhan [New Dispensation] 44, 46
Non-Mercurial Pills for Syphilis 68
Nowel-Smith, Harriet 184, 295
Numeralization of diets 125–6
Numshivia 2, 3
Nushkhajat 62–3, 271
Nutton, Vivian 117

O

O'Flaherty, Wendy Doniger 232–3, 305
Obeysekere, Gananath 230
Olabibi/Olaichandi 190–1, 206, 297
Olautha 187–92, 295, 297–301 [see also *bishuchika, naamutha*]
Orissa 50, 60
Orwell, George 68, 269, 272
Ovington, John 1

P

Pabna 62
Pahari, Subrata 203, 261, 274, 301
Pal, Nabinchandra 4
Pala Dynasty 231
Palamau Jail 53
Palit, Chittabrata 19, 21, 25, 261, 262, 266, 267, 284
Palmer Vadley 95, 278
pana [water-hyacinth] 140–1, 252–3, 288–9
Paricharika 47
Parke-Davis 246, 309
Pasteur 133
Pati, Biswamoy 19
Patiya 40
Patna 3–5, 99
Paton, Adell 11
Paul, Beharilal 61, 74
Philippines 128
Pigg, Stacy Leigh 10
Pinto, Sarah 67, 181, 272, 295
pitta 152, 230
Plague Manifesto 161, 292
Plague Regulations 160, 165, 290
Pollock, Sheldon 30, 254, 267
Porter, Roy 8, 14
Porter, William Henry 95, 278
Power 10–2, 14, 22, 24, 29–30, 78, 168–9, 254; bio-power 9, 24–5; state 20, 148, 150, 168, 192; 298 Rituals of 67; Body's 114, 118, 120, 133–4, 158–9, 162, 174, 193, 195, 198, 250, 254; Localized 134; Divine 161, 206–7
Prahasan (as genre) 105, 281
Prameha 24, 220, 228–30, 232, 303
Prameha Kalyan Bati 241, 307
Prasad, Srirupa 114
Pratirodh Shakti [*Swabhabik Rog Badhak Shakti*] 158, 160–1, 285–7, 291
Predisposing Causes (*purvavarti*) 98, 114–16, 158, 194
predisposition 112, 113, 114–8, 120, 127, 135

Pro Bono Publico' 63
Prosopography 22, 36, 59, 268
Publicly performed contests 44
Pune 147, 149
Punjab 76, 148, 149, 156, 264
purdah 24, 25, 44, 165
Puri 4–5
Pyne, Tarachand 5

Q

Quackery [quacks] 7, 26–7, 35, 64–6, 69, 86, 189, 201–4, 208, 221, 278
Quaiser, Neshat 85, 271, 275
Quran 233

R

Rae Bareli 50
Rafdhar, R. E. 95, 278
Rahman, Hakim Majibar 99, 279
Raina, Dhruv 11
Raj High School 64
Raj, Kapil 11, 263
Raja of Darbhanga 50
Raja of Nadia 138
Raja Pratapchand 36
Rajkristopur 66
Rajshahi 93, 96, 97, 98, 172; Government Hospital, 115
Ramanna, Mridula 11, 19, 263, 265
Ramnath 2, 3
Rand, W. C. 147
Rangalal Daktar 63–4, 66
Ray, Durgacharan 66
Ray, Devendranath 97, 114, 116, 122, 133, 156, 282, 283, 287, 290, 291
Ray, Kabita 11
Ray, Kartikeyachandra 138
Ray, Rajat Kanta 22
Raychaudhuri, Tapan 109, 281
Recovery of lost manhood [manliness, effeminacy] 118, 159–60, 166, 239, 241–2, 291
Reddy, Gayatri [gender as performance] 236, 306
Resistance 12–3, 20, 30, 158, 168, 176, 193, 195, 254, 266
Rev. Holland 56
Rhizomes [rhizoid reality] 213–4, 217, 228, 230, 232, 247, 258, 302
Risley, H. H. 7, 262, 271
Robinson, Francis 29, 267
Roja 45
Romantic [Romanticism] 140, 185, 288, 298
Rome 113
Rose, Nicholas 25, 267
Roy, Bikramadityo 72
Roy, B. C. [Bidhan Chandra] 35, 57
Roy, Binodbihari (also Ray) 93–4, 96, 98–9, 275, 278
Roy, Charubrata 57
Roy, G. C. [Gopaul Chunder] 35, 296
Roy, Kamakhyaprasad 72, 107, 272, 281
Roy, Rajkrishna 105, 106, 281
Roy, Satyakrishna 98, 278
Roy, Srirupa 21, 266
Roy, Tapti 77
Roy, Taraknath 117
Royle, J. F. 82, 83, 275
Russell Henry Chittenden 122–3, 283
Rutherford, Thomas Corrie 156–7, 291, 293–4

S

S. K. Roy & Co. 102, 280
sadhu 51–2
Salisbury 133
Salsa 103, 243–6, 282, 308

Sambuddha [Amulyakumar Dasgupta] 127, 285
samskar Bharat Samskar Sabha, 136, 196; *desh-samskar*, 47, 137; *gram-samskar*, 135, 137, 140; *samaj-samskar*, 135–7; *shahar-samskar*, 135
Sanatan 62
Sandiford 61
Sangwan, Satpal 18, 265
Sankramak Rog 117, 145
Sankramak Shoth 114–6 [see also Epidemic Dropsy]
sankraman 113–7, 145
Sannipathic Jwar 153
Sanskrit College 3, 80
Santipur 136, 211
Sanyal, Durgacharan 224–5, 304–5
Sanyal, Pulinchandra 96, 97, 121, 199–202, 220, 272, 278, 283, 300, 301, 303, 309
Sarbadhikary, Soorjo Coomar 39
Sarkar, Bhubanmohan 105–6
Sarkar, Nikhil (Sripantha) 75, 273
Sarkar, Sumit 135, 140, 158, 224
Sarsaparilla 243–5, 308
Sattwa-guna 117, 123
Saudamini 47
Scheper-Hughes, Nancy 12, 263, 266, 307–8
School Book Society 79, 181, 187
Scottish Church College 204
Searle, Charles 197, 295, 300
Second Anglo-Afghan War 50
Sedgewick, William 95, 278, 282
Semen 123, 215–8, 221, 225–7, 229–37, 240–1, 243, 306 [see also Spermatorrhoea]
Sen, Binodlal 89, 196, 227, 276, 299, 304, 305, 306
Sen, Dinesh Chandra 185–6
Sen, Haimabati 109
Sen, Harimohan 117, 119–20, 135, 137, 193
Sen, Hemchandra 159
Sen, Hur Chunder 88, 218
Sen, Jatramohon 47, 53
Sen, Kalimohan 94, 297
Sen, Keshabchandra 43, 136
Sen, Ramkamal 79
Sena Dynasty 231–2, 305
Sengupta, Nibaranchandra 70–4
Sengupta, Sachindranath 72, 107, 272, 281
Seth, Jadabchandra 4–5
Seth, Umacharan 3, 4
Shah, Duddu 78
Shahbad 50, 74, 272
Shahjahanpur 5
Shakti Sindhu Rasayan 243
Shapin, Steven 17, 265
Sharangadhar 231, 305
Shastras 81–2, 145, 274
Shastri, Shibnath 44, 136, 269–70, 277, 288–9
Sheel, Alok 147, 148, 290
Sheikh Misser 62
Shen k'uei 215
Shen-kui 215
Shepherd, Brown 159
Sherpur Dispensary 88, 218
Shevandavadum 2
Shibsagar 43, 46, 50
Siddha 10, 226, 303; saint, 205; Shaivite, 231
Simpson, W. J. 150, 153–7, 160, 169–70, 254
Singapore 57
Singh Rajput, Swaroop 60
Singh, Dhrub Kumar 179, 294, 296
Singh, Maharaja Ranjit 38
Singha, Kaliprasanna (Hutom) 44–6, 53, 138, 203, 267, 270, 281, 288
Sinha, Sandeep 7
Sircar, Mahendralal 32, 194, 195, 200, 269, 277, 298, 300
Sircar, Nalin Behary 154
Sircar, Shyamacharan 5

Sircar, Sir Nil Ratan 35, 43, 57–8, 69–70
Sister Nivedita (Margaret Noble) 163, 166, 292
Sitapur 50
Sivaramkrishnan, Kavita 76
Siyyar ul-Mutakhkhirin 40
Skinner, Quentin 21, 266
Smith, D. B. 85
Smoult, W. H. 128, 286
Sobhan, Abdus 89, 205, 276, 301
Sobhan, Moulvi Abdus 89, 205, 276, 301
Solemani Talenama 233, 305
Sondhya Bhasha 226
Sontag, Susan 241, 307
South Africa 57
Spermatone 221, 303
Spermatorrhoea 218–9, 221, 225, 228–9 [see also semen]
Sreemani, Panchanan 4–5
Sri Lanka 57, 305
Srikail 54, 56–7
St Augustine 234
state medicine 7, 13–14, 18, 25, 32, 62, 76, 104, 150
Sthanik Shakti [endemic influence] 134, 137
Strenshyam Master 2
subaltern [also as in Subaltern Studies] 12, 35, 120, 130, 148, 170–2, 176, 254
Sub-Assistant Surgeon 3–6, 45, 59–61, 80, 84–5, 92, 95, 249, 259
subjectivity 22, 24, 121, 124, 155, 157
Subordinate Medical Service 6, 58, 61, 95, 193, 278
Suchokrodondi 40
Suddhachar [*sadachar*] 145
Sudhakar Batika 221
Sukhanand 60
Sukra dhatu 218
Sukrameha 218, 221, 226, 228–30, 232, 241
Sulemani, Shamsuddin J. 204, 301
Sumathipala 215, 303
Sur, S. N. 141
Surat 1; Factory, 2; Plague, 291
Surgeon General 61
Sushrut Jadhav 215–7, 243, 303, 308
Susruta Samhita 190, 215, 218, 230, 237, 305
swadeshi 135, 140, 158, 159; Movement, 103, 135
Swami Aghorenath 52
Swami Vivekananda 52, 143, 161–3, 166–9, 172, 177, 292
Swami, Basharanando 52
Swami, Bishuddhanando 52
Swapna-dosh [*swapnadosh*] 218, 221, 228–9, 232, 236, 241
Swarna-ghatita Sarsa-Vita 243
Swasthya Dharma Panjika 53, 144
Swasthya Samachar 31, 71, 127, 131, 187, 286–7
Swasthya 92, 93, 97, 113, 120, 121, 139, 142, 144, 153, 156, 160, 161, 309
syndrome 213–5, 217, 247, 256–7, 302–3

T

Tabtabi, Ghulam Hussain 40
Tagore, Debendranath 44
Tagore, Prasannacoomar 204
Tagore, Rabindranath 22, 90, 132, 140, 158, 185, 186, 266, 296, 297, 307
Taliqa Kobiraj 63, 271
Tambiah, Stanley 173, 293
tartar emetic 45
technology of selfhood 25, 251
Thackrah, Charles Turner 181, 295
The Englishman 38, 154

The Lancet 216
Theosophical Society 52
Third Gurkha Regiment 50
Tibb-e-Nabi 167, 293
Tirhut 50, 62
Tissot, Samuel-Auguste 215–6, 235, 257–8, 306
totka 89, 172, 276
Transactions of the Medical and Physical Society (also *Transactions*) 79, 80
Tribedi, Ramendrasundar 88, 189–90, 297
Tripura 54
Troilongo Swami 52
Trollope-Kumar, Karen 307, 326
Tytler, John 77, 273

U

Ukil 41
Unani/hekimi 9–10, 26–7, 63, 67, 76, 80, 83, 85, 91, 99–100, 113, 148–9, 191, 203, 240, 263, 271, 273, 276, 281, 290
universal body 182
Upstart 66–8, 70, 106
Urban Lifestyles 105, 137–8
Urban, Hugh 227
Usa and Aniruddha 233

V

Vancloster de Roza, Domingo 3
Vaughan, Megan 10–12, 22, 24, 263, 283
Vedic remedy 68
Vernacular Licentiates in Medicine and Surgery (VLMC) 85
Vernacularization 1, 25, 30–1, 33, 77, 85, 87, 168, 170, 176, 177, 253, 254
Vidyasagar, Iswarchandra 43–4, 48
vital force 117–9, 282 [see also *jeevanishakti*]
Vrindavan 42
Vyam [both Manasik and Daihik] 119–24, 137, 141, 143, 283, 289

W

Wade, John Peter 2, 184, 261, 295
War Service 56
Ward, William 78, 274, 292
Waring, Edward J. 128, 286
Water Hyacinth Removal Week 141
Watson, Sir Thomas 115, 119, 283
Wazullah 62
weakness 105, 109, 114–5, 118–9, 121–4, 129, 159, 162, 213, 215, 218–21, 224, 237, 241–3, 246–7, 258, 285, 307 [see also *durbalata*, debility]
Wear, Andrew 81, 274
WHO 215
Wig 214–5, 302
Wigglesworth, Michael 234, 306
Wilson, H. H. 82, 83, 84–5, 275
Wilson, Janice 93
Wise, T. A. 60, 82, 83, 267, 270, 275
Worboys, Michael 18, 133, 265, 287
Wujastyk, Dominik 112, 197, 284–5, 299

Y

Yap 214, 302
Yoga 44, 231, 305, 308

Z

Zachariah, Benjamin 21, 266, 285, 289, 303